15.00

D1260575

# The Visual World
# of the Child

# The Visual World of the Child

ELIANE VURPILLOT
*Professor of Psychology, University René Descartes, Paris*

Foreword by Jerome Bruner
*Watts Professor of Experimental Psychology, University of Oxford*

Preface by Paul Fraisse
Translated from the French by W. E. C. Gillham

INTERNATIONAL UNIVERSITIES PRESS, INC.
New York

LCN 75-790
ISBN 0-8236-6749-9

Originally published in French under the title
*Le Monde Visuel du Jeune Enfant*
© Presses Universitaires de France, 1972

# Translator's Acknowledgements

My thanks are due firstly, and mainly, to my wife who gave detailed help throughout the preparation of the manuscript; Dr David Wood read a late draft in its entirety and made very many useful suggestions on rephrasing; Mrs Phyllis Preston gave invaluable help in disentangling meaning when my French language competence proved inadequate; and, finally, Mlle Vurpillot herself has earned my gratitude for her patience in answering my queries.

W.E.C.G.

# Foreword

Many will have occasion to be delighted with the appearance in English translation of this excellent volume, for it serves several functions and does so with great distinction. To begin with, it is an extraordinarily comprehensive account of the growing field of research on the development of perception and attention in young children. Its comprehensiveness comes not only from the author's breadth of scholarship, but also from her hospitality to new and emerging trends in research. In these pages one will find not only the conventional topics of space and object perception and the constancies, but also a very valuable and thoughtful account of work on eye-movements in relation to perceptual organisation. But it is not just a compendium either. For here too are succinct accounts of major theoretical positions on perceptual development from Lashley and Hebb to Piaget and such Russian investigators as Zaporozhets and Zinchenko. She misses little and manages to be fair-minded and clear in her accounts of research and of the theoretical positions from which they derive.

Not least among the book's virtues is its attempted integration of different points of view, an integration achieved by detailed examination of experimental evidence. It is unusual to find a writer in this field who attempts to explore such diverse literatures as the Russian work on orienting, Piaget's efforts to explicate perceptual development, Gibson's efforts on behalf of a theory of differentiation, and my own brand of functionalism – all in the interest of sorting out that which might constitute common ground and that which, properly, is open to adjudication by further research or further theoretical inquiry. It is this spirit that gives the book so pervasive a fair-mindedness.

There is one special gift to be found in this volume that I particularly appreciated. It is the excellent account of the author's own research using similarity and difference judgments as a method for determining the structure of children's perceptual organisation – her own work, and a considerable amount of related work of which I had not been coherently aware before reading her book when it first appeared in French.

Dr Vurpillot, it should be noted, is uniquely well suited to serve not only as a reporter of work in progress, but also as an 'honest broker' where points of view are concerned. She has worked not only with her colleagues in Paris, but also in such disparate scientific 'sub-cultures' as the Gibsons' laboratory at Cornell, at the Center for Cognitive Studies at Harvard, and among the Piagetians. My diplomatic channels yield the same story as I came to know when she was at Harvard in my laboratory: she is a good and a tough diplomat who not only brings the message from elsewhere, but sees to it that it is understood. Shortly before she came to Harvard, Professor Piaget told me that the only time Dr Vurpillot becomes pessimistic is when she gets hungry, and it is a state easily repaired. There is a probing, buoyant quality about Dr Vurpillot's account of work on perceptual development that suggests she was well nourished during the composition of this volume! It is this empirically based buoyancy, her good sense for theoretical issues, and her gift of clarity that make these pages notable.

JEROME BRUNER

*Oxford*
*October, 1974*

# Preface to the French Edition

From the moment of his birth the child opens his eyes on the world. No mother is so naive as to think that her baby's perception is the same as her own. But the baby's progress is so spectacular, the anthropomorphism of the adult so compelling, that we are all tempted to believe that the visual world of the infant becomes, in the space of a few months, similar to ours.

Yet even the reader who is aware of such a danger will discover, in studying the present book, that he still has something to learn in this respect, since it describes for us several stages of development which continue up to adolescence. One might ask how that can be possible. After all, the optic and retinal system is complete at birth; and surely perceptual Gestalten are established within the space of a few years?

In fact our visual world is not some sort of photograph, more or less fine-grained, but the result of a slow process of construction, which creates for us a world of objects, similar or different, interdependent, and meaningful. *The Visual World of the Child* studies the characteristics of this process of construction and demonstrates in an exemplary manner the methodology of modern psychology. The expansion of psychology in the twentieth century stems from an epistemological revolution which has exposed the vanity of a psychology based on introspective data, and the fertility of a psychology of behaviour. Historically, animal psychology has been the catalyst of this change but it is developmental psychology which has demonstrated its utility. In endeavouring to understand the child, one is forced to recognise that introspection, be it that of a Bergson or a Proust, is of no use. Although the child learns to speak quite quickly – and what he says is as significant as what he does – yet he tells us nothing about his mental experience. There is no developmental psychology which is not rooted in a psychology of behaviour, a view endorsed by Piaget himself. But the psychology of behaviour is not to be identified with behaviourism where the 'ism' represents the transition from a method to a theory which recalls the basic tenets of Watson. It does not necessarily involve a return to S-R theories of behaviour. Certainly all behavioural psychology starts with the study of situations and responses with the intention of explaining S-R sequences. But S-R theories too often do no more than report these sequences or explain them only in terms of mechanistic models conceptualised as the intervening variables.

The present volume does not approach the subject in this way but seeks to define how the child perceives through the investigation of what determines his response.

Explanation is not simple and operates, simultaneously, at several different levels. For example, how can one understand psychological development without taking account of neurophysiological development? Research findings, such as those concerning the role of maturation or the specialised structures identified by Hubel and Wiesel, are clearly taken into account by Mlle Vurpillot. But she also uses essentially hypothetical models such as Köhler's satiation theory or the constructivist schemas of Hebb.

This work recognises the role both of specific learning and of general learning with its multiple transfer – but always considered in a dynamic perspective where set, and style of approach, are the determining factors.

Cognitive organisation makes its appearance in the establishment of the invariance of objects and their identification. Its development is manifested in the perception of relationships and the discovery of the criteria of identity and difference.

All of these potential abilities are realised through perceptual activity which at the beginning is stimulus-bound but which becomes more and more dependent upon strategies consistent with representations and internal models.

Mlle Vurpillot demonstrates this development for us by drawing upon a wide range of contemporary research to which she herself has made a substantial contribution. She cites only evidence which is derived from systematic observation or from experimental studies. This very necessary discipline does not lead to the sort of extravagant theories which satisfy those minds more concerned with the aesthetic appeal of a thesis than its truth. The visual world of the child that she describes for us does not correspond to those rich pages of a Renaissance atlas where lions and giraffes decorate an Africa where only a few coastal towns are marked. Neither is her description like a large-scale map which does not omit a single footpath or the smallest hamlet. No area of psychology is yet capable of such exhaustive description. But it does present maps which resemble those produced by explorers of the nineteenth century. They located with precision the major features of human and physical geography with, sometimes, greater detail in those areas where their exploration had been more complete.

This book involves us in the excitement of investigation where, at every stage, the basic hypotheses come up against the complexity of reality. And it gives us a useful illustration of the contemporary methods and approaches of the psychologist.

PAUL FRAISSE

# Contents

Foreword by Jerome Bruner                                      *page* 9
Preface to the French Edition by Paul Fraisse                      11
Introduction                                                       21

PART ONE   THE ROLE OF VISUAL STRUCTURES IN THE
ORGANISATION OF SPATIAL RELATIONSHIPS

1   The Evolution of Perceptual Structures
    I The Discrimination of Embedded Figures                       32
       1 *The Nature of the Problem*                               32
       2 *Personal Research*                                       38

    II The Perception of Reversible and Ambiguous Figures          47
       1 *Some Experimental Data*                                  47
       2 *A Comparison of Two Interpretations*                     49

    III The Phenomena of Closure                                   52
       1 *The Identification of Familiar Forms*                    53
       2 *Primary and Secondary 'Good' Forms*                      55
       *Conclusion*                                                59

2   The Spatial Relationships Between Structures in
    Three-Dimensional Space
    I Perceptual Constancies                                       66
       1 *Development of Size Constancy*                           66
       2 *Development of Form Constancy*                           70
    II The Perception of Verticality                               73

3   The Perception of Form Orientation
    I The Differentiation of Forms Presented in
      Different Orientations                                       75

    II Recognition of an Identical Form in Different
       Orientations                                                81

    III Interpretations of Children's Performances                84
       1 *The Role of the Spatial Frame of Reference*              84
       2 *Observations of Animal Behaviour:*
         *Lashley's (1938) Interpretation*                         85
       3 *Köhler and Retinal Orientation*                          86
       4 *Interpretation in Terms of the Existence of*
         *Specialised Neurones*                                    87

16    *The Visual World of the Child*

5  *Hebb's Theory and Sequential Exploration*      88
     *Conclusion*      96

4  Intrafigural Spatial Relationships
   I  Topological and Euclidean Relationships in the
      Representation of Forms      98
      1  *Data Obtained on Stereognostic Tasks*      98
      2  *Data Obtained with Drawn Reproductions*      100
      3  *Discussion*      101

  II  Intrafigural Relationships and the Perceived Form      103
 III  Part-whole Relationships      105
      1  *The Localisation of a Part within a Frame of
         Reference*      105
      2  *The Perception of the Displacement of a Single
         Element in a Configuration*      110
      3  *The Perception of Differences Caused by the
         Permutation of Components*      114

      *Conclusion of Chapters 2, 3 and 4*      121

5  Perceptual Organisation and the Processes of
   Identification and Differentiation: The Child's
   'Syncretism'
   I  The Predominance of the Whole or of the Parts      125
      1  *The Concept of Syncretism*      125
      2  *Experimental Evidence*      126

  II  The Absence of Articulation Between the Whole
      and the Parts      132
      1  *Part-Whole Confusion*      132
      2  *The Rigidity of Perceptual Organisation: the
         Exclusive Perception of the Whole or of the Parts*      134

      *Conclusion*      145

PART TWO    THE ANALYSIS OF VISUAL STRUCTURES IN
TERMS OF THEIR PROPERTIES

6  The Role of Verbal Mediators in Discrimination
   learning
   I  The Role of the Abstraction of a Dimension of
      Differentiation in the Transfer of Discrimination
      Learning      154
      1  *Transfer Involving the Conservation of the
         Relevant Dimension*      155

2 *Learning Involving Reversal and Non-reversal Shifts*                                                             155

II Theoretical Interpretations                                              159
  1 *The Single-stage Connectionist Model*                            159
  2 *The Intervention of Language in Discrimination Learning*                                                           161

7 Selective Attention

  I Observing Responses and Discrimination Learning          175
  II Selective Attention                                                      181
    1 *Mackintosh's Hypothesis*                                          182
    2 *Transfer Along a Continuum*                                       186
  III Gibson and Gibson's Theory of Perceptual Differentiation                                                          188
    1 *Outline of the Theory*                                               189
    2 *The Influence of Repetition on Performance in a Differentiation Task*                                      192
    3 *The Effects of Perceptual Pretraining on Learning Involving Reversal Shift*                           193
  IV Learning a Dimension or Learning a Prototype            195

8 The Emergence of Differentiators

  I Data Concerning the Order of Appearance of Differentiators                                                          201
    1 *Data from Discrimination Learning Experiments*       201
    2 *Data from Comparison Experiments: Detection and Differentiation*                                          203
    3 *Data from Choice-preference Investigations*            209
  II The Interpretation of these Results                              211
    1 *In Terms of a Relative Dominance of Dimensions of Differentiation*                          211
    2 *In Terms of the Acquisition of Cognitive Structures*                                                              211

  Conclusion of Chapters 6, 7 and 8                                  213

PART THREE   STRATEGIES OF EXPLORATION AND CRITERIA OF JUDGMENT

9 An Examination of Some Parameters of Visuo-Motor Exploration

  I The Extent of the Exploration                                      221
    1 *Spontaneous Visual Exploration in Familiarisation and Recognition Tasks*                          221

18 *The Visual World of the Child*

2 *The Investigation of the Extent of Visual Exploration
in a Task of Perceptual Differentiation* 223
3 *Task Adaptation* 226
4 *The Effects of Insufficient Exploratory Activity on
Performances of Identification and Differentiation* 229

II The Distribution of Visual Fixations 232
*The Concentration of Fixations and Information
Value* 233
2 *The Heterogeneity of the Concentrations of
Fixations as a Function of the Spatial Areas
of the Stimulus* 233

III Strategies of Exploration 235
1 *Strategies of Comparison in Relation to
Judgments of 'Same' or 'Not the Same'* 236
2 *The Influence of Reading on Strategies of
Exploration* 243
3 *The Influence of Sensori-motor Variables* 246

IV The Registering of Information: the Duration of
a Visual Fixation 251

10 The Role of Perceptual Activity in the Genesis of
Representational Structures

I The Theory of the Image 258
1 *Wekker's Hypotheses* 258
2 *The Role of Perceptual Exploration in the
Construction of the Image* 261

II Tactile Models and Visual Models 263
1 *Recording Tactile Exploratory Activity* 263
2 *Data Relating to Intermodal Transfer in
Children* 264

III The Influence of Training on Exploration 267

IV Graphic Reproduction and Exploratory Activity 269

V Discussion and Interpretation of the Data Reported 271

*Conclusion of Chapters 9 and 10* 273

11 Identity Criteria of Equivalence and Difference

I The Relationship Between Differentiation and
Identification 278
1 *Physical Identity and Perceived Identity* 279
2 *The Meaning of the Term 'Identity' in Some
Perceptual Tasks* 280

3 The Logical Relationship of Identity 285

II The Verbal Response 'The Same' 286

III Relative sensitivity to Differences and Similarities 288

IV Experimental Data on the Acquisition of the
Identity Relationship 289
 1 *Paired Comparison Tasks* 289
 2 *Comparison Tasks with the Responses 'Same'
 and 'Not the Same'* 292

General Conclusions 312
Bibliography 338
Index 365

# Introduction

A human being survives to the extent that he adapts to an environment which presents him, at the same time, with the necessary materials for the satisfaction of his needs and the danger of destruction. For this reason everyone needs to achieve sufficient understanding of the world and of himself to be able to grasp the significance of the information which he encounters and anticipate the results of his own actions. An adapted human being is capable of judging if the reality situation is favourable to him – in which case he will act in order to maintain it – or unfavourable, and then the action taken will have the aim of changing the situation into a better one. In other words he must interpret all the information which is available before predicting what the outcome of the current situation would be if he did not intervene, to anticipate how it would change if he undertook one or another course of action, and to evaluate what consequences such outcomes would have for him.

Adaptation implies, therefore, the conjoint involvement of multiple processes. Evaluation of the current situation comes under the heading of perception, whereas the conception of previous states and anticipation of possible changes is the province of representation. The storage of observed relationships between sequences of events, on the one hand when the individual is a passive spectator, and on the other hand when he intervenes (and according to the manner in which he does it), is the domain of memory in general and learning in particular. Finally, intelligence is involved at the level of strategies and decisions when it is necessary to choose from amongst all the information available that which is relevant, and from amongst all the possible courses of action that programme which it is preferable to adopt. There is no act of knowing that does not bring all these processes into play and none of them is completely independent of the others.

Perception can appear to play the dominant role because it is necessary to organise information before being able to store it, make predictions or take intelligent decisions. But, on the other hand, the strategy selected and previously acquired knowledge influence the information-search and, in consequence, direct perception.

All information concerning the nature of the physical world and its current state passes through the intermediary of the individual's sensory receptors. The environment is a permanent potential source of stimuli but the only evidence of their existence lies, for a particular individual, in a concomitant modification of the activity of the cells of his neural receptors. The sensitivity of these differs considerably from one species to another and, to a lesser extent, from one individual to another in the same species. It follows, therefore, that an identical modification of the external world can bring about a neural response in one organism but not in another; this is the case, for example, with those high-frequency sounds to which bats are sensitive, but not humans. Thus the range of potential data to which each organism can have access is determined by the capacities of the receptor systems. The experience of the same world, of an identical situation, being based on the information we can extract from it, differs from one individual to another and even more from one species to another; in the last analysis it is individual and incommunicable.

While the sensory organs constitute the direct means of communication between an organism and its environment, and the information gathered by them forms the raw material with which all knowledge is going to be constructed, yet the nature of the nervous system is far from determining on its own what form the knowledge will take.

The contacts between an individual and all the potential information contained in the world do not have the same frequency of occurrence; furthermore the quality and quantity of information gathered differs from one organism to another. In the same species, with equal receptor capacity, one can observe a uniformity of learning in those individuals who belong to one subculture and live together in a restricted and relatively homogeneous environment, and, at the same time, a differentiation of learning between subcultures situated in very different environments. The differences between environments are, at once, geographic and social; and in the formation of concepts the nature of the surrounding countryside – urban or rural, coastal, desert, tropical or temperate – is involved as much as manufactured objects or social norms. To this it must be added, however, that the development of means of communication – by actual transport or by audio-visual transmission – in conjunction with demographic expansion, has reduced the distance between people, has placed the same information at everyone's disposal, and has induced cultural uniformity. Thus the tendency in our time is towards a reduction of cultural differences between educated people.

The nature and frequency of encounters with the environment, together with the sensitivity of the sensory receptors, jointly determine, therefore, what information a person has available in order to construct 'his' world. This information reaches him in the form of physical energy, or stimulation, to which the receptor nerve cells respond in chain reaction; this is essentially raw material which has to be processed. However, man's central nervous system is endowed with an innate capacity to organise nerve impulses into structured units. Fortunately the number of separate messages which the sensory receptors can record and transmit greatly exceeds the five to nine units of information which the human central nervous system appears to be capable of processing simultaneously. Above all, knowledge would seem to be the organisation of information into structures: perceptual, representational, mnemonic, intellectual. The multiple schemas acquired by the individual can, as appropriate, coexist independently one with another or link up to form structures of hierarchical complexity. Correspondingly, the nature of the nervous system sets the limits within which organised systems of cognitive structures can be developed.

The object of this book is to study the manner in which the child learns through the intermediary of the visual modality. Compared with the human adult, the child is limited in his cognitive activity in many ways, and above all by his biological immaturity. As with skeletal and muscular growth, it seems that the maturation of the central nervous system continues up to adolescence, but with a rhythm which differs according to the substructures involved and which becomes progressively slower with age. The younger the child the greater the influence of this factor. The immaturity of the nervous system is manifested by limited sensitivity of the receptors, inadequate neural connections and restricted storage capacity. The amount of data recorded is more circumscribed, is imprecise and is transmitted more slowly. At the same time the connections are neither numerous nor complex, so that few relationships are established between what is learnt, and these relationships mainly involve those elements which are close together. This immaturity is evident also at the level of the storage of recorded data. We do not yet know enough about the matter of cerebral traces to be able to say what the physiological basis of memory is; we only know that memory span increases with age and is almost non-existent at birth. Its growth is therefore almost certainly bound up with neural maturation.

Biological immaturity also affects the organs of motor activity and limits indirectly the range of information to which a child has access. Until he learns to walk, the young child can only operate in a very restricted radius in front of him and cannot change the location of this restricted territory at will, but has to be carried by an adult. Even later, his height and limited muscular power constitute significant handicaps. Finally, the imprecision of sensori-motor coordination adds to the spatial limitations of the field of activity, thus making it difficult to establish the laws of correspondence between the child's own actions and the reciprocal modifications of the environment.

Thus one can expect that, at first, the primary cognitive structures will involve only a few units of information and that spatial and temporal proximity will be the necessary condition for their integration. Simple chains of sensory stimuli and motor responses, in the form of motor habits or sensori-motor schemas, and perceptions limited to the set of stimuli within one modality – experienced in a given moment – could constitute these primary structures. As neural connections multiply and as the range of recall and processing extends, isolated structures, incomplete and limited to the present moment, link up and become organised into more complex wholes which encompass not only current information but what has been recalled – past information – and what is anticipated – information about the future. These new structures, which can be called secondary, finish by joining up and fitting in with each other until all knowledge belongs to a single, logical and coherent system.

It is reasonable to assume that the primary structures are essentially determined by the characteristics of the central nervous system since they are concerned with basic, simultaneously experienced sensory data. Without being independent of these characteristics, and therefore linked with maturation, the secondary structures are more vulnerable to the influence of the vagaries of the environment, both physical and human. The capacity to organise and to categorise appears to be innate, common to all human beings, but the number and the content of the categories depend on the nature of the physical environment and the cultural norms of the human group to which the child belongs.

Limited by his biological immaturity and by the, as yet, restricted experience he has gained at first hand of relating his expectations to the results of his actions, the child finds himself subject to the powerful pressure of the human environment which tends to impose on the young the cognitive structures developed by their elders.

It seems clear that a particular concept cannot be transferred as an organised whole from one individual to another; though the models of the adult serve as a guide, the child must nonetheless construct his own conceptual system. Furthermore, the acquisition of concepts is a dynamic process: the more numerous they become, the more likely they are to organise themselves in terms of a particular system and the less chance have other systems, initially equally feasible, of achieving realisation. The individual only seeks that information which is relevant to the proof or disproof of his own hypotheses, which are based on the concepts he has available; the pre-existing structures to some extent determine future structures. Only the awareness of incongruity puts in question the validity of previously acquired concepts and thereby calls for their modification. A society's system of concepts evolves slowly; correspondingly the child, endowed with the same type of nervous system, living in the same physical environment and continually presented with models of cognitive structures, arrives at maturity furnished with a conceptual system analogous to that of his fellow citizens.

In the course of his development he manifests, at each stage, a form of adaptive behaviour. But the form of his adaptation changes with age to the extent that, biologically, he becomes more adult, as his experience increases, and as he conforms to the cultural norms of his environment.

It is difficult for an adult to imagine that there exist other modes of adaptation than his own. His criteria of judgment appear self-evident to him and, when the performance on a task is what he expects, he is always tempted to conclude that it has been attained by the procedure he would have followed himself. Even if he allows that the child's plans of action and decision criteria are different from those of the adult, whilst still being a satisfactory form of adaptation, the greatest difficulty remains, namely, being able to infer the criteria to which the child conforms from the behaviour that is observed.

The very earliest child psychologists sought to define the child's visual world – in what respects it differed from that of the adult and how it changed as the child grew older. Their understanding of children was derived from the information available to them, but they selected their data and investigated it within limits fixed by the technical resources and the current theories of their time, as much as by their own experience and their personal motivation. In addition the interpretations of evidence differed from one author to another and were sometimes in flat contradiction.

In writing this book we have attempted to bring together a wide range of research on the behaviour of young children relevant to their visual perception of the physical world and, from the range of explanatory hypotheses which have been put forward, to identify those which meet most of the factual evidence. The realisation of this intention is itself limited by the capacities of the author, her personal experience and the ethos of her intellectual environment.

Also, like all attempts at understanding, what we have tried to do is itself very imperfect.

The research findings that have been selected consist of data obtained in carefully controlled situations, situations in which the subject produces a performance which enables the experimenter to understand how he has perceived and resolved the problem presented. A wide range of research has been selected with regard for these criteria, but the map of the child's behaviour that could conceivably tell us something about his visual world, remains incomplete.

Research concerned with babies, which has greatly expanded in recent years, is reported and discussed elsewhere (Vurpillot, 1972). We content ourselves here with a brief exposition of behaviour at two stages of development which are of particular significance: at birth and around the age of three months. A primary characteristic of the neonate is that of an organism whose capacities for sensory reception greatly exceed his capacity for response (Bruner, 1968). Whereas he is able to discriminate visually between stimulus patterns in terms of a number of variables, he can only respond with specific sensori-motor behaviours such as sucking, looking and hand closure, which do not match the fine gradations of his sensory capacities, or with random activity.

The neonate is capable of visual discrimination in terms of brightness, colour and degree of heterogeneity (amount of black and white contrast) of the stimulus, provided that the physical differences are gross. Thus his attention displays a preference for moving and boldly contrasting stimuli. The immaturity of his visual system is such that, lacking visual accommodation, he can only see clearly objects situated at a specific distance, and successive stimuli must be of sufficient duration, and sufficiently spaced, if they are not to be confused or to pass unnoticed. Figure-ground discrimination is evident at birth and would appear, therefore, to be innate; it does not seem to be a case, as Hebb (1949) has postulated, of the simple perception of something undifferentiated, since the neonate responds differentially to patterns of the same area and of equal reflectivity but on which the design and arrangement of the black and white parts vary. At the moment it is impossible to determine the degree of perceptual organisation involved and, consequently, at which stage of figure-ground discrimination (Wever, 1927) to place the neonate.

The period around the age of three months is characterised by a series of changes the origin of which can be found in the progress of neural maturation. Thus, visual accommodation is now perfect, visual pursuit operates in all directions, eye/hand co-ordination becomes evident at the same time as the occipital alpha rhythm, and the 'quieting' response appears. In short, all behaviour is typified by a degree of co-ordination which was absent, or very limited, until that time – progress in which the growth of neural connections and the acceleration of the processes of transmission in the brain undoubtedly play a central role.

Retinal maturation brings with it an increase in sensitivity which is apparent as much at the level of the absolute thresholds of response to light as it is in terms of perceptual acuity. This sensitivity continues to improve throughout the first year, though more slowly, paralleling the progress of receptor maturation.

It is more difficult to establish a link between the level of maturation and the awareness of spatial relationships which marks the beginnings of the perceptual constancies of shape and size, similarly between the level of maturation and the appearance of a perceptual organisation obeying the laws of Gestalt. On the other hand, the temporal expansion of recall, which manifests an increase in the persistence of a cerebral trace, fits in very well with an explanation in terms of cerebral maturation. Conditionability and habituation, which only become clear around the age of 2–3 months would also, therefore, be linked to organic changes.

To summarise: cerebral maturation continues after birth and reaches a significant stage between 2 and 4 months; until then certain behaviours cannot be established because of the sluggishness of cerebral processes and the limited number of connections. From this point everything changes and the interpretation of the development of behaviour becomes increasingly difficult and uncertain. Up to that time observable changes are more quantitative than qualitative, and their connection with anatomical and physiological changes relatively obvious. Once a level of maturation is reached which makes possible the appearance of new behaviours, then these are themselves going to have an influence on development. As a result, although the maturational process continues to unfold, it becomes more and more difficult to discern in the changes that one observes those which are directly imputable to maturation and those that must be attributed to the practice of these behaviours.

Research investigations involving babies, particularly numerous on the neonate and the infant of 4–6 months, become comparatively rare beyond these ages. When it comes to the experimental study of children from 1 to 3 years, a great deal remains to be done. One finds interesting observations, piecemeal research limited to certain themes, but no coherent set of connected, organised investigations concerned with the study of cognitive performance. Our relative ignorance concerning this period of childhood must be attributed largely to an absence of satisfactory techniques of investigation. Although from the age of 2 years a child, typically, already has an extensive vocabulary, our language codes are not the same and the implicit assumption that the use of a word by a child implies that he has the concept which the word represents is a source of misconceptions. Too often, to avoid this difficulty, the experimenter falls back on tasks and techniques developed in work with animals, which lead him to interpret the child's responses in the same way as those of the rat. In consequence, in the present volume, only the data on children from 3 to 7 years will be analysed in detail.

Not all the factors involved in the perceptual and cognitive development of children are studied in the pages that follow; notably those variables relative to the influence of the social environment do not have the place they warrant, partly because experimental investigations in this area are as yet few.

One final point: the selection of the evidence presented by the author, like the manner in which it is organised, is representative of her personal conceptual system as much as of reality.

# PART ONE

## The Role of Visual Structures in the Organisation of Spatial Relationships

# Chapter 1

# The Evolution of
# Perceptual Structures

Figure-ground discrimination can be demonstrated at birth (Kessen, 1967; Salapatek, 1968); the factor of uniform destiny appears to be operative at 5 weeks, and those of proximity and continuity somewhat later around the age of 6 months. Visual stimuli are therefore perceptually organised by the infant by the second half of the first year of life. Yet the primary perceptual structures which make up the visual world of children of 3 and 4 years of age, those which they operate and identify, appear to be rigid, indivisible, unanalysable and unarticulated.

For the child of 6 to 8 years the perceptual structures have lost much of their rigidity; the child of this age can break these structures down into parts, abstract certain of their characteristics and attend to one part whilst disregarding the others. Equally, different perceptual units can be combined, each one serving as a whole to the smaller units of which it is composed and, at the same time, as a component part of the comprehensive structure. It does not seem crucially important to us to decide whether there has been a transition from rigid primary perceptual structures, or whether the 7-year-old child can carry out intellectual operations involving perceptual structures which are the same at all age-levels, but which the 3-year-old child shows himself incapable of. It is a matter of theoretical preference, or perhaps the choice of words. To the present writer, who considers perception as a form of knowledge, the search for a precise boundary between what is perceptual and what is not is a pseudo-problem.

We are simply concerned to investigate how the child's ability to act on his perceptual structures develops with age, and the effects of this evolution on the processes of identification and differentiation.

The purpose of the present chapter is to specify how the components of a line-figure drawing are organised in perceptual units; the extent to which children of 4–7 years of age can break them down into their components and reassemble them in new forms as in solving embedded-figures problems; to what degree they can link up isolated perceptual units by means of imaginary lines in order to identify the more complex structures of incomplete figures; and finally to see if they can pass rapidly from one structure to another when these are equipotential (reversible figures).

## 1   THE DISCRIMINATION OF EMBEDDED FIGURES

Those puzzle pictures in which you are asked to find a particular object from amongst the multitude of lines of a complicated drawing are a well-known example of the techniques of conceal-ment. The difficulty of the puzzle is due to the fact that the object to be found coincides with none of the units in which the drawing as a whole is organised perceptually. In order to succeed it is there-fore necessary to go beyond the objects spontaneously perceived, to disregard them as such and to consider the whole drawing as a mass of lines; this has then to be analysed and new groupings of the components attempted in order to create a structure identical to the model.

## 1   *The nature of the problem*

(*a*) *Historical review.* The technique of the discrimination of em-bedded figures would seem to be a good way of studying perceptual organisation, provided that non-representational figures are used and that the drawings are made up of a restricted number of lines so that their geometric relationships can be strictly controlled. In this way it is possible, by presenting different figures which have to be abstracted from the same complex line-drawing, first to verify the predictive value of Gestalt theories of organisation, and secondly to study the possibilities of perceptual structuring in terms of the physical properties of the stimuli and the develop-mental level of the subjects. If in fact the laws governing the organisation of figures are valid, they must make it possible to predict those structures into which the lines of a given complex figure will organise themselves; and any problem where the solu-tion coincides with the discovery of one of these structures (as, for example, in problems of overlapping figures) should be solved rapidly and, furthermore, by the youngest children. Conversely, the discovery of a figure which does not coincide with one of these structures (as is the case in embedded-figures problems) should be impossible until a child's developmental level permits him to act on his perceptual structures and, if not to modify them, at least to bypass them.

Numerous investigations have shown that the normal adult solves overlapping figures problems easily and rapidly. Presented with a complex geometric design and asked to describe it, all adults break it down into the same figures: the segregation into perceptual structures is thus the same for all, at least within the same culture. Only brain-damaged adults (Poppelreuter, 1917, 1923) fail to perceive the overlapping figures in a complex line-figure drawing.

Gottschaldt (1926) has shown that the repeated presentation of stimulus-patterns is insufficient to bring about their organisation into perceptual structures. The aim of this investigation was to demonstrate that associationism, as a theory, was unable to explain the phenomenon of perceptual organisation, whilst Gestalt theory accounted for it perfectly. The technique and, particularly, the material developed by this research-worker have been used many times since then, and the name of Gottschaldt is inextricably associated with embedded-figures problems; thus any account concerning the resolution of such problems must review briefly the original experiment.

A figure of type A (a hexagon, for example) is presented a certain number of times in one-second exposures, the subject having the task of memorising it. After several different line-figures have been presented in this fashion, a second series of line-figures (type B) is presented, each being exposed for two seconds, and the subject asked to describe them. The figures of type B have been constructed in such a way that one part of each of them is exactly identical to one of the figures of type A, but according to the laws of Gestalt theory, this part cannot constitute a perceptual unit (fig. 1). If the laws of associationism applied, the probability of perceiving a figure of type A amongst the lines of a figure of type B should be greater the more frequently A has been seen beforehand. However, even though a type A figure is included in each of the figures of type B, its presence is reported by an insignificant number

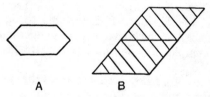

A               B

Fig. 1. Example of embedded-figure problem (Gottschaldt, 1926).

of subjects – less than 10 per cent and this proportion remains the same, whether the type A figure has been presented three times or 520 times. Gottschaldt concluded from this that only the physical properties of the stimulus determine its organisation into figures. The components of a figure of type A present objective relationships of proximity, orientation and length which bring about the perception of a figure (a hexagon, in the example given). When the components of this hexagon are added to others in order to make up a new figure of type B, the relationships between the components of the hexagon are less salient than those which govern the new structure B, and it is these latter that determine which figures will be perceived in B. A number of experiments of the same kind, carried out by other workers, have basically substantiated and further refined Gottschaldt's results (Djang, 1937; Hanawalt, 1942; Francès, 1963) whilst ascertaining more clearly the limits of their generalisation.

Gottschaldt's research was concerned with the spontaneous perception of figures in a complex line-drawing. Other psychologists have subsequently used Gottschaldt's original figures in order to study the plasticity of perception. When a figure of type A is presented side by side with the corresponding figure of type B and the subject is asked explicitly to find A in B, adults are rarely unsuccessful. The main variation is in the speed with which the task is accomplished, but in this respect individual differences are considerable and, in particular, women are consistently slower than men (Thurstone, 1944; Witkin, 1950; Andrieux, 1955).

(*b*) *Predictions concerning perceptual organisation.* Geometrically and conceptually speaking, a line is an infinite assembly of points which it is possible to consider separately; and the number of elements into which a line-drawing can be broken up is also infinite, as are the number of possible combinations between these elements. Perceptually, however, this is not the case since a line-drawing 'organises itself' into a limited number of perceptual structures. The Gestalt theorists predict that these structures, which we shall call *primary structures*, are essentially determined by the laws of 'good' continuity and 'good' form (closure, symmetry, internal equilibrium). It is possible to derive from these laws certain principles which enable us to predict into what primary structures any complex line-figure will be organised:

1   All the lines of a figure are involved in the construction of the primary contour structures (PCS).
2   No line or part of a line can belong to more than one primary

structure. [The sum of the components which make up the primary contour structures is equal to the sum of the components which make up the figure in its entirety.]

3 A line belongs in its entirety to a single primary contour structure; [the different segments of which it is made up cannot be used in the composition of several primary contour structures].

4 The primary contour structures are preferably symmetrical or at least as regular as possible.

5 The number of primary contour structures must be the fewest possible.

The laws postulated by Wertheimer (1923) are concerned essentially with the lines of a figure, but the surface of the paper which these lines enclose is also undoubtedly involved in the perceptual organisation. Thus we must add one supplementary principle:

6 Each white area of paper entirely surrounded by the lines of a figure and not crossed by another line constitutes a primary area structure (**PAS** or **MO**).

In the embedded figures problems (Gottschaldt's figures) the solution involves going beyond the primary structures to create *secondary structures*.

A secondary contour structure (SCS) is made up of lines, or segments of these, borrowed from one or several primary contour structures (fig. 2); the same line or the same segment of a line can belong at the same time to a primary structure and to one or several secondary structures.

A secondary area structure (SAS or AMO) is formed by the juxtaposition of several primary area structures (fig. 3).

From these formulations a fundamental difference is immediately apparent between secondary contour structures and secondary area structures. Whilst the secondary contour structures can only be made up of elements borrowed from several primary structures and depend therefore upon the preliminary dismemberment of these, the secondary area structures require no modifications of the corresponding primary structures, a simple addition being sufficient.

Complex line-figures can be divided into two groups, according to whether the relationships between the basic contour structures are those of overlap or juxtaposition (fig. 2).

In overlapping figures, the primary contour structures cut across each other at several points; the lines which make up these outlines continue, in the same direction, beyond the point of intersection.

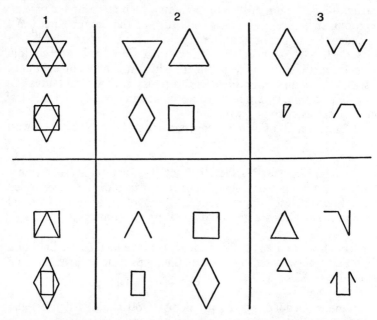

Fig. 2. Examples of the analysis of complex line-drawings (column 1), into primary (column 2), or secondary (column 3) contour structures (Vurpillot and Florès, 1946). In the top two rows of column 1 the figures are overlapping, in the bottom two rows they are juxtaposed.

Furthermore, the area enclosed by one of these primary contour structures can only be a secondary area structure.

In the case of juxtaposed figures, the primary contour structures only have points of contact and do not intersect. In particular instances one of them can constitute the outline of the complex figure, which puts it in a privileged position and tends to make it the

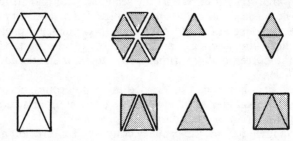

Fig. 3. Examples of the analysis of juxtaposed figures into primary or secondary surface structures (Vurpillot and Florès, 1964).

frame of reference for the other components of the figure. This privileged, or reference, structure always encloses a secondary area structure, but in certain cases another primary contour structure can enclose a primary area structure.

*(c) Hypotheses concerning the evolution of development.* Following on from these distinctions between the different components which are involved in embedded-figures problems, one could expect that such a task should demonstrate clearly the rigidity of perceptual structures in children from 3 to 4 years.

The young child perceives in a complex line-drawing a group of figures, clearly individuated, which he cannot analyse. It is therefore easy for him to find in the line-drawing the figure identical to a given model when this is coincident with one of these primary perceptual structures (overlapping figures problems). If, on the other hand, the model is not identical with any of the latter (for example, in enclosed figures problems) the child is unable to put it together from components abstracted from several of them. It follows: (1) that his performance, excellent in the first instance, will be poor in the second; and (2) that his incorrect responses will consist of designating a primary structure as the solution of a problem which demands the identification of a secondary structure.

As the child frees himself, progressively, from the influence of primary structures, the proportion of correct responses to enclosed-figures problems increases.

Several investigations have verified that part of this hypothesis concerned with performances involving -abstraction. When the problems entail searching for enclosed figures, the younger the children the greater the number of failures (Witkin, 1950; Ghent, 1956a). Indeed, it appears that before the age of 6 success is exceptional, no matter how much time the child is allowed (Ghent, 1956a). On the other hand, approximately 70 per cent of 4-year-olds are successful in identifying overlapping figures (Piaget and Stettler, 1954; Ghent, 1956a; Vurpillot, 1964a; Vurpillot and Florès, 1964). The percentage of successes varies a little according to the nature of the material (fig. 4); the greater the number of lines in the drawing, the more numerous the figures, the more points of intersection there are, the more errors and omissions are observed. Ghent (1956a) obtained, with the same 4-year-old children, an 84 per cent success rate with overlapping geometric figures and only a 53 per cent success rate with overlapping representational figures (fig. 4). In the latter case the points of intersection are significantly more numerous and irregularity of the forms more frequent. The factor of representation does not seem to account

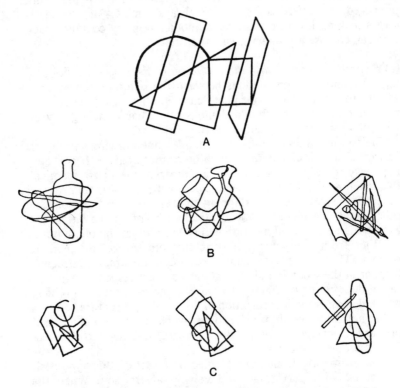

Fig. 4. Examples of line-drawings used in the investigation of overlapping-figures problems.
  *A* : complex figure used by Piaget and Stettler (1954).
  *B* : complex representational figures (Ghent, 1956a).
  *C* : complex geometric figures (Ghent, 1956a).

for the observed difference because, with material of the same type, Oléron and Gumusyan (1964) obtained a higher success rate with figures representing familiar objects than with geometric forms.

## 2   *Personal Research*

The author's personal contribution has involved the systematic study of the interaction between the levels of organisation of the surface area and contour of the figures which have to be identified and the influence of the technique of reproduction employed. Furthermore we have attempted to validate the hypotheses proposed by an analysis of the incorrect responses as well as by measuring the percentage of correct responses.

(*a*) *Technique.* A succession of experiments have been carried out, all following the same experimental procedure. A problem consists of the presentation of two line-figure drawings, a model to the left, and a complex figure to the right. The instructions given emphasise these points: that the figure to be found forms only a part of the complex figure and that it must be exactly the same as the model. If the child is not satisfied with his answer he can tackle the same problem again; no time-limit is imposed.

It follows from these instructions that the task is a double one: it involves reorganisation because certain lines in the complex figure must be abstracted from the others and reassembled in a new structure, and also comparison since the structure produced in this fashion must be physically identical to the model. Failures can occur therefore at two levels, that of organisation and that of the judgment of identity. But these two levels are themselves hierarchically organised. With a good capacity for organisation a child may do one of two things: he can respond correctly or, of course, fall into the error of giving a response based on equivalence instead of identity between the model and the reproduction. But if his level of organisation is inadequate, a response based on identity is impossible and the choice is limited to structures more or less equivalent to the model.

Two techniques of reproduction have been employed. Reproduction by tracing is derived from Thurstone (1944). The child, using a thick red pencil, has to go over those lines of the large figure which reproduce the model. This technique therefore requires the child to find the *contour* of the small figure in the larger one. In reproduction by colouring, the child has to fill in, with a red pencil, all of that *area* of the larger figure which is identical to the model.

(*b*) *Validation according to the number of successes.* Two experiments (exp. I and exp. II) have involved the systematic investigation of the ascending order of difficulty of a series of problems as a function of the interaction of the following factors:

—the discovery of primary structures or the construction of secondary contour structures;
—complex figures made up of juxtaposed or overlapping figures;
—open or closed simple figures;
—the level of organisation, primary or secondary, of the area of the figure to be found.

Six groups of problems were prepared, characterised by different types of organisation, which could be reorganised on two different levels (figs 5 and 6).

## 40   *The Visual World of the Child*

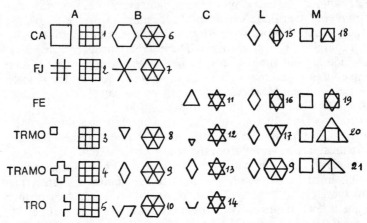

Fig. 5. The 21 embedded-figures problems of experiment I (Vurpillot and Florès, 1964).

The columns correspond to the five series of problems. In series A, B and C, differing simple figures have to be found in the same complex figure. In series L and M the same simple figure has to be found in different complex figures. The rows correspond to the categories of problems defined as a function of the type of organisation of the components required for a correct response.

*Primary level of organisation*: The discovery of primary contour structures PCS.

1 *CA problems*. The simple figure, or model, is identical to a complex figure of the juxtaposed type.
2 *FJ problems*. The model is identical with a primary structure (PCS), other than the 'frame', in a complex figure of the juxtaposed type.
3 *FE problems*. A model is identical with one of the primary structures (PCS) of a complex figure of the overlapping type.

*Secondary level of organisation*: The construction of secondary contour structures (SCS).

4 *TRMO problems*. The contour of the model is not identical with any primary contour structure of the complex figure, but the area enclosed is identical with a primary area structure (PAS).
5 *TRAMO problems*. The contour of the model is not identical with a PCS of the complex figure, but the area enclosed comprises the sum of several primary area structures (SAS).
6 *TRO problems*. The contour of the model is an open figure,

identical with no primary contour structure of the complex figure.

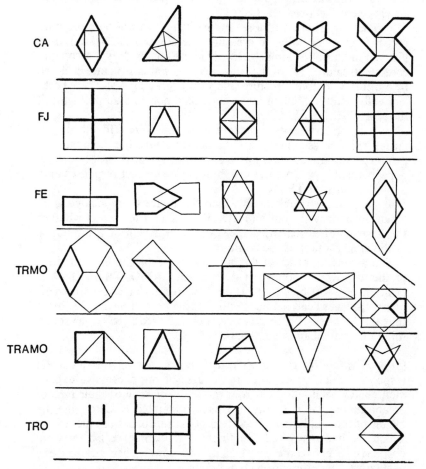

Fig. 6. The 30 embedded-figure problems of experiment II. The correct response indicated by *thick lines* (the model reproduced on the complex figure).

On the basis of the foregoing analysis (pp. 34 and 35), the following predictions were made concerning the relative difficulty of the six categories of problems.

1 The first three categories of problems, which require the identification of a primary contour structure, will be easier than the other three, which involve the construction of a secondary

contour structure. In other words, at the same age-level, the number of successes should be greater for the first three categories, and success in the last three should appear only when a certain stage of development has been reached.

2 The construction of a secondary structure will be more difficult if it involves both the area and the contour (TRAMO), than if it is a matter of a primary area structure enclosed by a secondary contour structure (TRMO) or of a secondary area structure enclosed by a primary contour structure (FE, CA, FJ). A TRAMO type problem will, therefore, obtain fewer correct responses than problems of the types TRMO, FE, CA and FJ.

3 A secondary contour structure will be more difficult to construct than a secondary area stucture, thus the combination primary contour-secondary area should be easier than the reverse. A problem of type CA will thus obtain more correct responses than a problem of type TRMO.

4 As to those problems in which the figure to be located is an 'open' secondary structure (TRO), it is difficult to predict whether the absence of an enclosed area would be a help or a hindrance in the construction of the contour.

The ascending order of difficulty expected on the basis of these predictions was as follows: CA, FE, FJ, TRMO, TRAMO – the position of TRO being uncertain. The results of the two experiments that were carried out verified these predictions, and showed that the absence of a completely enclosed area (TRO) was something of a handicap (see figs 5, 6, 7 and 8).

(c) *Validation by the analysis of errors.* All of the incorrect responses which occurred in the course of our successive experiments have been analysed from the point of view of their type of organisation; that is to say, we have attempted to determine, by means of the child's pencilled attempts at reproduction, the way in which he had organised the lines of the complex figure, what obstacles he had come up against, and how he had resolved the particular difficulties in each problem.

Only one category of errors will be described here, namely those which involve giving as the answer a primary contour structure when the correct response is a secondary contour structure. Table 1 gives the proportion of errors which involved tracing a primary contour structure, whether a 'frame' or a juxtaposed figure within a complex structure of that type, or an overlapped figure within a structure of overlapping figures, in four experiments involving problems of types TRAMO and TRO.

Errors due to tracing primary contour structures make up about

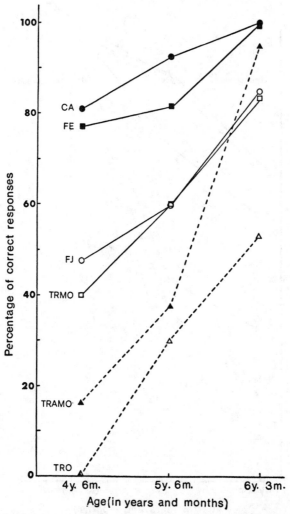

Fig. 7. Evolution with age of the proportion of correct responses in each category of problems in experiment I (Vurpillot and Florès, 1964).

See the text for the definition of the categories; the ascending order of difficulty across the six categories is CA, FE, FJ, TRMO, TRAMO, TRO (Kendall's W (1948), significant at the ·01 level).

two-thirds of the total number of errors between 4 and 5 years and persist at all age-levels. Their significant diminution, at 6 years in experiments I and II, at 5½ years in experiment III, and at 5 years

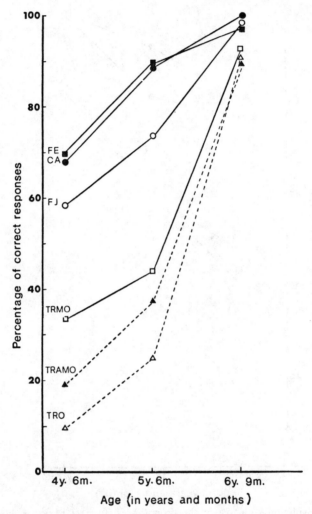

Fig. 8. Evolution with age of the proportion of correct responses in each category of problems in experiment II.

See the text for the definition of the categories. With the youngest children, the discovery of primary contour structures (CA, FJ and FE) is easier than the discovery of secondary contour structures (TRMO, TRAMO, TRO). (F=95·81 at 4y.6m.; F=170·02 at 5y.6m.; both significant at the ·0005 level.) The problems of type FJ are more difficult than those of type CA at 5y.6m. (F=9·47 significant at the ·01 level). There is an ascending order of difficulty from TRMO to TRAMO to TRO (F=18·78 at 4y.6m.; F=16·78 at 5y.6m.; both significant at the ·0005 level).

in experiment IV, coincides in each case with a marked increase in the number of correct responses.

Table 1   *Proportion of errors due to tracing primary structures in TRAMO and TRO problems (experiments I, II, III, and IV)*

| | Ages | | | | | | Number of problems |
|---|---|---|---|---|---|---|---|
| | 4–5 yrs | | 5–6 yrs | | 6–7 yrs | | |
| | N | PCS % | N | PCS % | N | PCS % | |
| Exp.  1 | 156 | 58·3 | 115 | 47·0 | 36 | 11·2 | 8 |
| Exp.  11 | 214 | 69·2 | 172 | 69·2 | 24 | 45·8 | 10 |
| Exp. III | 96 | 56·2 | 75 | 40·0 | 21 | 23·8 | 5 |
| Exp. IV | 252 | 66·7 | 133 | 33·1 | 134 | 23·9 | 13 |

PCS=percentage of errors involving primary contour structures amongst the total number of errors. N=gross number of errors. Experiments III and IV differ from experiments I and II only in the number of problems and subjects involved.

Experiment V attempted to investigate the interaction between the organisation of the contour and the organisation of the surface-area in a complex figure as a function of the bias towards one or the other organisation brought about by the technique of reproduction employed.

Thurstone's technique (1944), which requires the child to trace over the lines of the model in the complex figure with a red pencil, draws attention to the contour of the figure which has to be found. The technique which requires the child to colour in that part of the complex figure occupied by the figure to be identified, must, on the other hand, emphasise the internal surface-area of that figure. In experiment V, twelve problems were tackled in succession by the same children using both techniques (Vurpillot and Florès, 1964). These problems were so formulated that, in four of them, the contour of the figure to be identified is that of a primary contour structure, whilst the construction of the surface area is at the secondary level of organisation; in another four the reverse is the case (i.e. primary surface area, secondary contour); and in the remaining four the contour and the surface-area enclosed by the figure to be identified have to be constructed by the sort of activity denoted as the secondary level of organisation (fig. 9).

Table 2 summarises the main results of experiment V; since the relative difficulty of the different problems was the same at all ages, the results of the fifty children from 4 to 6½ years have been combined.

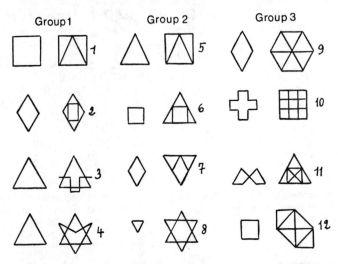

Fig. 9. The twelve problems of experiment V (Vurpillot and Florès, 1964). There are four problems of group 1 (1st column), four of group 2 (2nd column), and four of group 3 (3rd column).

The results of the experiment are clear; when the figure to be identified presents a primary level of organisation of contour and a secondary level of organisation of the surface-area, performance is better by the tracing technique (sign test significant at the ·01 level, within subjects); when the figure to be identified pre-

Table 2

| Level of organisation involved in the discovery of the figure to be identified | | Percentages of correct responses obtained with each method | |
|---|---|---|---|
| Contour | Surface-area | Tracing % | Colouring % |
| Level  I(CA or FE) | Level II(AMO) | 87·0 | 63·0 |
| Level II(TRMO) | Level  I(MO) | 66·5 | 83·5 |
| Level II(TRAMO) | Level II(AMO) | 13·0 | 28·0 |

There are four problems and 50 subjects, that is 200 responses to each category of problems. MO=primary surface-area structure; AMO=secondary surface-area structure.

sents a primary level of organisation of the surface-area and a secondary level of organisation of the contour, performance is better with the colouring technique (sign test significant at the ·01 level, within subjects). When the level of organisation involved is secondary for both the contour and the surface-area, performance is better with the colouring technique.

It is possible to draw two conclusions from these data. The methods selected clearly induce different sets, and the relative difficulty of the problems seems to be determined largely by the level of organisation of the part (contour or surface) which the technique selected enhances (tracing for the contour, colouring for the surface). Moreover, and as had been predicted in the analysis of the problem, the secondary level of organisation of contour presents greater difficulty than that of surface-area. The problems of the third category are clearly easier to resolve by colouring, thus focusing attention on the surface-areas involved, than by tracing, which draws attention to the contour.

It can be concluded from this series of experiments concerning the discrimination of embedded figures that the laws of organisation of a complex figure in terms of a number of simple perceptual structures are valid as early as the age of 4 years. When the figure to be identified coincides with one of the primary structures predicted in terms of these laws, children succeed in the great majority of cases from the age of 4 years. However, when the figure to be discovered coincides with none of the primary structures of the complex figure, success is found only after about 6 years of age. When the child fails, he tends to select one of the primary structures; the younger he is the more systematically this occurs.

## II THE PERCEPTION OF REVERSIBLE AND AMBIGUOUS FIGURES

Theoretically, a collection of stimuli should be capable of being organised in a multiplicity of ways. This is not the case with perception, and typically a single form of organisation is manifested, the form of which can be predicted in terms of Gestalt theory. Nonetheless, there are some situations, more or less artificial, in which the laws of organisation predict two forms of segregation into figures. This is the case with the so-called reversible figures, in which the roles of figure and background are held alternately by different areas of the same picture.

### 1 *Some Experimental Data*

When one particular form of perceptual organisation can be predicted in terms of Gestalt theory, the figures perceived are extremely stable; if, on the other hand, the application of these laws is compatible with several different forms of organisation, then perception becomes unstable and the various figures are perceived alternately. The number of changes observed varies with the fixation time and the age of the subjects, but the data obtained by different investigators are often contradictory. According to Köhler (1940, p. 68), using two subjects and the classic segmented circle, the longer the period of fixation, the more rapid the alternation between perceptions became. However, using the Schroeder staircase, Bruner, Postman and Mosteller (1950) found, on the contrary, a slowing down of alternation with time. The physical characteristics of the stimulus figure (Graham, 1929; Porter, 1938), the set induced by the instructions (Bruner, Postman and Mosteller, 1950), or by reinforcement (Schafer and Murphy, 1943), the personality of the subject (Guilford and Hart, 1931; Porter, 1938), to quote only a few examples, are all factors which influence the probability of the manifestation – and persistence – of one form of organisation rather than another.

Two categories of reversible figures are to be distinguished on the basis of whether or not representation plays a role in the segregation. In the segmented circle figure the organisation into other figures is independent of any identification; the determination of the most appropriate area to constitute the figure (black rather than white, narrow segments rather than wide ones) is simply a function of the structural properties of the figure.

This is not the case when the same figure can be identified in two quite different ways: the wife or the mother-in-law, the rabbit or the pirate (Leeper, 1935), a tree or a duck (Elkind and Scott, 1962). In these cases, representation plays an important role and enters into conflict with the structural properties of the figure. The case of representational reversible figures will, therefore, be dealt with later in this book, when the relationship between perceptual organisation and the identification of figures is being considered (Chapter 5).

Relatively few investigations have been devoted to the perception of reversible figures by children. The classic technique is not appropriate for young children. It involves instructing the subject to continuously fixate the centre of the reversible figure and to press on one morse key for as long as he perceives one figure-ground organisation and another morse key when the second organisation takes the place of the first. Consequently one has to rely upon the child's verbal responses, and by this means to compare the number of times one or the other form of organisation is reported, in a given period of time.

All other things being equal (width of the segments of the circle, their orientation, instructions, etc.), adults more often perceive the black part rather than the white part as the figure (Botha, 1963). This predominance of black over white is not found in children from 3 to 5 years (Johannsen, 1960; Botha, 1963). These two authors obtained comparable results using quite different techniques. Johannsen (1960) used a method which involved making a comparison between a model and one from a series of six figures, cut out in brown paper, which represented the silhouettes of well-known animals. The models, sixty in number, were more or less ambiguous versions of the six animals represented in the series from which a choice had to be made. The silhouette of each animal was reproduced either in black on a white background, or in white on a black background, at five levels of visual masking, the masking giving it a speckled appearance and an imprecise outline. The author compared the number of correct identifications obtained for each level of masking, on the one hand with the black models on a white background, and on the other hand with the white models on a black background. As expected, the number of correct identifications decreased as the degree of masking increased, but no difference was apparent between black figures and white figures, the discrimination of one being no easier than the other for children from 3 to 5 years.

Botha (1963) employed a method of induced set. During a training session he presented two types of stimuli, either a black cross or a white cross, each on a grey background, for brief exposures of two seconds. For group A the black cross appeared twenty-one times, the white cross seven times; for group B the reverse was the case. The test stimulus was a classic segmented circle, with black and white segments all of equal size and identical to those of the crosses used in training. During the test period the child was asked to say what he saw; it was found that the figure presented least often during training, whether black or white, was the one most often reported (twenty times as against ten) by the experimental group of thirty 5-year-old children. These results confirm those of Johannsen (1960): the black figure on a white background is not dominant for young children. Botha interprets the preference for the figure seen least often during training as being due to a build-up of inhibition proportional to the number of presentations of the same stimulus.

## 2   *A Comparison of Two Interpretations*

To a certain extent, reversible figures allow us to contrast Köhler's interpretations with those of Piaget.

Köhler (Köhler and Wallach, 1944) attributes the reversal between figure and ground to the phenomenon of satiation. Prolonged inspection of the same figure brings about a progressive increase in the resistance of the neural receptors to the 'figure current'; beyond a certain critical value, the flux of the current is reversed and, as it always goes in the direction of figure to ground, what was the ground becomes the figure and what was the figure, the ground. Köhler and Wallach (1944) postulated that figure-ground reversal should be produced more easily in tissue slightly satiated in a permanent fashion, which led them to predict a slowing down with age of the rate of alternation between opposing perceptual organisations. Indeed, they put forward the hypothesis that at birth the degree of permanent satiation is almost nil, in which case the rate of alternation between figure and ground would be extremely rapid and would slow down progressively as the level of permanent satiation increased.

For his part Piaget (Piaget and Morf, 1958, pp. 71–74) considers reversible figures as the manifestation of a 'certain capacity for preconcepts . . . to combine or divide with a small margin of freedom demonstrating the subsequent action of additions and losses' (Piaget and Morf, 1958, p. 71). He gives as an example a figure formed by a black screen $A'$, with a circular hole $A$ cut in the middle, which is filled by white card. Two perceptions are possible according to whether $A$ or $A'$ plays the role of the figure: it is possible to perceive a white disc on a black background, or a black surface with a hole cut in it and placed on a white background. If we take Piaget and Morf's designation[1] of the figure as $Fi$, the background as $Fo$, the interior of $A$ as $In$, the interior of $A'$ as $In'$, the boundary between the two as $Fr$ and the whole $A+A'$ as $E$, the reversible transformation can be expressed by the following equation (Piaget and Morf, 1958, p. 72):

$$(A=Fi=In+Fr)+(A'=Fo)$$
$$\rightleftarrows (A=Fo=In)+(A'=Fi=In'+Fr)$$

Such an equation can be put through different transformational operations and by this means a set of equations can be obtained which are logically correct but some of which are not perceptually possible. Thus one can obtain $In=E-Fr-Fo$, which would associate the boundary $Fr$ to the background; however, we know that, perceptually, the contour always belongs to the figure. An example of this kind is used by Piaget to emphasise the partial nature of the

[1]*Translator's note.* The French abbreviations have been retained here to facilitate reference to the original.

isomorphisms which exist between logical structures and perceptual structures. 'There does exist a perceptual capacity for separation or combination which is in part reversible and, because of this, assimilable to a preoperational schema. But . . . this capacity is limited and . . . the so-called reversible figures are thus merely inverted, since certain forms of reversibility . . . are, in fact, excluded' (Piaget and Morf, 1958, p. 73).

Reversible figures are only a privileged instance of the perceptual reorganisations possible within a particular field of centration, but, for Piaget, it is always a matter of structures derived from perceptual activity, capable of attaining a certain degree of automation but remaining, nevertheless, inflexible compared with the reversible mobility of operative activity. The abrupt and involuntary reversal of the relationship between figure and ground is attributed to the results of previous perceptual activity. Viewed as an index of perceptual mobility and plasticity, the product of perceptual activities, the alternation between configurations perceived in the same field of centration can only increase with age.

Here then are two authors who predict opposing directions of development, one from a neurological model (Köhler and Wallach, 1944), the other from a logical model (Piaget and Morf, 1958).

All the available data show very clearly that the plasticity of perceptual organisation increases with age, whether it is a matter of identifying a figure both as a whole and as a collection of parts (Dworetzki, 1939; Elkind, Koegler and Go, 1964; Elkind and Scott, 1962) or of identifying it differently according to which part takes the role of the figure – all of which is consonant with Piaget's interpretation. It is by no means certain, however, that Köhler and Wallach's (1944) interpretation can be rejected without hesitation.

A reference to the relevant literature (Köhler and Wallach, 1944; Köhler and Fishback, 1950), reveals that one of the basic requirements for the influence of satiation is the perfect topographical coincidence of the cerebral areas excited by the two configurations of successive stimuli. To test Köhler's theory it is therefore necessary to put it in the situation for which it seeks to account, select the physical stimuli accordingly and specify a fixation point. Some investigators have done this and one of them (Hochberg, 1950) has been able to demonstrate a modification of the rate of alternation of the figure-ground structure of a segmented circle, after prolonged inspection of a black (or white) cross on a grey background; the results obtained are in accord with the theory of satiation, provided that the sensitising figure and the test figure present the same geographic distribution of black and white areas. In short, if one allows, as Köhler and Wallach (1944) do not, the existence of a directional effect from the figure current, the results of Hochberg's (1950) experiment are compatible with the effect of satiation, in adults.

The hypothesis of the existence of permanent satiation and of its augmentation with age is particularly difficult to verify (and, as far as we know, there is no experimental evidence to support or controvert it). In none of the experiments reported in the preceding pages was a fixation point imposed on the children during the perception of ambiguous figures. On the other hand, we know that figural after-effects decrease with age between 5 and 11 years, only to increase again from 11 to 18 years (Pollack, 1960). However, Köhler and Wallach (1944) predicted an inverse relationship between the degree of permanent satiation and the intensity of the figural after-effect. The descending part of the developmental curve obtained by Pollack would therefore verify the predictions of Köhler and Wallach. In order to explain the ascending part of the curve, Pollack invoked the influence of a second factor which he conceived as a process of association between the cerebral trace of the inspection figure and the neural excitations relative to the test figure, a factor which would slow down the rate of alternation. Piaget himself (1961, p. 241) envisages a possible association between a homeostatic process of a physiological nature and a perceptual activity linked up between successive perceptions. Any development in this activity would accelerate the passage from one perception to another and would moderate the effect of the physiological process. As to the nature of the latter, it is, he says, the province of the psycho-physiologists to investigate this and to verify whether it is a matter of satiation as proposed by Köhler or of some other process.

### III   THE PHENOMENA OF CLOSURE

The law of closure is one of the laws of organisation put forward by the Gestalt school, but, as Bobbitt (1942) has observed, the term 'closure' is not defined in the same way by all those who have used it. Koffka (1935) sees in the phenomenon of closure a particular instance of the law of *pragnanz*, that is to say, the tendency of the forces operating in the perceptual field to seek equilibrium. A closed form would be more stable, better balanced, than an open form, and would therefore be perceived preferentially (Wertheimer, 1923). For Wertheimer (1923) and Koffka (1935) the role of the law of closure is relatively limited; when dealing with an organisable figure, whether composed of open or closed figures, all other things being equal, the general tendency is to 'prefer' to perceive closed figures. But when the law of closure finds itself in competition with the law of uniform destiny, the latter is dominant (Wertheimer, 1923).

The term 'closure' has been used by numerous authors who have given it a rather different meaning. Several of them have established a relationship between the phenomenon of closure and the processes of reasoning (Helson, 1926; Reiser, 1931; Ogden, 1932; Botzum, 1951; Mooney, 1954 – to name only a few). It would seem that whenever a psychological phenomenon presents a certain degree of incompleteness, there is a tendency on the part of the organism to suppress the lacunae, by the process of either perceptual or conceptual reorganisation. From this point of view, which seems to have been adopted by the majority, closure would be defined in perceptual terms by the tendency to organise as a complete and structured whole, elements which are more or less isolated (Bobbitt, 1942). The missing parts are not actually seen, but what is present becomes integrated in a more complete form and identified as a consequence of this. Defined in this way, it is difficult to consider closure as a purely perceptual phenomenon, independent of intellectual activity and relevant antecedent experiences. Consequently, one can expect it to be manifested more and more clearly as the child grows older.

## 1 *The Identification of Familiar Forms*

The proportion of correct identifications of drawings which are made up of discontinuous lines doubles between 5 and 14 years, then no longer varies with age; the most rapid progress takes place between 5 and 9 years (Rey, 1947).

Gollin (1960, 1961, 1962, 1965, 1966, 1967) has devoted a whole series of researches to the identification of incomplete drawings representing objects well known to children, such as a shoe, an umbrella, a telephone, an elephant, etc. (fig. 10). Each model was drawn at five levels or degrees of continuity of the contour: from level 5, at which the contour was continuous, to level 1, at which the contour consisted of segments separated by large gaps. Each drawing was presented for three seconds and the child instructed to say what it represented. In the first experiment (Gollin, 1960) eleven models were presented at the five levels, starting with the most incomplete drawing and finishing with the one with a continuous contour. As he had predicted, the younger the child, the more complete the drawing had to be for correct identification. In subsequent experiments Gollin studied various means of improving children's performance. Thus a preliminary training programme involving fifty drawings derived from ten models led to a certain degree of aptitude for the recognition of incomplete drawings in children of $3\frac{1}{2}$ years. These same drawings re-presented to the children a week after the training period were recognised at a level where the contour was less complete. This improved capacity for recognising incomplete drawings was apparent, to a lesser degree, with models which had not been seen during the training period (Gollin, 1960).

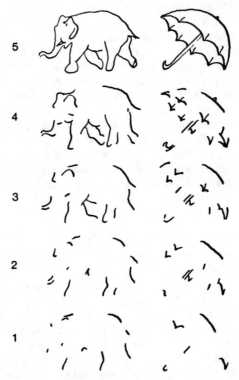

Fig. 10. Example of incomplete drawings (Gollin, 1960).

*In descending order*: the same drawings at decreasing levels of continuity of contour, from level 5 (continuous) to level 1 (the most discontinuous).

Gollin subsequently employed another training technique, using only drawings from levels 3 or 5 of continuity of contour, these being derived from twenty models. Some of the subjects saw, in succession, the twenty drawings at level 3, attempted to identify each one and had their attempt confirmed or corrected by the experimenter. Then the same twenty drawings were presented at level 1 for the child to identify again. Training for the other subjects took place with the level 5 drawings (continuous contour). Training on the drawings of median discontinuity (level 3) greatly improved subsequent performance on different (more discontinuous) versions of the same models (level 1), whilst training on drawings with a continuous contour (level 5) was much less effective. The effects of training were greater in 5-year-old children than in those of $3\frac{1}{2}$ years (Gollin, 1960).

A second series of experiments (Gollin, 1961, 1962, 1965) examined both the role of the time interval separating the training period from the test performance, and the duration and intensity of that training. The test performance, evaluated in terms of the number of correct identifications made of drawings at level 1 of continuity, seemed to vary as a function of the degree of reactive inhibition developed by the subjects during the training period[1] on the drawings of level 5. Thus 8-year-old children needed a learning series of twice the length required by adults in order to attain the same level, which, Gollin suggests, implies the formation of greater reactive inhibition. It follows from this that the test performance is much inferior in children when it follows almost immediately after (one minute delay) the training period, whilst a delay of twenty-four hours allows the inhibition to dissipate. In adults, test performance is the same, whether it is measured one minute or twenty-four hours after training (Gollin, 1962). If the formation of reactive inhibition is induced by introducing ten overlearning series, the effect of the delay between training and test is then the same in adults as in children (Gollin, 1965).

In summary, Gollin concludes that, having reached the same level of learning performance, all the subjects have learnt the same thing and are therefore capable of producing the same test performance, once the reactive inhibition engendered by the training session has dissipated. However, the degree of this inhibition is proportional to the duration of the learning period: the longer it is, the longer the delay between training and test must be for the desired results to be optimal.

## 2 Primary and Secondary 'Good' Forms

Piaget and Stettler (1954) have devoted a long article to the perception of 'good' forms by children through the use of imaginary lines, and have interpreted their results as a function of the development of perceptual activity. They asked children in the age-range 3–9 years to identify various geometric forms presented, sometimes

[1] Which amounts to serial learning with anticipation.

Table 3   *Changes in performance when identifying drawings of level 1*

|        | Children of 8–9 years | | Adults | | |
|--------|-----------|---------|------------|---------|---------|
| Delay | Un-trained | Trained | Un-trained | Trained | Over-trained |
| 1 minute | 6·48 | 5·33 | 8·56 | 10·40 | 8·93 |
| 1 day | | 8·93 | | 11·27 | 13·87 |
| 2 days | | 11·40 | | 12·40 | 11·47 |
| 8 days | | 9·87 | | 10·53 | 11·40 |

Performance is measured by the number of drawings identified correctly from the twenty of level 1 of continuity when the delay which separates the training period from the test varies between 1 minute and 8 days (Gollin, 1965).

individually, sometimes overlapping, and where the contour was either a continuous line, a dotted line, or a broken line with large gaps. Thus, for example, a circle of 21 mm diameter might be represented by five arcs of a circle each 5 mm in length; and a square, of 35 mm each side, by its four corners (4 mm for each side of the angle). Children from 2 to 3 years were quite capable of identifying a circle, a square or a triangle when they had continuous contours and were presented individually but they could not do so when there were several overlapping forms. In this latter case, however, it was difficult to distinguish the part played by a failure to understand the instructions from an actual inability to analyse a complex figure in terms of simpler structures. But by the age of 4 years, the children identified overlapping forms with continuous contours in three-quarters of the cases.

When these same geometric forms had a discontinuous contour, 3-year-old children completely failed to identify them, and it was only at 6 years that all of the forms were identified without error, on individual presentation. Neither the absolute size of the figures nor the size of the gaps in the contour appeared to be of any importance. It would, however, be imprudent to conclude that before the age of 4 years children are incapable, under any circumstances, of recognising incomplete forms. The degree of familiarity with the forms presented certainly plays a role, and the younger the child the more important this is. When a child has had prolonged training in the discrimination of a triangle from a circle, both drawn with a continuous contour, he is capable, as early as the age of 2 years, of differentiating both forms and of selecting one, when the contour is represented by no more than six black dots (Gellerman,

1933); a performance, let us note, which rats are quite incapable of, although they discriminate as well as children do between line figures of continuous contour.

In Piaget and Stettler's (1954) experiment, the youngest children treated each angle, each segment of a line, like an individual figure independent of the others. The lacuna separating two visible segments of a line was not perceived as the imaginary part of a longer line which took in the visible segments and the lacuna in the middle. The evocation of imaginary lines does not seem to be manifested until 6 years of age. If, instead of presenting a single incomplete figure on its own, two such figures overlapping were presented, the youngest children responded as for individual figures in that they interpreted each segment separately, while the oldest children linked up the various segments into unitary structures. The most common error was that of organising all the lines into a single, comprehensive, irregular figure, either open or closed.

Closure is not always operative, therefore, as the Gestalt theorists had predicted, in the sense of making a form regular and symmetrical. Consequently Piaget has used the results of this investigation to make the distinction between 'good' primary forms and 'good' secondary forms. Only the first of these results from a field effect, that is to say the interaction between the elements perceived in a single field of centration,[1] defined by a visual fixation. In the case of drawings made up of continuous lines, visual pursuit can follow a line through its entire length and thus circumscribe the complete contour of a figure. The perceptual activity of exploration is facilitated by continuity of contour, which would explain the identification of overlapping figures as early as the age of 4 years.

By comparison, in figures made up of discontinuous lines, each segment involves a visual fixation, the movement from one to the other constituting a sort of bond; in order to assemble the content of successive fields of centration into a coherent, structured whole, the child must carry out a construction in the proper sense of that term; the segments must be joined together by a progressive selection which presupposes an anticipation of the complete form; the visual movements must be co-ordinated in terms of a strategy which predicts the maintenance of direction in the exploration, the use of movements and transpositions and also the relationship with multiple points of reference. This act of construction brings into play all the child's perceptual activities and the progress observed with age in the identification of incomplete figures simply follows

[1]The 'field of centration' (Piaget, 1961), like the 'sensory tableau' (Piaget, 1936), corresponds to the content of the proximal stimulus.

the development of the perceptual activities of movement, anticipation and referencing.

Mooney (1957a) presented children in the age-range 7–13 years with a series of figures derived from Street's (1931) completion test. The figures were made up of black and white areas, as in highly contrasted photographs, deprived of all half-tones and so emphasising extremes of light and shade. Mooney used fifty prints representing human faces, classified according to the age and sex of the person represented and the degree of masking involved; in addition twenty prints were prepared in the same way but representing no particular object. The children had the task of grouping the seventy cards into seven categories: boy, man, old man, girl, woman, old woman, and 'unidentifiable'. The number of correct identifications increased with age, going from 36 per cent at 7 years to 72 per cent at 13 years. At all age-levels, the relative order of difficulty of the different prints remained the same and differences between individuals were considerable.

Piaget and Stettler (1954) used as experimental material pieces of card in the shape of rectangles, circles, triangles, etc., which had irregular pieces cut out of them, and asked the subjects to draw each piece of card as it had been before it had been cut into. Although the normal adult perceives the piece of card, in almost every instance, as a regular geometric form which has a piece missing, the youngest children filled in the lacunae in an entirely idiosyncratic manner (fig. 11) and tended to transform the whole into a familiar and representational form. It was only from the age of 8 years that children were successful in this task. This sort of problem presents a supplementary difficulty in that the edges where the piece has been cut out constitute a real and visible contour which the child, in order to reconstruct the 'good' form, must ignore in favour of an imaginary line. The conflict is thus acute and in this case the child completes the figure in terms of those forms which are most familiar to him and, at the same time, the best fit to the form he is actually dealing with. The form which he constructs is accordingly irregular and representational, rather than than regular and geometric.

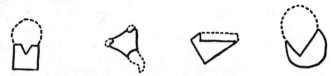

Fig. 11. Examples of 'cut-into' figures completed by children (Piaget and Stettler, 1954).

The results of Piaget and Stettler (1954) are in agreement with those of Gollin (1960, etc.) in showing that the identification of figures with large areas missing is not possible below a certain level of development. The role of perceptual activity postulated by Piaget appears to account in a satisfactory manner for the increase in success-rate with age as well as for the observed errors; and the fact that the older the child the more effective certain forms of training become (Gollin, 1960) would confirm this interpretation. Training is related both to the discovery of those distinctive features of each model which reveal its identity and the possible strategy for the solution of the problem presented. This strategy is related to the activity of exploration and the organisation of the perceived components of the figure; training can, therefore, only be effective to the extent that there exists in the child at least the beginnings of perceptual activity, and training will be correspondingly more effective as the capacity for perceptual activity becomes greater. The limited effectiveness of training in the identification of figures with continuous contours – level 5 (Gollin, 1960) – is due to the fact that their identification does not demand the intervention of perceptual activity.

The experimental material used by Mooney (1957a) appears heterogeneous in comparison with that of Piaget or Gollin; the break in the contour is achieved by the partial abolition of the boundaries between figure and ground and the removal of various parts, such as the eye, characteristic of the form to be identified. This is a much more difficult task, but a process of exploration, anticipation and organisation would still seem to be the key to correct identification. Contrary to this expectation the number of correct identifications made by adults is the same when the cards are presented tachistoscopically as when they are presented in free field vision (Mooney, 1957b). Furthermore, the force with which a form suddenly imposes itself and the impossibility of recalling it voluntarily is reminiscent of the effects of insight and of the reversibility of figure-ground segregation so dear to Gestaltists.

CONCLUSION

Some general conclusions concerning the development of perceptual organisation in children emerge from the research which has been described and discussed.

The first of these is a qualification as to the extent the available experimental results can be generalised. Almost all of the investigations have used two-dimensional line-drawings, so that the perceptual organisation has involved line-figures and not objects.

However, it is by no means certain that the perception of objects which are three-dimensional, and therefore susceptible to relative displacement, would obey exactly the same laws of organisation as line-figure drawings. Moreover, it can be assumed that the organisation of the world of objects is achieved earlier than in the case of line-drawings, notably owing to the factor of the parallax of movements which are not involved in the perception of figures (Gibson, 1950, 1967; Walk and Gibson, 1961). It is also likely that line-drawings tend to be perceived as pictorial representations of objects and that the topological relationships perceived between figures are derived from the topological relationships perceived between real objects.

A second conclusion concerns the validity of the laws of organisation of Gestalt theory. These laws permit the prediction of the unique structures into which the lines and surface areas of a line-drawing will organise themselves and in terms of what pattern of topological relationships (overlapping, superimposed, etc.) these structures will be articulated. With some qualifications, these laws seem to have universal validity and account for the performances of children from the age of 4 years. Below this age-level the available data are as yet insufficient for an answer to be given to the questions of the innateness of these laws and the development of the relative significance of the different principles of organisation such as proximity, continuity, uniform destiny, etc. (Rush, 1937; Bower, 1965a, 1967a). It is difficult to specify, in the results obtained, the part played by the principle of organisation under investigation and that of the methodology employed (choice of experimental situation, type of measurement used, etc.).

If we take into account the limited amount of evidence, the particular characteristics of the material (line-drawings) with which it has been obtained, and the large number of variables, more or less controlled, which are involved, it appears that the organisation of the stimuli which a line-drawing presents – into a number of perceptual structures – cannot be reduced to a 'field effect' in the Gestaltist sense of that term. The physical properties of a line-drawing render certain forms of organisation distinctly more likely than others but do not determine in a univocal and invariant manner during the course of development what will be perceived and how it will be perceived. Thus the dominant figural character of black, which determines the segregation of two areas of black and white of the same size and shape, into a black figure on a white background, appears only after the age of 5 years (Johannsen, 1960; Botha, 1963).

But if experience is involved in perceptual organisation, the universal and precocious application of its laws makes it impossible to attribute the principles of organisation to environmental factors and the frequency of association of certain stimuli alone, as certain empirical psychologists have tried to do, for example Brunswik (Brunswik and Kamiya, 1953: Brunswik, 1956) in the case of the law of proximity.

Hebb's (1949) hypothesis, in terms of the genesis of cell-assemblies, could account for the development with age of perceptual organisation; it lends itself particularly well to the interpretation of a progressive articulation between the whole and the parts. It makes it possible to predict the construction, during a first stage, of isolated units, each limited to the elements perceived in a visual fixation. Later, as a result of visuo-motor exploration, the initial groupings are combined into more comprehensive ones, which allow an alternation between the perception of the whole and perception of its parts (the phase sequence). In a sense Hebb is proposing a concomitant neurophysiological model of the interrelationship of the perceptual structures with the subject's exploratory activity. In another area, Hebb's ideas fit some data which have only recently become available. The privileged role of the line, as seen in experiments on the stabilised retinal image (Pritchard, Heron and Webb, 1960), has led Hebb to regard the line as an innate perceptual structure, the basis of subsequent, more complex structures. The investigations of Hubel and Wiesel (Hubel and Wiesel, 1959, 1962, 1963, 1965, 1968, etc.) on the retinal fields of the cat and the monkey have demonstrated the existence, from birth, of neurones of the striate cortex specialised in the perception of straight lines and boundaries. If these results are also valid for man, one would be able to see in these neurones the physiological basis of innate perceptual structures. The prospects opened by the research findings of Hubel and Wiesel and Hebb's hypothesis would appear very exciting; as yet, however, Hebb's model remains unverified and Hubel and Wiesel's investigations have only been concerned with animals. Furthermore, if there is one area where it is necessary to guard against the facile generalisation from animal to man it is that of innate patterns of behaviour.

A third general conclusion relates to the emergence between the ages of 5 and 8 years, according to the characteristics of the tasks, of a degree of plasticity in perceptual organisation. The period from 5 to 8 years has been noted by many authors as one during which distinctive and important behavioural changes take place in the child. From the point of view of perceptual organisation the change takes the form which will now be described.

Before this key period, the laws of organisation are dominant

and they alone determine, within the limits of the physical properties of the stimulus, what structures will be perceived; when several
forms of organisation are possible in terms of the laws of segregation (ambiguous or reversible figures), only the most probable one
is seen; in the case where they are equipotential, as in certain
reversible figures (e.g. a circle with equal segments), the alternation
between percepts occurs at a very slow rate. When the laws of
organisation only predict one structure, the ability to break down
the primary structures and use their components to make new
forms, does not appear until the age of 5 to 6 years, as our experiments with embedded-figures problems have shown.

Consequently, it is reasonable to assume that around the age of
6 years, children become capable of utilising a secondary level of
perceptual organisation which can be distinguished from the
primary level in several respects.

At the primary level, a line-drawing is organised in a rigid manner into structures whose form is determined by the laws of Gestalt.
Each component of the figure (line or surface area) belongs to only
one of those structures of which it constitutes a part. The relationships between structures are essentially topological.

At the secondary level a component (line or surface area) can
belong at the same time to several structures, which makes possible the construction of new units. The same line, or surface area,
the same group of lines, can then play two roles simultaneously,
that of the structure comprising all the parts, and that of a sub-
structure included in the main structure. To the topological
relationships between primary structures are added, or substituted,
hierarchical, inclusive relationships between primary and
secondary structures.

At the same time, it must not be forgotten that primary structures are always more pervasive than secondary structures and
that, beyond a certain level of complexity, secondary units can be
constructed, in the proper sense of the term, piece by piece, by
means of an appropriate strategy, but can no longer be perceived
directly (Gottschaldt, 1926).

The appearance of a secondary level of organisation indicates
the involvement of intellectual processes and appears to correspond
exactly to the operation of what Piaget calls perceptual activities
(Piaget, 1961).

The primary level constitutes the effects of centration, in which
perception amounts to the relationships between those elements
seen in a single field of centration determined by a visual fixation.
The secondary level enables the subject to link up, into a structured
whole, elements perceived in several successive fields of centration.

It is then essentially a matter of a temporal-spatial integration of parts linked by movements and by being placed in relationship with each other.

At this secondary level, the subject is also capable of employing imaginary components and of integrating into the same perceptual structure real and imaginary parts, such as, for example, the lines and lacunae of an incomplete figure, thereby displaying, in addition to the movements, an activity of schematisation and anticipation.

It is certain that these various perceptual activities begin well before the critical age of 6 years, even if the accession to the secondary level of organisation seems to take place suddenly. The recognition of incomplete figures is seen as early as the age of 2 or 3 years in certain cases (Gellerman, 1933; Gollin, 1960) when the figure is a well-known one and the lacunae in the contour are small. One can only speculate as to the point at which recognition is just a matter of the elements concerned with no imaginary lines involved. In consequence, it would seem to be all the more reasonable to support Piaget's (1961) hypothesis according to which perceptual activity is precocious but is at first only effective within very restricted spatial and temporal limits; progress with age, above all else, is a matter of the extension of the range of perceptual activities.

*Chapter 2*

# The Spatial Relationships
# between Structures in
# Three-Dimensional Space

At a very early stage in his development the child organises the stimuli emanating from the physical world into a limited number of distinct perceptual structures. And very soon he becomes aware of the relative spatial situation of the physical objects underlying the perceived structures, and organises his actions accordingly. But only gradually are the spatial relationships evidenced by his activity integrated into a coherent space, the nature of which changes in the middle of the second year with the emergence of the symbolic function. A primary perceptuo-motor space, the dynamic elaboration of which (Galifret-Granjon, 1964) depends on a reflex and later a manipulative adaptation, is confined within the limits of the activity itself; within this space objects are permanent and invariant, connected spatially in the feasible set of displacements (Piaget, 1937). A secondary, representational space begins to develop when the symbolic function is established. Representational space develops by stages, like the perceptual space to which it relates; it is topological before being projective and Euclidean (Piaget and Inhelder, 1948), that is to say, the transformations modifying the proximity, the contiguity and the order of spatial elements will be taken into account before alignments and metric characteristics.

Representational Euclidean space is not truly established until around the age of 9 to 10 years (Piaget and Inhelder, 1948); until then the child makes use of incomplete, and more or less independent, systems of spatial relationships in which the subject himself occupies a privileged position. The achievement of representational Euclidean space comes about when the incomplete systems are integrated into a unitary conception of space, when a system of general reference in which the subject occupies a position just like any other object, is substituted for a system of egocentric reference.

The development with age of the spatial relationships which connect objects in three-dimensional space, has given rise to few experimental studies. In so far as perceptual phenomena are concerned, object invariance is acquired during the course of the first year and, as far as one can quantify such things in babies, perceptual constancies seem well established from the very beginning. On the other hand, the ability to anticipate what appearance object O will present in situation B, knowing how it looks in situation A, and the spatial transformation which will bring object O from A to B, appears relatively late. The evaluative processes employed by the adult and by the child from 4 years of age make demands on their capacity for representation, and the observed development with age in the appraisal of perceptual constancies could well be due to this.

The ease and rapidity with which graphic material can be produced has meant that spatial relationships and their development with age have been studied much more frequently in two-dimensional drawings than in three-dimensional space. Thus we have a large amount of data on the perception and reproduction of line-drawings. In order to gauge at what level of spatial organisation a child is operating, he is asked to reproduce a model line-drawing on a sheet of paper, or else to select, from amongst a number of line-drawings, the one which is identical to the model, or to say whether or not two drawings are identical. In these last two cases the material presented for comparison differs from the model by a spatial transformation of the type involving rotation or translation, either of the whole figure or of one of its parts. These two alternatives are far from equivalent and the type of spatial relationships to which the child is able to refer in order to give his response are not exactly the same; we shall, therefore, deal with them in two separate chapters (Chapters 3 and 4).

A line-drawing is always perceived as one or a number of distinct figures, situated within a frame of reference constituted either by the edges of the sheet of paper on which it is drawn, or by a closed figure which surrounds it. When the 'frame' contains a single figure, its displacement leaves its topological relationship with the frame invariant, and so can only be detected by recourse to metric relationships or to egocentric retinal references. However, when several figures coexist within a frame, the displacement of one of them can modify its topological relationships with the others.

If the use of topological relationships precedes that of metric relationships, the perception of the displacement of one part must occur at an earlier age, when there are several figures, than when there is only one. It would, however, be imprudent to regard the degree of difficulty in perceiving a displacement as simply a function of the type of relationship (topological or metric) involved. When a line-drawing can be broken down into several perceptual structures, these constitute a configuration and maintain with it the relationships of parts to a whole. The displacement of a part can, therefore, appear as a difference to the extent that it modifies the form of the configuration whilst the system of topological relationships remains invariant.

I   PERCEPTUAL CONSTANCIES

By the end of the first year of life, the objects the child perceives in his environment are permanent and invariant. Indeed, even at two months a baby does not respond to an object solely in terms of the size and form of the retinal projection it activates; of particular note is the manifestation of size constancy, admittedly somewhat rudimentary, as a function of the perceived size and the distance of the object (Bower, 1964, 1965b).

Although researchers are in agreement in placing the appearance of perceptual constancies sometime during the first year, the theoretical explanations which they propose lead them to predict different patterns of evolution with age. Gestalt theorists have seen in perceptual constancies a process of automatic equilibriation, conceived as a field effect and therefore independent of the subject's experience. Empiricists have insisted on their cognitive and therefore evolutionary character. Finally, Piaget postulates the intervention of two mechanisms, one involving the automatic integration of perceptual indices, the other compensatory adjustments regulated by perceptual activity. The first group was concerned to show that perceptual constancies can be demonstrated very early and do not change with age; the second group has insisted on the modifications brought about by the subject's experiences (the degree of familiarity, the representationality of the object, the personality of the subject); whilst the third predicts an evolutionary development from underestimation in the child, due to insufficient compensation, to overestimation in the adult, due to over-compensation.

1   *Development of Size Constancy*

Size constancy has been investigated in adults and children by the psychophysical method of determining a point of subjective equalisation between a standard object near to the subject and variables at some distance (or vice versa). Such a technique has the great advantage of enabling quantitative evaluation of the degree of constancy to be obtained, so making possible the production of curves of development as a function of age; on the other hand it does have important limitations. Firstly, it can hardly be used with very young children, and apart from Beyrl (1926), who employed subjects in the age-range 2–10 years, almost all investigators have been satisfied to start at 4 or 5 years; in consequence there is very little evidence on children under the age of 5 years. Secondly, misjudgments of the standard, the effect of the central tendency and serial errors, which are impossible to exclude in this sort of investigation, change with age. Finally, constancy is measured by means of a judgment of comparison; the obtained response therefore depends not only on what the child has perceived but also on his criteria for making that decision. For all these reasons, it is difficult to disentangle from the observed changes those which amount to changes in constancy itself.

A review of the literature concerned with size constancy in children shows considerable disagreement between different authors, which can be attributed entirely to differences in the experimental situations (Piaget and Lambercier, 1943a, 1943b, 1956; Zeigler and Leibowitz, 1957; Jenkin and Feallock, 1960; Denis-Prinzhorn, 1961).

For one group of researchers, the youngest subjects under-estimate, this under-estimation decreasing with age, with exact constancy appearing at about 7 years and followed, from the age of 10 years, by a degree of over-estimation which increases up to adulthood. This evolution from an under-estimation to an over-estimation is only found when the object is no more than a few metres distant. As the distance between the observer and the object increases, constancy decreases and this decrease is more marked the younger the child (Beyrl, 1926; Zeigler and Leibowitz, 1957; Harway, 1963). Thus, in Beyrl's study, the standard object was a disc 10 centimetres in diameter, situated 1 metre from the subject. The disc judged equal to the standard by a child of 2 years was 12 cm in diameter when the distance was 2 metres, but at 11 metres the disc judged equal was 18 cm in diameter. For a child of 7 years the disc judged as equal to the standard was between 10–11 cm in diameter at 2–5 metres distant, and a little over 12 cm at 11 metres distant. From the age of 10 years, variation in distance between 1 and 11 metres is no longer a significant variable and constancy is almost perfect.

When the variables are presented one by one and the point of subjective equalisation obtained from a series of paired comparisons, the resulting degree of constancy is a combination of the degree of real constancy and the degree of misjudgment of the standard object. The standard object tends to be over-estimated relative to the variable object; the object which is at some distance from the subject and which is at first under-estimated relative to an object near the subject tends, with age, to be increasingly over-estimated. When the proximal object serves as the standard, its over-estimation compensates for that of the distal object; however, when it is the distal object which takes the role of the standard, the two over-estimations are summed. In the latter situation the over-estimation appears earlier and attains a greater magnitude than in the former (Piaget and Lambercier, 1943a, b, 1951, 1956).

When constancy is measured by a technique of paired comparison between a standard object and a series of variables for selection, presented simultaneously, the effects of the central tendency are very marked and, in the same subject, constancy varies with the composition of the series. When the standard object is the same size as the median object of the series, constancy is perfect (Burzlaff, 1931; Lambercier, 1946a); in changing the end-points of the series, and therefore the size of the median unit, the subjective point of equalisation is, at the same time, displaced. This always tends to be around the median value and the younger the child the more marked this central tendency is (Lambercier, 1946a, b).

The observed degree of constancy also varies with the instructions that are given, but the influence of this factor increases as the child grows older. Rapoport (1967) established an experimental setting in which she was able to adjust the size of a variable triangle, situated at 8 or 10 m from the subject, the standard triangle being 3 m from the subject. There were two alternative instructions: objective instructions to give to the variable the same real size as the standard (correct to two decimetres), and 'phenomenal' (or 'apparent size') instructions to give to the variable the appearance of the same size as the standard. In children between the ages of 5 and 7 years, no difference was found as a result of the different instructions; from the age of 9 years, constancy was greater with the 'objective' instructions and the discrepancy between the two situations increased with age. The apparent size did not change with age, whereas the objective size increased, but even in this condition the investigator did not find any over-constancy.

The same author investigated size constancy in children from 5 to 10 years using an original technique which avoided dependence on a verbal report of the judgment made (Rapoport, 1969). Five toy railway tracks were placed side by side on a table and at right-angles to the child. On each track a locomotive drew a tender carrying an isosceles triangle. The trains were situated at distances which varied from approximately 0·45 m to 6·40 m, and all the triangles differed in size. The child had to make the trains come towards him, one after another, by pressing a button – beginning with the one that carried the largest (or the smallest) triangle and continuing with the one that carried the largest triangle of those that remained, etc. A pre-test made it possible for the experimenter, in each child's case, to retain only those triangles which could be discriminated in terms of size, at the same distance, whatever this happened to be.

In order to succeed, the child had to take into account both the apparent height and the distance; an errorless performance would correspond to perfect constancy, whilst errors which involved the selection of a triangle smaller but nearer would indicate some influence of the height of the retinal projection and, therefore, an under-estimation. In this experiment all the subjects under-estimated; it was more marked in the children than in the adults but did not change between the ages of 5 and 10 years.

Distance constancy or space perception at variable distances evolves with age as does size constancy. At distances of less than 4 m, an area near to the subject is over-estimated by 5-year-old children compared with one further away; this under-constancy gives way to perfect constancy around 9 years of age, then to over-constancy in the adult (Denis, 1961; Wohlwill, 1963). When the distance is increased, over-constancy is no longer found but under-constancy is increasingly apparent the younger the child and the greater the distance.

Wohlwill (1963) concluded, on the basis of a detailed review of the literature concerned with size constancy, that certain situational variables are inoperative with children and have a very slight effect on adults; these variables are relative to the physical structure of the experimental setting, for example the regularity or irregularity of surface texture in distance perception (Wohlwill, 1963) or the introduction of intermediary objects conducive to the structuring of the visual field in size perception (Lambercier, 1946b). Other variables, however, do affect the degree of constancy, especially in the case of older children and adults, when they bring about an over-constancy. Amongst these factors Wohlwill cites the influence of the repetition of judgments, motivation, the intrinsic difficulty of the judgment, and the form taken by the instructions; an objective instruction which requires a response in terms of the actual physical height of the object is much more likely to lead to over-constancy than a phenomenal instruction which requires the subject to respond in terms of the apparent height.

It seems therefore that, as a perceptual phenomenon, approximate constancy is manifested at an early age, although under-constancy is the rule. In the very young child this constancy only applies within a restricted distance from the subject – about 4 metres – and accuracy falls away rapidly as the distance increases, the size of the retinal projection determining responses involving distant objects. As the child grows older the perceptual phenomena become increasingly subject to the influence of intellectual processes, and the changes in performance with age seem to us to be much more a matter of how the child approaches the task and interprets the instructions than of any perceptual change.

The data concerning form constancy, which has been studied much less than size constancy, suggest that its development is similar.

## 2   *Development of Form Constancy*

It is conventional to say that form constancy increases up to adolescence but decreases slightly after that. This view is mainly derived from an investigation by Klimpfinger (1933) which involved children from 3 to 14 years. However, more recent studies (Brault, 1962; Vurpillot, 1964b; Meneghini and Leibowitz, 1967) by no means confirm Klimpfinger's findings. The development observed by this author could be due in part to the characteristics of the experimental setting (Meneghini and Leibowitz, 1967); the stimulus selected as the standard was an ellipse with the larger axis one and a half times the smaller axis – a form which, more than any other, induces a high degree of constancy (Leibowitz and Meneghini, 1966); finally, and most important, the distance at which the variable was placed (5·40 m) was, for children, a considerable one – a factor which, on its own, would handicap young children. Maximum constancy is found earlier by Brault (1962) who puts it between 9 and 11 years. This author evaluated form constancy by a comparison between parts and measured the degree of constancy by the gap between this comparison, calculated from the physical size, and the same obtained from the perceived size of the identical parts, measured by adjustment. Vurpillot (1964b) and Meneghini and Leibowitz (1967) found a diminution of form constancy with age, the first author between the ages of 5 and 12 years, the others between the ages of 4 and 16 years. Vurpillot used irregular, non-representational forms, situated 4 m from the subject, Meneghini and Leibowitz an ellipse 1 m or 5 m from the subject; both established a subjective point of equalisation between the standard object and the variables for selection which comprised projections of the standard in various orientations.

At 1 m, constancy was almost perfect at $4\frac{1}{2}$ years, then decreased regularly with age; at 5 m it was much more uncertain and did not change with age; and the more the standard was tilted, the worse constancy became (Meneghini and Leibowitz, 1967). As in the case of size constancy, the nature of the instructions only influenced older children; at 5, 7 and 9 years the variable judged equal to the standard was the same with 'objective' instructions (indicate the projection identical to the actual object, situated in the fronto-parallel plane) as with 'phenomenal' instructions (indicate the projection which corresponds to the apparent form of the standard). It was not until 11 years that responses differed according to the nature of the instructions, constancy then being superior with objective instructions (Vurpillot, 1964b). Thus, with objective instructions, constancy increased from a minimum at 9 years, whilst with phenomenal instructions it decreased with age up to 12 years. The influence of the degree of tilt only made itself felt from the age of 7 years. At 5 years a child differentiates an inclined stimulus from a fronto-parallel stimulus, but does not differentiate between different orientations – possibly because he does not perceive them, possibly because he does not perceive them as being significant. From the age of 7 years, the child's responses are determined by the orientation of the standard, but he is incapable of representing to himself how the form will look when placed in the fronto-parallel plane: he is unable to anticipate its appearance in one plane from its appearance in another (Piaget and Inhelder, 1948; Vurpillot, 1964b). He responds, therefore, according to the apparent form, whatever the instructions happen to be. It is only at 12 years that he attains a level of representation which is adequate to allow him to reconstruct another aspect of the stimulus, from the data available.

The interaction between perception and the child's capacity for abstraction could explain the evolution of form constancy as a function of phenomenal instructions, whilst the development of the capacity for representation would account for the observed evolution when instructions are objective.

When constancy is being evaluated, the proximal stimulus contains, at one and the same time, information about the size of the retinal projection of the standard, the area which it occupies, its texture density gradient,[1] and the form of its contour, together with information about the densities and texture gradients of the background, of the other objects, the dimensions of the retinal projections of the latter, and so on. The automatic composition of all these indices is sufficient to constitute a visual perceptual world, isomorphic to the physical world and in which perceived objects are invariant (Gibson, 1950, 1966).

[1]The density of optical texture is the cyclic alternation between weak and strong luminous intensities at the level of the retinal projection of a surface area. When this surface is inclined in relation to the observer the density of the optical texture increases in a continuous fashion with the distance which separates the observer from a particular part of the surface: it is this which is described as the gradient of texture density (Gibson, 1950).

The very young child responds to this visual world without analysing it, and therefore without seeking to isolate within the proximal stimulus that which is relative to one or another spatial characteristic of the objects perceived. Furthermore he is quite incapable of representing mentally what sort of change in this perceptual world would follow from a modification of the physical world – such as the rotation of the standard around an axis. Objective instructions and phenomenal instructions have the same value for him and lead to the same response since he can only perceive the actual situation. The data from numerous investigations are in general agreement in showing that, within a radius limited to a few square metres around the child, perceptual constancies are very accurate at an early stage of development which suggests an automatic, pre-programmed composition of information.

From the moment when the child becomes capable of imagining what sort of perceptual change would follow the spatial displacement of an object, he takes into account in his predictions all that he knows concerning this particular object, or has observed in analogous situations. He evaluates and compensates for probable error, and it is then that objective instructions induce over-constancy in evaluating the size of neutral objects such as triangles or steel rods. This over-constancy can also be found in the perception of forms when these are neutral or irregular (Guignot, Macé, Savigny and Vurpillot, 1963).

However, instructions to respond according to the appearance of the object (phenomenal instructions) become ambiguous and necessitate a choice between several responses as soon as the child is able to analyse all the information contained in the proximal stimulus and to respond in terms of only a part of this. But the dissociation between the information concerning the form of the retinal projection and that which relates to the distance and degree of incline of the object from the fronto-parallel plane, is only a partial one. Consequently the subject fluctuates between various possible responses and has only limited confidence in his judgment; inter- and intra-individual variability is considerable and bimodal response distributions are often found.

It seems to be easier, however, to disregard what one knows in fact, and to respond mainly according to the retinal projection when the judgment concerns form rather than size. The decrease in form constancy observed as the child grows older, when the instructions are phenomenal (Vurpillot, 1964b; Meneghini and Leibowitz, 1967), could be explained by the progress of the ability to analyse and abstract the properties of the stimulus.

Another interpretation is proposed by Meneghini and Leibowitz

(1967) who attribute this decrease to the gradual replacement of perceptual experience by conceptual experience. Without a system of concepts, and as yet with a limited ability to manipulate verbal symbols, the young child would identify the objects which surround him in terms of his perceptions alone; for him the perceptual constancies of size and, particularly, of form play an adaptive role and introduce an essential stability into his visual world. This role loses its importance as other modes of organising experience are added to perception.

## II THE PERCEPTION OF VERTICALITY

The existence of terrestrial attraction means that, for all inhabitants of the earth, the choice of a Euclidean system of reference is not entirely arbitrary. The vertical axis which coincides with the direction of this attraction, and therefore with the longitudinal axis of the body of a person in a standing position, is of privileged significance and is usually employed as one of the three orthogonal axes of reference.

In young children the perceived vertical tends to be assimilated to the longitudinal axis of the body, without taking account of the possible divergence between the latter and the line of terrestrial attraction, so that the determination of a visual vertical varies with the position of the body and tends to be parallel to its axis (Wapner and Werner, 1957). As the child grows older, the two systems of reference, the egocentric system relating to the body's axis, and the representational system independent of the subject, become dissociated. The disparity between the two systems can be measured by the angle of the difference between the apparent visual vertical and the apparent localisation of the body axis (Wapner, 1968). A bar of light can be adjusted in the dark, either to appear vertical (apparent visual vertical), or to appear parallel to the body axis, whilst the subject is seated on a chair, leaning either to the left or the right at an angle of 30° from the true vertical. A systematic error is found in the adjustment of the visual vertical, an error which changes direction between 13 and 15 years. From 7 to 13 years, the bar of light is tilted in the same direction as the body (Aubert effect, 1861), whilst from 13 to 15 years it is tilted in the opposite direction. The estimation of the direction of the body axis gives rise to a systematic error which takes the form of an exaggeration of the actual tilt of the body. This error decreases between the ages of 7 to 12 years and then increases from the age of 13 years. At all ages the disparity as measured by the gap between the two adjustments is greater than the physical disparity (30°) and the difference increases with age. As the child grows older, the two localisations are differentiated and the position of the perceived vertical separates itself from the perceived axis of the body.

# Chapter 3

# The Perception of Form Orientation

The sensitivity of the individual to differences in orientation develops with age, and the general assumption is that this evolution occurs in two different directions according to whether the task involved is one of differentiation or of recognition.

## I THE DIFFERENTIATION OF FORMS PRESENTED IN DIFFERENT ORIENTATIONS

All investigators agree in reporting that young children tend to judge the same forms as identical, whatever their orientation. However, the age from which a differentiation can be made between figures on the basis of their orientation depends very much on the materials employed. Furthermore, one has to consider to what extent a confusion between forms that are identical, but in a different orientation, stems from the non-perception of a difference due to sensory incapacity, or from a categorial judgment which gathers into a single, equivalent class, forms which are perceived as invariant, whatever their relation to a frame of reference.

Before going on to sample the many investigations concerned with the discrimination of the same form in different orientations, the vocabulary used in describing these orientations will be defined in terms of the spatial transformations which make possible the movement from one figure to another.

An initial distinction must be made between simple rotations in a single plane and inversions or rotations in space. In dealing with inversions we shall employ the nomenclature used by Fellows (1968):

—inversions of type V obtained by a rotation of 180° around a horizontal axis;
—inversions of type H obtained by a rotation of 180° around a vertical axis;
—inversions of type VH obtained by a rotation of 180° around a

horizontal axis followed by a rotation of 180° around a vertical axis. Geometrically an inversion of type VH is equivalent to a simple rotation of 180° through a single plane.

Some inversions can give rise to mirror images when the forms to be compared are presented in a certain way. When both figures are side by side (horizontal presentation), only in the case of a type H inversion does it mean that one of the figures will be the mirror image of the other. When they are placed one above the other, it is the type V inversion which brings about the formation of mirror images (fig. 12).

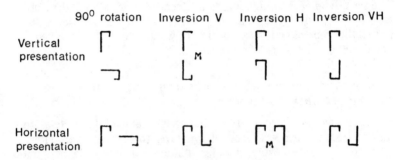

Fig. 12. Spatial transformations employed in the evaluation of the perception of orientation.

The letter M indicates those cases where the type of transformation and the manner of presentation create mirror images.

If one takes account of the relative spatial situation of the two forms which are being compared, mirror images constitute a special case, one in which the congruence of the two figures can be obtained by a simple rotation of 180° through space, around a horizontal or vertical axis. In all other cases of inversion, in order to be able to superimpose one figure on another, it is necessary to add a lateral transposition to the simple rotation in space.

Confusion between similar letters of the alphabet, with some degree of inversion, is considered to some extent responsible for difficulty in learning to read; consequently there have been many investigations dealing with lower-case letters such as *p* and *q*, *b* and *d*, *d* and *q*, *p* and *d*, *n* and *u*, etc. Such errors, usually called 'reversals' are particularly numerous in beginning readers of 5–6 years (Monroe, 1928; Johnson, 1957); they decrease gradually with age but it is by no means rare to find them in children up to the age of 9 or 10 years (Monroe, 1928; Schonell, 1942).

Paired comparison tasks involving isolated letters have shown that up to the age of 6 years discrimination is good except for the reversible letters *b, d, p* and *q* (Smith, 1928; Hill, 1936). It is to Davidson (1934, 1935) that we owe the first analyses which classified such confusions as a function of the axis around which the rotation occurred, and which enabled one letter to be transformed into another. Errors of inversion of type V and VH are eliminated by about a mental age of 6 years, whilst inversions of type H persist up to a mental age level of $7\frac{1}{2}$ years. The particular difficulty of detecting inversions of type H is confirmed by many authors such as Vernon (1957) and Fellows (1965). Given the horizontal arrangement of letters in books of Western cultures, inversions of type H necessarily give rise to mirror images.

The relative difficulty of detection of inversions of type V and H is clearly evidenced in the researches of Newson (1955), Rudel and Teuber (1963), and Huttenlocher (1967a, 1967b).

Newson (1955) gave a form comparison problem to a hundred children aged 5 years and found that in general they were unable to distinguish a non-representational figure from its mirror image. The same confusions were apparent when the task involved copying a figure. In a second experiment, Newson replaced the comparison task with a problem which required the identification of one 'odd' object from amongst a series of similar objects (oddity problem). The series was made up of identical figures one of which was in a different orientation from the others. Errors in the detection of the 'odd' figure were much more frequent when the inversion was of type H than with any other transformation (V, VH or R). The difficulty of the task seemed to depend entirely on the type of transformation employed; the mirror images were particularly difficult to distinguish, the other changes of orientation were equivalent. No other factor, such as the symmetry (or otherwise) of the figure, the ratio of length to breadth, compactness, representationality, or the number of parts, had a systematic effect on performance in this particular task.

Rudel and Teuber (1963) gave a group of children, ranging in age from 3 to 9 years, a discrimination learning task involving two similar figures in different orientations; these were presented side by side, and a specific response paired with each stimulus. The discrimination between a vertical and a horizontal rectangle, and between an upright and an inverted U (transformation type V), was established very easily. However, the distinction between two oblique rectangles inclined at an angle of 45° – one to the left, the other to the right – or between two U's on their sides with their open ends to the left and to the right (transformation H) was only learnt with great difficulty. Rudel and Teuber proposed the hypothesis that the spatial situation of the characteristic which makes it possible to differentiate two forms affects the relative ease of discrimination. Thus two U's differently oriented can only be distinguished on the basis of the position of the opening in the figure. When the U's are on their sides and reversed, one open to the left, the other to the right, the distinction is between left and right; however, when one U is upright and the other upside-down, the distinction is between upper and lower. But the recognition of the upper as opposed to the lower part of a figure is much more important for adaptation to the physical world than the distinction between right and left. Besides which, if the distinction between right and left is seen as a function of the lateral dominance of the central nervous system (Orton, 1937; Hecaen and Ajuriaguerra, 1963) one would expect that those figures which only differ in terms of having the same part to the right or to the left would be easily confused until the age when dominance is clearly established.

Several authors (Sekuler and Rosenblith, 1964; Huttenlocher, 1967a, b), think that the difficulty in discrimination is more a matter of the type of transformation which is involved between one figure and another than of the particular characteristics of the figures themselves (opening to the left or the right). Huttenlocher (1967a) repeated Rudel and Teuber's experiment, with 5-year-old children. She used a horseshoe figure in four orientations, these being presented in pairs, either side by side, as in Rudel and Teuber's experiment, or one above the other (fig. 13). The children were slower in learning to discriminate the mirror images (pairs 1, 2, 7 and 8) than those which were not mirror images (pairs 3, 4, 5 and 6). However, whether they were mirror images or not, the learning which involved figures open towards the top or towards the bottom (3, 4, 7, 8) was more rapid than with those figures open towards the left or right (1, 2, 5, 6).

In a paired comparison task given to children from 4 to 5 years of age, Wohlwill and Wiener (1964) confirmed that differentiations between type H inversions were much more difficult than between type V inversions, in the horizontal presentation. Their material, consisting of symmetrical geometric figures (fig. 14), was constructed in such a way that the influence of several structural variables of the stimulus could be studied.

The material comprised two series of eight figures, series 1 differing from series 2 only by the addition of small details inside the contour. Within a series, half the figures were closed forms, the other half open forms; in half of series 1 the interior detail was placed in the lower part of the stimulus figure, in the other half it was placed in the upper part (of the figure in normal orientation). Three

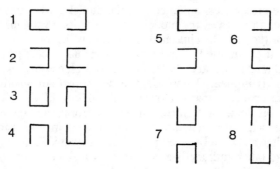

Fig. 13. Figures used to investigate discrimination between different orientations of the same figures (Huttenlocher, 1967b).

On the left (1, 2, 3, 4) horizontal presentation; on the right (5, 6, 7, 8) vertical presentation.

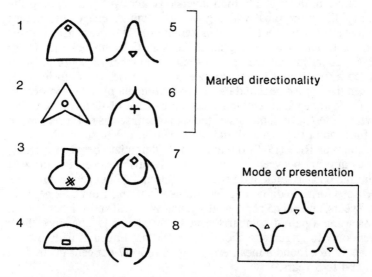

Fig. 14. Sample of figures used in a paired comparison task (Wohlwill and Wiener, 1964).

Figures 1, 2, 5 and 6 are described as being of marked directionality by the authors.

For half the subjects the figures were presented with a vertical axis of symmetry; for the other half the axis of symmetry was horizontal (a 90° rotation from the former).

*Bottom right*: mode of presentation; *at the top*, the model; *below*, the variables for comparison.

figures were presented simultaneously, the model above, and below, side by side, a replica of the model and one of its inversions, either of type V or type H. The child had to indicate which of the variables was identical to the model, and the experimenter recorded the accuracy of the response and its latency. The presence or absence of interior details influenced performance no more than whether the figures were open or closed. However, the nature of the inversion (V or H) was important; the number of errors was significantly greater when a distinction had to be made between inversions of type H (mirror images) than between inversions of type V. This confirms the results of other authors (Newson, 1955; Rudel and Teuber, 1963; Huttenlocher, 1967), but the duration of the response latency was the same for both types of inversion.

As far as most investigators are concerned, therefore, it appears that the difficulty of distinguishing between different orientations of the same form depends very much on the type of spatial transformation which is involved in moving from one to the other. Rotations are easier to differentiate than inversions, and within this group the most difficult are those which give rise to mirror images (inversions of type H in the horizontal presentation). However, using forms similar to letters of the alphabet, Gibson, Gibson, Pick and Osser (1962) found no differences between the number of confusions between a model and its inversion and the number of confusions between the same model and its rotation through a plane of 45° or 90°.

The age at which children become capable of distinguishing between different orientations of the same form seems to be very much a function of the material and the type of problem selected.

Thus for Rice (1930) the ability to differentiate between orientations appears between 5 and 6 years. With the same kind of task, Gibson, Gibson, Pick and Osser (1962) found 45 per cent confusions between forms in different orientations at 4 years, around 22 per cent at 5 years, and only 5 per cent at 7 years. Wohlwill and Wiener (1964), also using a paired comparison task, but a simpler one since there were only two figures to choose from and not fifteen as with Gibson *et al.* (1962), found a mean error rate of only 17 per cent in children from 4 to 5 years.

Gellerman (1933) taught two 2-year-old children to discriminate an equilateral triangle with its base horizontal from various negative stimuli, and then measured the degree of generalisation of this learning. When the positive stimulus, the triangle, was rotated 60°, the child put his head on one side in order to restore to the projection on his retina the orientation on which he had been trained, and responded positively to it provided that the negative stimulus was other than a triangle. But if the experimenter presented, side by side, the original triangle and one the same but rotated through 180°, then the child did not know to which one he should respond. In other words, he was well able to recognise a triangle in different orientations but did not differentiate between these orientations.

It would seem to be difficult to attribute the errors of young children to a failure to differentiate perceptually between orientations without taking into account the difficulties inherent in the task with which they are presented. A paired comparison task demands of the child that he should explore all of the alternatives presented and compare them one by one with the model; this involves the implementation of a relatively complicated strategy which the young child does not possess but which apparently can be induced by appropriate training. Thus, by means of a slow and gradual period of training, Bijou and Baer (1963) succeeded in reducing the number of confusions between mirror images of a geometric form to less than 10 per cent in children from 3 years of age.

Some of the contradictions apparent in the work of different authors concerning the relative precocity of discrimination between different orientations of the same form must be attributed to the non-equivalence of the tasks involved. In a perceptual differentiation task the figures are presented simultaneously and all the child has to do is to show that he does not perceive them as the same. At this level a successful performance is possible if the sensory patterns are different. In a paired comparison task, the child must not only differentiate between the available choices but also select the one identical to the model; to the task of differentiation is added the task of identification.

As Over and Over (1967) have demonstrated, discrimination learning is even more difficult than paired comparison. In their study all the 4-year-old children and half the 6-year-olds were unable to achieve a discrimination learning between two oblique lines inclined in opposite directions, whilst almost all of them, both 4-year-olds and 6-year-olds, were successful in a paired comparison task employing the same figures.

II RECOGNITION OF AN IDENTICAL FORM IN DIFFERENT ORIENTATIONS

A common assumption in the literature is that children, being much less aware than adults of the spatial situation of objects, lacking a structured frame of reference, will be superior to their elders in the recognition of forms presented in an unusual orientation. Such a view is derived in the main from anecdotal evidence – the most common being the observation that children from 3 to 4 years often turn over the pages of picture books upside-down – together with a small number of studies carried out many years ago. Under scrutiny these observations and studies show themselves to be much more ambiguous than is generally realised.

Let us deal first of all with the observations of children with picture books. For Stern (1909) the child experiences the same pleasure in looking at books whatever the position in which they are presented, but other psychologist parents (Fellows, 1968) do not necessarily agree. A personal observation, concerning a child of 18 months, showed evidence of a definite awareness of the orientation of a human figure. The child was turning over the pages of a book and suddenly came across the following two pages side by side: on the left-hand page was a drawing of a little boy standing, on the right-hand page a drawing of a clown doing a hand-stand. When she noticed the clown she turned the book round; the clown now had his head at the top, and the boy his head at the bottom; as soon as the child noticed the picture of the boy she turned the book round again. Several times in succession the child changed the position of the book so that the picture she was looking at was in the normal orientation. Yet one or two hours later this same child was turning over the pages of her book upside-down.

This simple observation suggests that turning over the pages of a book produces two kinds of satisfaction: one mainly sensory and cognitive, that of looking at and recognising pictures, and the other purely sensori-motor, that of turning the pages in regular rhythm. It is almost certain that this latter satisfaction is independent of the orientation of the book.

As to the early experiments concerning the recognition of forms in varying orientations, these do not show that the child is superior to the adult; on the contrary, the number of errors and the time taken in recognition were greater in children, but they were less affected by changes in orientation.

Thus Mouchly (Köhler, 1950) presented children with a card bearing drawings of familiar objects, two of which were identical and had to be selected by the child. These two objects were presented in three ways: in a normal orientation, upside-down (180° rotation compared with the other objects), and one upside-down with the other the right way up. Children of 4 to 8 years and adults were involved in the experiment and the number of errors and the response time were recorded. At 4 years performance was the same in all three conditions; the older the child the more clearly a difference became apparent in favour of the situation where the two drawings were presented in a normal orientation. Oetjen (1915) had children from 9 to 13 years and adults read nonsense words made up either of letters normally oriented or of letters rotated through 90°; the adults deciphered the words more quickly than the children but whilst for the latter the difficulty was the same whatever the orientation of the letters, the adults were slowed down by the abnormal orientation.

It would appear, therefore, that up to a comparatively late age the orientation of the stimuli, even when familiar, does not affect identification. However, the recent work of Ghent casts doubt on these conclusions.

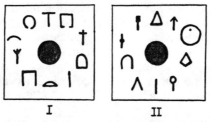

Fig. 15. Example of the material used in the recognition of figures in various orientations (Ghent, 1960).

In I, as in II, the test figure was shown, very briefly, in the central area marked by the black disc; the child had to choose from amongst the ten surrounding figures the one which was identical to the test figure. This was presented either in the same orientation, or in a different orientation from the figure to be selected.

Ghent (1957, 1960) measured, by means of tachistoscopic presentation, the ability of children from 3 to 7 years to recognise forms as a function of their orientation. In the first stage of her investigation she determined the exposure time at which each child was able to recognise 50 per cent of drawings of familiar objects presented individually. In the second stage the child was seated facing a screen which had on it an empty central area surrounded by the drawings of the objects. Some of these were presented tachistoscopically, one by one, in the central area, for the period of time determined in the first stage of the experiment, and in four different orientations: normal, and rotations of 90°, 180°, and 270°. The child had to indicate, from amongst the surrounding drawings, which one represented the same object as the one that had been flashed on the screen. The comparison of the number of errors as a function of the orientation of the stimulus showed that when this orientation was normal, recognition was better than for all other orientations. At 3 years there were twice as many correct identifications in the normal orientation as in any of the others; from the age of 5 years there was no longer any difference in performance as a function of orientation.

The orientation of the objects for selection was not a significant variable, the number of correct identifications being the same whether they were all in the normal position or rotated through 180° (Ghent and Bernstein, 1961).

### III INTERPRETATIONS OF CHILDREN'S PERFORMANCES

The numerous researches concerned with the differentiation between varying orientations of the same form or the identification of a form in different orientations have emphasised the inferiority of young children compared with their elders in these two types of tasks. However, research workers do not agree as to the ability of very young children to perceive the orientation of a form, or on the reasons for this poor performance. The principal interpretations which have been proposed will be outlined and evaluated in the light of the relevant research findings.

### 1 *The Role of the Spatial Frame of Reference*

The traditional, classic hypothesis postulates that the orientation of a form is only perceived in relation to a general system of reference. The child would not, therefore, distinguish between orientations of the same form until he had established a structured, representational perceptual space in which each point was fixed in terms of a Euclidean system of orthogonal co-ordinates.

In the terms of this interpretation, the child should perceive, very early, the form of a figure on the basis of a certain number of intrafigural relationships, which would enable him to recognise it when the invariance of these relationships is respected. As he developed, the child would gradually transfer to a primitively homogeneous visual space the heterogeneous characteristics of motor space. The notions of top and bottom, right and left, largely the outcome of an adaptation to the concept of terrestrial attraction, would be introduced and a stable system of spatial co-ordinates would be established. This would give objects a different appearance according to their orientation, and at the same time would lead to errors in the appreciation of the intrinsic properties of these objects and in their identification. The increasing effectiveness with age of certain perceptual illusions such as the over-estimation of a square standing on its corner compared with a square with its base horizontal, or of a vertical line compared with a horizontal line (Wursten, 1947) have been interpreted in this sense (Piaget and Morf, 1956).

The classic interpretation predicts therefore that the very young child would be unable to differentiate between orientations of the same form but would be quite capable of identifying a form whatever its position. Up to 1960 the psychological literature was in general agreement in reporting that if a child was successful to some extent in perceiving differences of orientation, he was nonetheless very inferior to the adult, whilst, conversely, he was superior to the latter when it was a matter of recognising a figure presented in a different orientation. Having a spatial system of reference was seen as a handicap in identification tasks.

However, as early as 1940, Köhler did not consider such an explanation to be adequate because, on the one hand, children from 3 to 4 years seemed to him to be already in possession of a well-structured perceptual space, while, on the other hand, children of 8 years (Mouchly, 1940) and even 11 years (Oetjen, 1915) still showed themselves as superior to adults in the recognition of inverted figures.

The reappraisal of earlier observations and the contributions of recent research in particular have demonstrated that the child is capable of perceiving and differentiating varying orientations of a form long before he has a coherent system of spatial relations. But this perception of orientation does not have the same stability and universality as that of the adult; certain orientations are easily differentiated, others not. As to the alleged superiority of young children over adults in the identification of forms in varying orientations, this has not been replicated in recent investigations.

## 2 Observations of Animal Behaviour: Lashley's (1938) Interpretation

According to Bingham (1913) a chicken is capable of learning to distinguish a triangle from another form but the discrimination is not transferred to a situation where the triangle, the positive stimulus, is presented upside-down. Bingham concluded that the chicken responded as a function of the relationship of the stimulus to its frame of reference and not of its actual form, which would imply that the chicken possessed a capacity to differentiate between orientations.

Lashley (1938) proposed an alternative interpretation of the results obtained by Bingham. He hypothesised the existence of three stages in perceptual development. In the first stage, the organism responds solely on the basis of the distribution of light and shade on the retina. Thus a triangle and its inversion project different images and are therefore discriminable. Bingham's chickens would be at this stage and would not be able to go beyond it. The weak point in such an interpretation is that, however slightly the chicken moved or inclined its head in looking at the stimulus, the distribution of light and shade would change on the retina; accordingly one could ask how the chicken arrived at an appropriate criterion for learning. At the very least it would be necessary to propose the supplementary hypothesis that the chicken has a certain tolerance to modifications of the projection of the stimulus but that this tolerance is limited to a few degrees' rotation.

In Lashley's second stage, the animal organises the stimulus perceptually and is sensitive to an intrinsic characteristic of the latter formed by a system of internal relationships. The animal abstracts the form from its context and becomes capable of recognising it and of responding to it no matter what its position. A corollary of this is that it would not make a distinction between different orientations. The young child is at this stage. The third stage assumes the acquisition of a supplementary abstraction, that of a spatial relationship between the form and its context.

Lashley's interpretation predicts, therefore, a total incapacity in the young child to differentiate between orientations, and this is contradicted by numerous experimental findings. The interest of his theory is that it allows for the possibility, in organisms low down the evolutionary scale, of the discrimination of orientations from amongst heterogeneous retinal stimulation. Progress in terms of the perceptual organisation of the patterns of stimulation into structured forms, identical in their internal relationships, would therefore deprive the organism of the possibility of differentiating them. The generalisation of such hypotheses to the child entails certain conclusions. One can postulate that the neonate does not yet possess organised perceptual structures, which would mean predicting a stage when the baby would differentiate orientations, like the chicken, followed by a stage where he was no longer able to differentiate them; but, in fact, nothing in the available data shows a deterioration in the ability of young children to differentiate in this way. Alternatively, one can postulate that form-perception is present from birth in human beings, and thus one is brought back to the classic model.

## 3   *Köhler and Retinal Orientation*

For Köhler it is necessary to distinguish clearly between the orientation of an object in perceptual space, that is in relation to the objects around it, and the orientation of the projection of this object in relation to its retinal co-ordinates. A normal orientation in perceptual space is compatible with an inversion on the retina; this is what happens when a person bends forward and looks between his legs.

He perceives the objects as the right way up and not upside-down, but at the same time sees them as having a strange, bizarre appearance. Vice versa, if in this same uncomfortable position the subject looks at a picture, upside-down like himself, the retinal projection of the latter takes up the normal orientation in relation to the retinal co-ordinates. The picture is then perceived as upside-down in perceptual space but does not present a special quality of strangeness (Köhler, 1940). Köhler concluded that recognition is hindered by an impression of strangeness and that the factor responsible is the orientation of the form relative to the retinal co-ordinates and not to perceptual space.

He added that, of course, the retinal orientation was involved only to the extent that it conditioned an orientation of the neural processes corresponding to the sensory excitation. What matters is thus 'not the *place* of retinal projection (and of corresponding processes in the brain) . . . but rather the relation between directions within the object and certain directions within the tissue . . .' (Köhler, 1940, p. 29). When this relationship changes, the visual characteristics of the object also change. Thus Köhler assumes that the tissue of the visual centre is permanently pervaded by a gradient which has a fixed direction. This gradient and its influence become progressively stronger as the child grows.

### 4 *Interpretation in Terms of the Existence of Specialised Neurones*
The analogy which is apparent between the performances of the octopus and those of the young child has led some investigators (Sutherland, 1963; Fellows, 1968) to put forward a common interpretation.

The young child (Rudel and Teuber, 1963), like the octopus (Sutherland, 1958), easily differentiates a vertical rectangle from a horizontal rectangle but tends to confuse two oblique rectangles at 45° and 135°. Both the child (Rudel and Teuber, 1963; Huttenlocher, 1967a, b) and the octopus (Sutherland, 1960a) confuse inversions of type H (right-left) more easily than inversions of type V (above-below).

Fellows (1968), who made a special study of the perception of form orientation in animals and children, proposed the hypothesis that, as with the occipital lobe of the octopus (Young, 1960), the striate cortex of the very young child contains a much greater proportion of cells specialised for the horizontal and vertical retinal field than for the oblique field. The manifest progress with age in the discrimination of obliqueness could, he suggests, be the result of two factors. Either the cells for the oblique field develop much more slowly than the others, or the child gradually acquires the techniques which will allow him to compensate for a physiological inferiority. In the present state of our knowledge it is difficult to discuss the relative merits of these two interpretations. We know that the dendrites of the cortical neurones have not reached full development at birth, but multiply and extend during the course of the first few months (Purpura, Carmichael and Housepian, 1960; Schadé and Baxter, 1960), but, on the other hand, we know that from the functional point of view, the classifying neurones of the new-born kitten have the same capacities as those of the fully-grown cat (Hubel and Wiesel, 1963a). It is, therefore, quite impossible to say whether Fellows' first hypothesis is correct or not. Even if it were, it is certain that, as in all other perceptual performances, the influence of the child's cognitive acquisitions is added to the progress due to maturation.

## 5   *Hebb's Theory and Sequential Exploration*

(a) *Hebb's hypothesis.* For Hebb (1949) the perception of a structured form results from a progressive integration of perceptions, initially independent, and corresponding to the various parts of this form. Each of these parts gives rise, at the level of the central nervous system, to the development of particular cell assemblies, and subsequently, as a result of visuo-motor exploration, these diverse assemblies are linked together and then integrated into a new, more complex assembly. The activation of the latter brings about the perception of the entire stimulus. Throughout the genesis of this assembly an effective visual exploration of the stimulus is considered indispensable. This exploration is far from being a matter of chance since, according to Hebb, certain parts of the stimulus have, more than others, the property of triggering the fixation reflex – this being the case, for example, with the angles of a triangle. These parts constitute poles of visual attraction and visuo-motor exploration is from one pole towards another. Once the initial cell assemblies are well integrated into a complex assembly corresponding to the whole stimulus, then actual visuo-motor exploration ceases to be indispensable; the activation of the complex assembly and therefore the perception of the whole can be brought about by a partial stimulation, in particular the visual fixation of just one part of the stimulus. During the stage when the form is being learnt, a succession of separate points of fixation on the various poles of attraction of the stimulus releases the sequential activity of the cell assemblies and the successive perception of the different parts of the stimulus. Once the structure of a complete form is established in a unique and complex cell assembly, a single fixation point is sufficient to bring about the perception of the whole, but at the same time as the nerve impulse is spreading through the circuit of the complex assembly, the perception of one part of the stimulus is succeeded by another. A sequential exploration, internalised from the stimulus, has taken the place of the actual visuo-motor exploration. Like the latter, it has a point of departure and follows a set pattern. The identification of the stimulus depends very much on the choice of the point of departure and the direction of the exploration. Not all the parts of a stimulus are equivalent for its identification; some of them are more characteristic than others and, if it is a matter of a single visual fixation, it is of some significance whether it is on one point rather than another.

A number of psychologists have attempted to verify Hebb's hypotheses by means of developmental studies. Up to the present, the direct recording of the visuo-motor activity of the baby has only been attempted by Kessen and his associates (Kessen, Salapatek and Haith, 1965; Salapatek and Kessen, 1967; Salapatek, 1968). The existence of poles of visual attraction, determined by the structural properties of the stimulus, seems to be confirmed by Kessen's first experiments; the points of visual fixation in neonates were concentrated around the angles of a triangle. But a visual exploration, following the sides of the triangle from one angle to another, such as Hebb had postulated, only appeared in a few of the neonates examined. More recent investigations (Salapatek, 1968) only partially confirm the results of earlier experiments: the neonates looked at the sides as much as the angles of a triangle, the centre as much as the contour of a disc.

(*b*) *The focal points.* Ghent has devoted a whole series of investigations (Ghent, 1956b, 1957, 1960, 1961, 1963, 1964; Braine-Ghent, 1965a, 1965b; Ghent and Bernstein, 1961; Ghent, Bernstein and Goldweber, 1960; Mandès and Ghent, 1963; Antonovsky and Ghent, 1964) to the verification of Hebb's hypotheses concerning the influence of internalised exploration in the identification of forms. She develops these hypotheses and defines them in the following way. In an identification task every individual engages in either an actual visuo-motor exploration, or an internalised exploration without visual displacement. This exploration follows a definite order which remains constant for the same form, although the point of departure changes with age. In very young children, from 3 to 5 years of age, this point of departure coincides with what Ghent calls a 'focal point', a privileged area of the stimulus, and exploration proceeds vertically, from top to bottom, starting at this point. Its determination is independent of any learning, being a function only of the physical characteristics of the stimulus. In older children and adults the 'focal point' loses its significance and exploration, actual or internalised, can go in various directions; however, the vertical direction of exploration, from top to bottom, remains preferred. The major change that appears with age relates to the origin of this exploration; whilst in the very young a focal point determined by the structural properties of the stimulus always constitutes the point of departure, in older subjects exploration tends to start in the upper part of the stimulus, whatever its characteristics.

For Ghent, the point of departure and the direction of the sequential exploration of the stimulus would totally determine the perception of the stimulus in a very young child, partially so in an older child.

We have seen that for the majority of psychologists the perceived orientation of a form is in relation to its frame of reference, the acquisition of which is therefore a necessary condition for the perception and differentiation of different orientations of the same form. Ghent (1961) thinks, on the contrary, that in the very young child the orientation of a form is perceived as one of its intrinsic properties. The actual visuo-motor exploration which has brought about the perceptual organisation of a form has, at the same time, determined its subjectively correct orientation. Ghent states that a stimulus is perceived as well oriented when the focal point, the origin of the actual exploration which is subsequently internalised, is located in the upper part of the visual field. However, when this focal point is in the lower part, there is a conflict between the 'privileged' direction of exploration, along the vertical from the focal point downwards, and the direction this exploration needs to follow – from the focal point upwards – if the stimulus is to be seen in its entirety. Because of this conflict the form is perceived as wrongly oriented, with its top at the bottom.

For unfamiliar forms, the situation of the focal point in the visual field determines the subjective orientation. In the case of familiar forms, it is the frequency of a specific part being located in the upper area of the visual field which determines the normal subjective orientation of the form. Every form has one or more structural points which determine the origin of its exploration and subjective orientation. In the case where this form is frequently presented in an orientation other than a 'good' subjective orientation, there will be a conflict between an 'upper part' which coincides with the focal point and an 'upper part' determined by the frequency of appearance in the upper area of the visual field; an acquired subjective orientation can replace a subjective orientation which is a function of the structural properties of the stimulus. For example, the point of an open acute angle appears to provide the required properties for attracting visual fixation and so to become the point of departure for the exploration of such a form. The 'correct' subjective orientation of this form would be an inverted V. But the learning of the alphabet involves the repeated presentation of V, that is, with the point of the acute angle at the bottom; in older children the form V is consequently perceived as correctly oriented, whilst in young children the opposite is true.

Although not possessing a general system of spatial reference, the very young child nonetheless perceives forms as oriented and is capable of differentiating their various orientations. Such an ability implies the existence of a frame of reference which Ghent puts at the retinal level. Because of the characteristics of the visual system, the upper part of the stimulus is always the lower part of the retinal projection of this stimulus.

Beyond the age of 5 years, the child begins to construct a system of general reference in which he occupies a position of the same value as the surrounding objects. The older child thus has available two ways of perceiving the orientation of a form: he continues to perceive it in a subjective orientation, determined by its intrinsic characteristics and the related sequential exploration, but at the same time is able to perceive and compare varying positions by reference to a system of spatial co-ordinates.

In order to demonstrate the validity of her hypotheses, Ghent and her associates carried out a series of experiments with children from 3 to 7 years. To begin with they attempted, successfully, to demonstrate that not all the orientations of an unfamiliar geometric figure are equivalent and that only one is perceived as 'correct'; that is to say, the upper part of the figure is clearly located in the upper part of the visual field and this 'correct subjective orientation' is the same for the whole of a particular age group.

Ghent (1961) constructed a series of figures with varying structural properties related to hypotheses about the nature of focal points. She presented to her subjects pairs of drawings of the same form, side by side, but with one of them rotated through 180°; she asked the child to indicate which of the two forms appeared to be upside-down, with its top at the bottom.

For the majority of the drawings the results were clear and coherent within each age group, which confirms that there is a very definite subjective orientation for unfamiliar forms. For certain of the forms this correct subjective orientation remained the same at all ages, but for others there was a change with age; thus a circle with a gap at the top was seen as upside-down by 86 per cent of 4-year-olds but as being the right way up by 81 per cent of 7 to 8-year-olds. The same experiment repeated with tachistoscopic presentation led to the same pattern of results (Ghent, Bernstein and Goldweber, 1960).

The fact that it is the youngest children who show the most marked preference for a particular orientation of the stimulus leads one to suppose that this is a function of the structural properties of the stimulus and not the effect of the influence of the cultural environment. The observation of the same preferences in Iranian and American children (Antonovsky and Ghent, 1964) confirms that the subjective orientation is independent of the cultural setting. This is only true for very young children, however, and the influence of learning and the environment is evident in older children. Thus V oriented like the letter of the alphabet is seen as upside-down by all the 4-year-old children, right way up by those of 7 years; Y has no subjective orientation at 4 years which it has for 100 per cent of 7-year-olds. Other developmental changes in subjective orientation would seem more difficult to interpret; why does a gap in the contour of a figure act as the subjective base for very young children and as the top for older children? If the focal point of a figure is, as Ghent suggests, the determinant of what is seen as the upper part of the figure, must we then assume that this focal point is the continuous part of the contour for the younger ones and the gap in the contour for the older children? If a focal point is really determined by the structural properties of the stimulus it would be better not to propose the hypothesis that these properties can change with age and, pending further investigation, to assume that the role of focal points diminishes with age. The change of preference must then be explained in terms of the intervention of other factors than the structural poles of visual attraction.

(c) *The role of the retinal frame of reference.* In order to verify that the subjective orientation of a form is in fact relative to a retinal frame of reference and not to its position with regard to the context, Ghent, Bernstein and Goldweber (1960) presented the same series of geometric figures and drawings of familiar objects to children who, bending forward, looked at them through their legs. The judgments made by pre-school children were completely at variance with those of older children and adults. For the latter the perceived orientation was relative to its context and, for example, a drawing of a person was judged the right way up when it was oriented like the other objects around it; thus it was given a subjective position, when its head was projected on to the upper part of the retina. The pre-school child however, judged the drawing as the right way up when its head was projected on to the lower hemi-retina and its feet on the upper hemi-retina.

This predominance of the retinal 'frame' as the system of reference in young children has been reported by other investigators. Thus, the younger the child, the more the subjective vertical approaches the vertical meridian of the retina, which accounts for the marked errors of judgment noted when young children are asked to adjust a rod to the vertical with their head on one side (Wapner and Werner, 1957; Wapner, 1968).

(*d*) *The direction of internalised exploration.* Postulating that when a figure is perceived as well oriented, it is because its focal point is situated in its upper part, Ghent analysed the experimental material in terms of the judgments made by children of 4 to 5 years and derived a list of the structural properties of the stimulus which determined the top or bottom of the figure as far as the subject was concerned. The spatial location of the figure or figures on the card, their relative size and the degree of contrast determined the subjective orientation. Thus when the card bore a single, simple figure – a line, dot or square, black on a white background or white on a black background – then this card was perceived as well oriented, the right way up, when the figure was situated in the upper part; this figure was treated as the focal point. When the line was equidistant from the edges, the card was seen as the right way up when this line was vertical, but badly oriented if this line was horizontal. When the card had two figures of unequal size on it, the smaller one had to be at the top for the card to appear the right way up. In a more complex figure, the focal point tended to be: a break in a line, the point where it changed direction, the intersection of two lines, or a change in the thickness of the line. When the card was made up of two equal areas, one black, one white, the black area became the focal point. Finally, a curve or an angle constituted the focal point in preference to a straight line, and in the case of open figures the focal point was situated on the continuous part of the contour, on the side opposite to the lacuna.

Thus a 4-year-old should manifest a preference for figures set out along a vertical axis of symmetry, rather than a horizontal one, with a focal point located in the upper part. This focal point should be black rather than white, small rather than large, or should coincide with an irregularity of the figure. If one proceeds from these principles, which are derived from children's judgments about the orientation of figures, it is possible to predict how one should orient other figures for the child to see them as the right way up or upside-down.

Ghent sees the results of this experiment as proof that internalised exploration starts from the focal point and proceeds in a vertical direction from top to bottom. Such a conclusion goes far beyond the data. What does such an investigation in fact show us?

Firstly it demonstrates the existence of a subjective orientation and that it is the same for all children at a certain age-level. An unfamiliar figure is thus perceived as having an upper and a lower part, independently of its situational context. Furthermore, this upper part would seem to coincide with certain physical properties of the figure: irregularity, relative size, relative contrast, etc. It is possible to designate as the focal part that area of the figure perceived as the upper part and to propose the hypothesis that it constitutes the point of departure for exploration, but it is a hypothesis that the experiment in question does nothing to verify.

However, two other series of experiments provide data which, without being decisive, are compatible with a hypothesis of an exploration in the vertical direction, starting at the focal point.

In the case of very young children, drawings of familiar objects were recognised more easily in tachistoscopic vision when they were presented in their normal orientation (Ghent, 1960). Ghent interprets this facilitation in terms of a congruence between the sequence of perceptual events arising out of the exploration of the figure presented and that of the perceptual events relating to similar forms seen previously (Ghent, 1960). When unfamiliar objects are involved, such as geometric figures, Ghent would expect to find an ordered sequential exploration from top to bottom starting from the focal point. If the figure were presented in the appropriate subjective orientation, that is if it were perceived as being the right way up with the focal point in the upper part, the internalised exploration would therefore involve a complete scrutiny of the figure. If, on the other hand, the figure were presented in another orientation, then the part situated above the focal point would not be explored and the chances of correct identification reduced accordingly. Whether it is a matter of familiar or unfamiliar forms, the number of correct identifications will be greater if the point of departure of the exploration is situated in the upper part of the stimulus. This starting point is a structural focal point for geometric forms, but for familiar forms it can be a focal point that is acquired through repeated experience.

On the basis of these hypotheses, Ghent predicted that, when seen tachistoscopically, geometric forms would be recognised more frequently when they were presented in their subjectively normal orientation. Accordingly, employing the technique used with familiar forms (Ghent, 1960), she presented to children in the age-range 3 to 5 years a selection of figures whose subjective orientation had been evaluated (Ghent, 1961). At 3 years the figures were more accurately recognised in the correct orientation; at 5 years performance was the same whatever the orientation (Ghent and Bernstein, 1961).

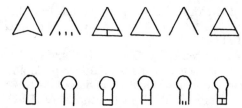

Fig. 16. The influence of the relative situation of the 'focal point' and of the distinguishing part of the figures (Braine-Ghent, 1965); in each row is a group of forms subjectively oriented the right way up ('focal point' at the top).

Figures in the same group can only be discriminated by their lower part.

In some other experiments, Ghent and her associates constructed material in which they deliberately situated the focal part and the distinguishing part of a figure in opposite areas of the stimulus. Groups of figures were constructed along the following lines. Within one group all the figures had the same focal point and identical sides (fig. 16), but differed from each other in the part opposite to the focal area; this part was therefore distinctive and alone made it possible to differentiate between the members of the same group. The existence of a focal area and of a clear subjective orientation was verified by reference to the preferences of a group of pre-school children.

The experimental task was that of finding, from amongst a number of figures (all members of one group), one identical to the stimulus figure which was presented in four orientations: subjectively 'correct', and rotations of 90°, 180° and 270°. In the subjectively correct orientation, the focal point was at the top, the distinguishing part at the bottom of the stimulus. The hypothesis was that if the internalised exploration started from the focal point, recognition would be better when the stimulus was presented in the subjectively correct orientation, but that if the internalised exploration started systematically from the upper part of the stimulus, then the best performance would be when the stimulus figures were upside-down, with the distinguishing part at the top and consequently always seen. The results obtained confirmed the predictions: children from 6 to 8 years (Mandès and Ghent, 1963), like adults (Ghent, 1963), correctly identified the stimulus more often when the distinguishing part was at the top than when it was at the bottom or to the side. In contrast, children of 3 years made more correct identifications when the focal part was at the top and the distinguishing part at the bottom than when the reverse was the case (Braine-Ghent, 1965a). In the latter situation, starting from the focal point and exploring below it, they were less likely to notice the distinguishing part. Children of 4 to 5 years performed like those of 6 years and older.

With the aim of verifying Ghent's hypotheses, Wohlwill and Wiener (1964) constructed their material (see p. 78 and fig. 14) in such a way that the figures could be divided into two groups, one with marked, the other with slight directionality. The term 'directionality' appears to apply to the subjective orientation. Thus the directionality of a figure would be marked when it had a very clear subjective orientation and slight when the subjective orientation was ambiguous. Across the experimental results, the degree of directionality appeared to bear no relation to the number of errors of comparison as a function of orientation, but the response latency was clearly less for figures with marked directionality. This effect was particularly marked when the directionality followed a vertical axis, the presumed path of the perceptual exploration.

CONCLUSION

Contrary to what had been suggested by earlier investigators concerned with the perception of orientation, children are aware from an early age of the differences in orientation of the same figure within a frame of reference. Where authors are in disagreement this is due mainly to the choice of experimental settings and differing techniques of appraisal. But the very young child does not show the same awareness of all differences in orientation; the degree of difficulty of a discrimination would seem to be determined by the type of transformation involved in passing from one orientation to another of the same figure. Thus inversions of type H, obtained by a rotation around a vertical axis, are much more difficult to differentiate than inversions of type V obtained by a rotation around a horizontal axis. The former involves a distinction between left and right, the latter a distinction between top and bottom; however, it is known that the child differentiates top from bottom earlier than right from left (Vereecken, 1961). Whichever transformation is involved in the formation of mirror images, these present a particular difficulty.

A discrimination between different orientations of the same form implies the existence of a system of reference. The first to be employed is at the retinal level; the different points of figures are located with reference to the vertical and horizontal meridians of the retina. To this egocentric system is added, much later, a representational system of reference in which the subject as well as the objects in his visual field are localised in terms of the same orthogonal axes.

Alongside an orientation related to a frame or system of reference there exists a subjective orientation, the intrinsic characteristic of the object or figure. We are indebted to Ghent for having demonstrated this phenomenon and the data she presents are extremely clear. However, the interpretation of these results which she proposes, couched in terms of the theories of Hebb, remains in need of verification. Before accepting this interpretation it would be necessary, in the first place, to demonstrate the existence of focal points. The recording of eye-movements makes it possible to determine the localisation of the first visual fixation of a figure and to evaluate the degree of attraction of each of its points. If one of these points regularly showed an attraction greater than the others it could be considered as the focal point of the figure in question. Next, it would be necessary to verify if, whenever this focal point was situated in the upper part of the visual field, the figure was perceived as the right way up, and *vice versa* that the figure was perceived as upside-down when the focal point was in the lower part of the visual field. Finally, it would be necessary to record the path followed by the eyes in the first explorations of an unfamiliar form, a period during which it is assumed the cell assemblies are constructed. From the observed path of inspection one could then deduce what the direction of the internalised exploration would be and verify, tachistoscopically, whether the siting in the upper or lower part of a figure of the focal point and of the area which differentiated the figure led to different performances in identification tasks, as Ghent has postulated (Ghent, 1963; Mandès and Ghent, 1963; Braine-Ghent, 1965a).

# Chapter 4

# Intrafigural Spatial Relationships

## I TOPOLOGICAL AND EUCLIDEAN RELATIONSHIPS IN THE REPRESENTATION OF FORMS

The form of an object or figure is often assimilated to the set of intrafigural relationships which remain invariant across displacements of the object (or figure) in space. The nature and number of relationships maintained vary according to the geometry employed – be it Euclidean, topological, projective, affine, etc. The physical world is described in Euclidean terms but, from the psychological point of view, the choice of a particular geometry depends on the subject's level of development. In the perceptual domain, the awareness of metric relationships is extremely precocious, since the child of 18 months moves and acts in Euclidean, sensori-motor space. This precocity, together with the limited nature of the infant's response repertoire, prevents the experimental demonstration of the transition from a topological perceptual space to Euclidean space. However, the relatively late emergence of representational capacities and the protracted evolution of representational space allow us to study these stages. If, as Piaget postulates, the order in which the various spatial relationships are acquired is the same in the areas of representation and perception, it would be sufficient to demonstrate the anterior appearance of the topological as against the Euclidean in representational space to infer that it had been the same in perceptual space.

Two methods have been employed in the study of intrafigural spatial relationships, reproduction by drawing and stereognostic perception, both of which make demands on the child's representational capacities.

### 1 Data Obtained on Stereognostic Tasks

The experimenter puts into the child's hand, one at a time, objects constructed in terms of certain topological or Euclidean relationships; the child feels the object – a screen preventing him from seeing it – and then reproduces it by drawing or chooses from a set of forms the one which represents the object he handled. It is therefore a form of investigation which involves relatively complicated operations since the information obtained is tactile-kinaesthetic, whilst the response is made by a comparison between this information and visual data, which necessarily involves an intermodal integration of sensory stimuli and the intermediary of a 'spatial image' of a visual nature (Piaget and Inhelder, 1948, p. 32). The objects are selected in such a way that some of them are similar topologically, yet quite different from the Euclidean point of view – for example, a square and a circle, or a ring and a disc pierced with a small hole.

Piaget and Inhelder (1948) observe that between $3\frac{1}{2}$ and 4 years closed forms are distinguished from open forms whilst two closed forms, such as a circle and a square, are confused. The differentiation between curvilinear and rectilinear forms begins at 4 years, but the square is not distinguished from the rectangle until $4\frac{1}{2}$, and it is not until 5 years that there is no longer confusion between a cross and a star. Piaget and Inhelder conclude that topological relationships such as open/closed, solid/pierced-with-a-hole, intertwining/superimposed, etc. are recognised before Euclidean relationships such as curvilinear/rectilinear, equality or inequality of the sides of a figure, the size of the angles, the number of angles, the intrafigural metric relationships, etc.

This precedence of the topological over the Euclidean has been contested, at least in part, by several authors (Lovell, 1959; Page, 1959) who have replicated Piaget and Inhelder's experiments using more elaborate materials. Thus Lovell (1959) did not find that his subjects had more difficulty in distinguishing a circle from an ellipse or a semicircle than an open form from a closed form. He put forward the hypothesis that the child chooses the object – for him identical to the one he has felt – according to the presence or absence of certain Euclidean attributes such as gaps, corners, holes, points, protrusions, hollows, etc. Pinard and Laurendeau (1966) also observed that indented figures, stars for example, were often reproduced as open figures, and they interpreted this in terms of an assimilation based on partial topological characteristics. In this case errors arose from the identification of the whole from a detail of the object which acted as the distinctive feature (Cramaussel, 1924; Vurpillot, 1962); the confusion between a model which was a closed figure and an open figure reproduction would be due to insufficient perceptual exploration. Pinard and Laurendeau (1966) provide detailed results obtained from a large group (600 children from 3 to 12 years) and using two series each of twelve forms (fig.

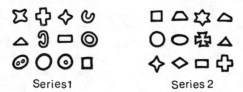

Series1                                Series 2

Fig. 17. The figures of series 1 and 2 of Pinard and Laurendeau (1966).

17). The forms in the first series differ in Euclidean and topological terms whilst all those of the second series are complete and closed, differing only in Euclidean terms. Pinard and Laurendeau went on to make two analyses of their results; the first consisted of comparing, for the whole group, the percentage of correct identifications obtained with each form; the second involved the analysis of the errors and the evaluation of the confusions that occurred.

If one simply compares successes, the results confirm those of Piaget and Inhelder. At all ages the topological forms (series 1) were identified more frequently than the Euclidean forms (series 2), but the difference is slight (mean success-rate of 79·9 per cent in the first series as against 71·9 per cent in the second series).

The second analysis was more productive. The investigation of sources of confusion revealed the following:

1 Errors in which topological features were respected were more frequent than those where they were not. As early as 3 years of age, when the child could not find the figure exactly corresponding to the object he had handled, he chose one homeomorphic to it.

2 The distinction between curvilinear and rectilinear was at least as precocious. Confusions between rectilinear figures, or between curvilinear figures occurred in 75 per cent of cases at the age of 3 years.

3 Amongst rectilinear forms, the distinction between indented (cross, star) or pointed (triangle) forms and those without indentations (square, rectangle) occurred at a very early age.

### 2   *Data Obtained with Drawn Reproductions*

The number of investigations of the ability of young children to reproduce material by drawing is considerable, but our techniques of analysis do not yet appear to be adequate for the wealth of information obtained by this means. Consequently, any attempted analysis of the data appears limited and unsatisfactory.

The twenty-one figures (fig. 18) devised by Piaget and Inhelder (1948) have been subsequently used by a number of authors who

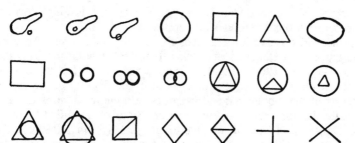

Fig.18. The 21 figures of Piaget and Inhelder (1948) used in the investigation of the relative importance of topological and metric relationships in copying line-figure drawings.

have refined the analysis of the reproductions thus obtained. Whatever the type of classification employed, all produce roughly the same results. The topological features 'open' and 'closed' are the first to be reproduced, between the ages of 3 and 4 years, and are in general better respected at all ages than those of class (Pinard and Laurendeau, 1966). In the reproduction of rectilinear figures the Euclidean relationships appear after the topological ones, but this superiority of topological relationships is not always found for curvilinear figures (Lovell, 1959).

## 3  *Discussion*

An analysis of the data from experiments using stereognostic and graphic techniques allows certain conclusions to be drawn concerning the development of spatial relationships.

It must be said first of all that some of the results which involved the copying of line-drawings are probably due partly to a deficiency of motor control in very young children. Furthermore, reproduction by drawing lends itself badly to a distinction between curvilinear and rectilinear. We know that the first scribbles are swirling or wavy in form (Lurçat 1962) and that spontaneous rectilinear lines appear long after curvilinear lines. This difference in facility between the movements that are involved in the execution of curved or straight lines remains for some time. At 4 years of age children still experience considerable difficulty in introducing an angular inflexion into a line they are drawing, which leads them to replace a broken line by a wavy one and an angle by a curve (Wittling, 1966). The handicap imposed on the child by the motor movement itself is, however, slight. The reproduction of the same models by means of rods is achieved some months earlier than their reproduction by drawing (Lovell, 1959), but the advantage is limited to the very youngest children and from the age of 4 years there is a high correlation between the two modes of response.

A second observation concerns the copying of figures which are overlapping, juxtaposed or enclosed and of regular or irregular form. Thirion (1969) sought to explain the reason for the limited progress observed between the ages of 4 and 5 years in the reproduction of the topological features of certain figures (figures 1, 2 and 3 of fig. 18, for example) and discerned signs of a conflict between the demands of Euclidean and topological systems. Because the very young child does not take into account Euclidean characteristics, which means that he does not bother to deal with the irregularities of contour of amoeboid forms, he is able to give all his attention to maintaining topological relationships. The older child, who is becoming aware of Euclidean characteristics, attempts to deal with these at the same time as topological ones; consequently the task becomes much more difficult and he is impeded by the awkwardness of his approach. The situation can arise, therefore, where topological relationships are sacrificed for the sake of metric relationships.

Ultimately a complex perceptual field can be described in terms of a particular number of simple figures of strong internal structure and united according to a particular system of interfigural spatial relationships. Even in the examples given by Piaget and Inhelder (1948, p. 77), it seems clear that the simultaneous reproduction of projective intrafigural characteristics (differentiation of a circle from a triangle) is possible without topological interfigural characteristics being reproduced (intersecting figures reproduced separately). At the same time, at the interfigural level alone, it would seem possible for metric characteristics to be taken into account whilst topological characteristics are ignored. Pêcheux (1969) had children in the age-range 4 to 6 years copy models composed of two simple figures of different sizes, which were touching or separate, with the smaller figure either inside or outside the other. At 4 years, in 27 cases out of 126, the differences in size were correctly reproduced but tangency was not respected (table 4).

The hypothesis that the topological system as a whole precedes the Euclidean system would appear to be too simple to account for the data actually obtained.

Two spatial relationships that seem, quite definitely, to precede the others are the topological distinction between 'open' and 'closed' and the Euclidean relationship of curvilinearity as opposed to rectilinearity.

In general, topological features seem easier to maintain than Euclidean ones, but once the child is aware of both types of relation-

Table 4 *Conformity to topological and metric relationships in copying drawings*

|  |  | Topological characteristic: Contact | | |
|---|---|---|---|---|
|  |  | Success | Failure | Total |
| Metric | Success | 73 | 27 | 100 |
| Characteristic: |  |  |  |  |
| Size | Failure | 10 | 16 | 26 |
|  | Total | 83 | 43 | 126 |

These results are derived from 126 responses of 32 children aged 4 years.

ships, the conflict brought about by the complexity of the model is not always resolved in favour of the first of these and, according to circumstances, the child chooses to sacrifice one or the other. It is not therefore a matter of a simple hierarchy within which all topological features must be maintained before a single Euclidean relationship is allowed.

## II INTRAFIGURAL RELATIONSHIPS AND THE PERCEIVED FORM

A recent experiment by Sinclair and Piaget (1968) suggests that the perceived form of an object is not simply the sum of the intrafigural relationships but also includes relationships with the retinal system of reference.

The authors presented children in the age-range 4 to 9 years with square pieces of card the sides of which were either vertical and horizontal (i.e. the card standing on its base) or oblique, by reference to the child (i.e. standing on a corner). With the child watching, the experimenter transformed a square on its base, A, to a square on its corner, B, by rotating it through 45°, and then asked the child if B was still a square, if it was the same card as A, and if it was the same size. The responses obtained showed an evolution in three stages during the course of which the criteria of identity were modified. For 4- and 5-year-olds, and even for half the 6-year-olds, figure B, the square on its corner, was no longer a square, was no longer even the same piece of card, and was not the same size as A. The simple rotation through a single plane had thus, at one and the same time, destroyed the individual and categorial identity of the object and changed its properties. In the case of 6- and 7-year-olds, the object conserved its individual identity, it remained the same piece of card and retained its dimensions, but it changed its category: it was no longer a square. Invariance was achieved, finally, around the age of 8 to 9 years – the object remained a square and the perceptual change was attributed to the displacement of the figure relative to a frame of reference.

The observed evolution could be interpreted in the following fashion. A square on its corner belongs perceptually to the category of diamond-shapes, and is much more like any of that group than a square on its base. The distinction between the two groups, squares and diamond-shapes, is based on the opposition of the verticality and horizontality of the sides of the former and the obliquity of the sides of the latter; verticality and horizontality are in this case relative only to the retinal axes of reference.

The child of 4 to 5 years, like those a few years older, perceives the transformation of A (a square on its side) to B (a square on its corner) as a change of form. The form being the dominant property of the object and the most certain means of recognition, it determines the invariance of the object. If the form changes, the object also changes – it is no longer the same and, in consequence, there is no reason why it should remain the same size and even less reason why it should keep the same name. The child of 7 years continues to perceive A and B as different forms and it is still on the basis of form that he makes his categorisations; consequently he refuses to give to B the same name as A, but, freeing himself from an egocentric frame of reference, he becomes capable of comparing A and B part by part and of recognising that each segment of A has exact correspondence in B. Paradoxically the child thus judges two objects as identical whilst at the same time refusing to put them in the same category. He is capable of analysing both figures from the point of view of their intrafigural relationships, and yet he still takes account of the relationship between the figure and the retinal meridians in deciding on its form. It is only when a system of reference external to the subject is added to the egocentric system that the child becomes capable of comparing the square on its corner with the square on its side and, simultaneously, distinguishing and relating the intrafigural relationships of each figure and their relationships with the system of reference. He is then able to isolate what remains invariant despite the considerable perceptual changes, and so classify the figures on the basis of this invariance. Although children are capable of recognising and naming a square from the age of 4 years, the concept of a square is clearly modified with age. It is possible to say, on the basis of those studies which used drawings in particular, that a square would be initially a closed figure with sides parallel to the horizontal and vertical meridians of the retina, which means that rectangles on their sides are included. The requirement of the sides being equal would be added next. But it is much later, around the age of 9 years, that the characteristics of horizontality and verticality to the retinal meridians would cease to be necessary. Only at this point would the form of a square amount to no more than the sum of intrafigural relationships.

## III  PART–WHOLE RELATIONSHIPS

### 1  *The Localisation of a Part Within a Frame of Reference*
Little research has been devoted to the experimental investigation of spatial localisation. Systematic observations of play activity with bricks have shown that very simple topological relationships such as directionality, or the localisation of an object in a fairly large open space, proximity, and inclusiveness, are already perceived and manipulated as early as one year of age (Brandner, 1938; Gesell and Amatruda, 1947).

From the middle of the second year a child can align blocks vertically as he builds towers; horizontal alignments appear later, both providing evidence of the capacity for maintaining a continuous direction. More precise topological relationships such as the middle, the ends, and intersection are reproduced between 2 and 3 years. Finally, a grasp of the relationships above-below, behind-in front, right-left, appears at about 3 years of age (Vereecken, 1961). The task devised by Van Zutphen, and quoted by Vereecken (1961), involves presenting the child with a card bearing a highly schematised drawing of a house (fig. 19). With the child watching, the experimenter places inside this house a piece of card representing the door and then, above this door, either a window or a chimney. He then asks the child to reconstruct a house identical to this model by means of the appropriate components. Success appears around the age of 3 years. However, if, instead of asking the child to position a door and a window or a door and a chimney at the same time, the experimenter takes a single object – a window for example, and asks the child to copy his positioning of it inside the outline of the house, errors are much more numerous. In fact, in the latter case the relationship of the window to the house is not simply topological but already metric, since the child has the task of putting the window *nearer* the top than the bottom. On the other hand, when it is a matter of positioning the door and the window at the same time, the problem remains within the area of topological relationships: the two components are inside the contour, the window is above the door, the door touches the contour, the door does not touch the window.

The left-right relationship appears later, after the age of 3½ years.

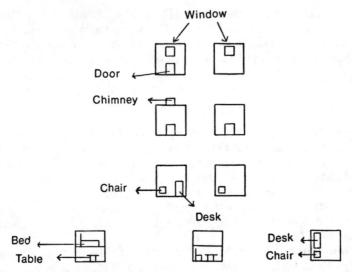

Fig. 19. Example of Van Zutphen's experimental material (Vereecken, 1961).

Another of Van Zutphen's experimental tasks, very similar to the preceding one, requires the child to position a chair and a table within a frame representing a kitchen. In this case also the localisation of a single object in the left or right part of the frame is achieved with greater difficulty than when two objects are involved together. In these various experiments the spatial relationships to be reproduced are limited to one direction at a time – one object is situated with reference to another or to an outline frame, either in the vertical direction in the case of top-bottom, above-below relationships, or in the horizontal direction in the case of right-left relationships. One would expect that the localisation of an object by reference to two directions at the same time would be achieved much later. We know (Piaget and Inhelder, 1948) that representational space and the ability to locate any point in space in terms of imaginary rectangular co-ordinates are not achieved until around the age of 9 years.

However, when the setting is simple enough, children show themselves capable, as early as 5 years, of taking account of the spatial situation of components in the reproduction of a configuration. In the course of their investigation of the development of number, Piaget and Szeminska (1941) asked their subjects to give them as many counters as were involved in making up a model configuration of the following kinds: a row, a circle, a house, a cross, a square, a triangle and a diamond. From the age of $4\frac{1}{2}$ years the children obeyed the instructions by reproducing the model as exactly as possible by a series of one-to-one correspondences between counters. When the reproduction was exact, the positioning of the components was the same as that of the counters in the model, taking into account two orthogonal axes of reference.

It occurred to us that by selecting items not as neutral as counters and placing them within a real-life, familiar frame such as the windows of a house, the ability to localise one part of a whole whilst taking account of both horizontal and vertical directions, might be demonstrated at an earlier age. Vurpillot and Berthoud (1969) presented children with two front elevations of houses, side by side, the six windows of which were closed by shutters. The experimenter explained to the child that the windows in the same position in both houses contained the same pictures, then he opened the shutters of one window in the first house, showed the child what it contained, and asked him to open the window in the second house which had the same things in it. The experiment was carried out with two types

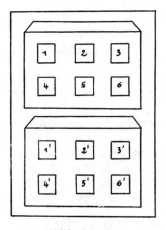

Wide houses
*Vertical comparisons*

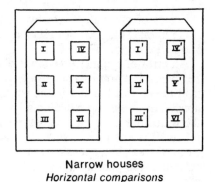

Narrow houses
*Horizontal comparisons*

Fig. 20. Material used in the localisation of a part (Vurpillot and Berthoud, 1969).

of houses: tall narrow ones situated side by side, and wide low ones situated one above the other. Even as early as $3\frac{1}{2}$ years, children did not give chance responses: exact localisations amounted to 34·3 per cent whilst chance alone would have predicted 15·6 per cent. At $5\frac{1}{2}$ years the proportion of correct responses exceeded 70 per cent. The errors that emerged can be separated into several categories and sub-categories. In the first category come the errors of symmetry; the child opened a window situated in the same row (narrow houses) or in the same column (wide houses), this window occupying not the homologous position to the model window but the symmetrical position in terms of the axis of symmetry of both houses.

Table 5   *Analysis of errors of localisation*

| | Ages (in years and months) | | |
|---|---|---|---|
| *Categories of errors* | *3y. 6m.* | *4y. 6m.* | *5y. 6m.* |
| Total number of errors | 189 | 156 | 81 |
| Errors of symmetry | 49·2% | 71·4% | 91·6% |
| Errors of perseveration | 27·3% | 10·2% | 1·2% |
| Other errors | 23·5% | 18·4% | 7·2% |

The percentages are calculated in relation to the total number of errors obtained at the given age-level. The errors of perseveration consisted either of always opening the same window, or of repeating the response which had just been successful (from Vurpillot and Berthoud, 1969).

Errors of symmetry were by far the most numerous since they made up half the total of observed errors at $3\frac{1}{2}$ years and almost all at $5\frac{1}{2}$ years (table 5).

An error of symmetry amounts to a localisation of the window to be opened in terms of a single axis of reference; the window selected is in the correct line but in the wrong column in the case of the tall houses, or in the correct column but in the wrong line in the case of the wide houses. It must be observed that the use of a single axis of reference is compatible with a certain number of correct responses since when a child opens a window chosen on the basis of this single reference, the probability is one in two that he will make a correct choice by chance alone. Table 6 shows that children of $3\frac{1}{2}$ years

Table 6   *Proportion of correct responses and errors of symmetry (percentage)*

| | Ages (in years and months) | | |
|---|---|---|---|
| *Response categories* | *3y. 6m.* | *4y. 6m.* | *5y. 6m.* |
| Correct responses | 34·3 | 49·3 | 71·8 |
| Errors of symmetry | 32·6 | 36·1 | 25·0 |
| Total | 66·9 | 85·4 | 96·8 |

The percentages are calculated from the total number of responses, 288 at each age-level (Vurpillot and Berthoud, 1969).

seem already able to take account of one axis of reference in 66·9 per cent of cases, and that these responses divide equally between those which are correct and those which are errors of symmetry; it is probable that at this age the correct responses are not derived from two orthogonal axes but from a single one. From the age of $4\frac{1}{2}$ years the number of correct responses exceeds the number of errors of symmetry which would seem to correspond to the beginning of the use of two axes of reference.

The proximity factor plays an important role in the determination of responses, particularly with the youngest subjects, but it operates as much by reference to the subject, when the child tends to open one of the windows nearest to him, as by reference to the model, in which case the child tends to open the window nearest to the model. Thus it is impossible to separate out completely the two forms of proximity. Finally, when the comparison between two houses involves vertical visual scanning (wide houses), the windows in the upper rows tend to be opened more frequently than those of the lower rows. The upper part of the visual field seems, therefore, to be preferred from an early age.

Two conclusions can be drawn from this investigation. The first concerns the developmental evolution of the spatial localisation of a single component in a rectangular frame of reference. Three phases can be distinguished: during the first one the children do not seem to take account of the position of the model window, they open any window at all, and sometimes the experimenter is obliged to check them during the first trial in order to prevent them from opening shutters on the model house as well as on the other. But the choice is not entirely a matter of chance, since the child prefers to open the shutters situated nearest to him.

In the second phase, marked by the predominance of errors of symmetry, the child takes into account a single axis of reference. Two-thirds of the children aged $3\frac{1}{2}$ seemed to be operating at this level already, at least in the experiment in question.

In the third phase the child finally employs both axes of reference, vertical and horizontal, at the same time.

The choice of the first axis of reference seems to be mainly determined by the direction of visual inspection according to how this moves from the model to the reproduction; the child opens a window in the correct row when visual scanning is horizontal (narrow houses situated side by side) or in the correct column when visual scanning is vertical (wide houses situated one above each other). This leads us to a second conclusion, concerning the role of eye movements in the determination of spatial references. Vereecken (1961) has put forward the hypothesis that the path taken by the movement of the eyes, when it follows the line of a frame of reference, or when it goes from one object to another, acts as a support for the reference system; the results of the present experiment would seem to be in accord with these predictions. However, it must be observed that the regular arrangement of the windows of our houses into rows and columns favoured a rectilinear visual trajectory. It would be interesting to ascertain whether this trajectory would remain horizontal or vertical in the absence of a frame of reference or when the components of the configuration were situated randomly or in oblique lines.

Finally, it appears that horizontal and vertical visual displacements are not equivalent. This is not new; what is new, however, is the extremely precocious manifestation of a preference for the upper part of the visual field which, according to previous investigations (Piaget and Vinh-Bang, 1961a) did not seem to be in evidence until 7 years of age. On this point supplementary research is required, and the interpretation of our results needs to be verified.

## 2   *The Perception of the Displacement of a Single Element in a Configuration*

The experiment of Vurpillot and Berthoud (1969) shows that from the age of $3\frac{1}{2}$ years children are capable of taking into account simple spatial relationships between the components of a configuration. It might be supposed, therefore, that the displacement of one of these components would be perceived as a difference, at an early age, at least in the case of regular and 'strong' configurations in the Gestaltist sense of the term.

Three configurations, A, B and C, were constructed using nine identical components (drawings of daisies). The first, A, was a circle; in the second, B, the circle was disarranged – some of the daisies were still arranged in an arc whilst the others were scattered; in the third, C, all the components were placed irregularly (fig. 21). On the basis of these configurations, twelve pairs of drawings were constructed, four of the pairs being identical and eight different. A difference consisted of the displacement of a component towards either the exterior or the interior of the configuration. In configuration B the displacement involved either a component situated in the middle of the arc of the circle ($B_1$) or the component which terminated the arc of the circle ($B_2$). Thus it can be assumed that the displaced component is part of a less regular configuration in $B_1$ than in A, in $B_2$ than in $B_1$, and in C than in $B_2$. Children in the age-range $3\frac{1}{2}$ to $5\frac{1}{2}$ years were asked to say whether the two configurations making up a pair were the same or not.

This experiment produced two main results (Pineau, 1969;

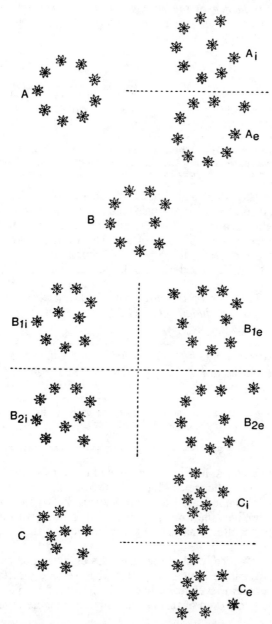

Fig. 21. Configurations used in the investigation of the perception of a displacement of a single component (Pineau, 1969).

Table 7   *Influence of the configuration on performance (correct judgments of difference), as a percentage*

| Age (in years and months) | 3y. 6m. | 4y. 6m. | 5y. 6m. |
|---|---|---|---|
| Circle A | 0 | 31·25 | 64·58 |
| Disarranged circle $B_1$ | 0 | 20·83 | 60·42 |
| Disarranged circle $B_2$ | 2·8 | 16·67 | 45·83 |
| [1]Potato C | 0 | 14·58 | 43·75 |

The results are expressed as a percentage of the correct responses 'not the same'. There were forty-eight responses in each case (after Pineau, 1969).

Vurpillot, Lécuyer, Moal and Pineau, 1971). Firstly, as had been predicted, the displacement of a single component brought a 'difference' response more often, the more regular the configuration – that is, in children from $4\frac{1}{2}$ to $5\frac{1}{2}$ years of age. However, displacements towards the interior seemed to be perceived much more easily than displacements towards the exterior (table 8).

Table 8   *Influence of the direction of the displacement (correct judgments of difference), as a percentage*

| Age (in years and months) | 3y. 6m. | 4y. 6m. | 5y. 6m. |
|---|---|---|---|
| Towards the interior | 1·04 | 31·25 | 83·33 |
| Towards the exterior | 0 | 8·33 | 21·87 |

The results are expressed in percentages on the basis of the responses of twenty-four subjects at each age-level. There were ninety-six responses in each case (after Pineau, 1969).

The first of these results can be interpreted in terms of the law of uniform destiny (Wertheimer, 1923) which predicts that the displacement of a single component of a group disturbs the organisation of the field and modifies the form perceived. But on its own this law does not seem to offer a satisfactory explanation of the data, for several reasons.

At $3\frac{1}{2}$ years, practically all of the responses obtained are 'same' – whatever configuration is presented and whatever the direction of the displacement. However, according to the results of Vurpillot and Berthoud (1969), children of this age are already capable of localis-

[1]*Translator's note.* Not the familiar oval *pomme de terre*, but the knobbly sweet potato or *patate* – hence its use here as a descriptive term.

ing particular elements, at least in one direction. Moreover, it seems strange that the displacement of a single component of a circle, a displacement which destroys the best form that we know, should not be perceived at this age, whilst the baby differentiates regularity from irregularity (Fantz, 1965a, 1967; Lang, 1966) and when even the jay (Hertz, 1928) can easily locate a point outside a circle – to give just two examples.

It must be assumed, therefore, that 'same' responses given to pairs that differ are not all the result of a failure to perceive differences; in any case the children's spontaneous remarks confirmed that a displacement perceived and referred to by a phrase such as 'that one's untidy', for example, did not prevent a child from giving the response 'same'.

The observed difference in performance between displacements towards the interior and towards the exterior is even more difficult to interpret, and several factors would seem to be involved. Let us take the case of the circle: according to the law of uniform destiny, the configuration is disturbed as much by an exterior as an interior displacement. But if one examines the two figures Ae and A it can be seen that in Ae the displacement introduces one marked point of inflexion and two slight ones into the contour, whilst in Ai the contour now presents three distinct points of inflexion. In terms of information theory, the difference between A and Ai is more marked than between A and Ae. A comparison between the number of points of inflexion in the contour is much less convincing for the other configurations, but a new factor can be invoked. Owing to the limited surface area of each configuration, the interior components are close together and tend to form partial structures. Thus it can be seen that in B there is a single interior component, whilst there are two in $B_1i$ and $B_2i$, and one again in $B_1e$ and $B_2e$; in the same way Ce has three interior components whilst Ci has four. It is possible that the interior component or components of a configuration attract the attention of young children more than components on the contour; if their density changes, a difference is perceived; if it remains invariant, so does the configuration. A difference situated on the contour would only be perceived if the gaze shifted from the powerful attraction of the central area (Vurpillot, 1968) and the child proceeded to a complete and methodical exploration of the figures.

It can be assumed that, in a situation which appears quite straightforward, the physical properties of the stimulus determine the area of gaze attraction; if the perceptual exploration is very limited, only this area is inspected, and a displacement is only perceived if it modifies the content of this area; finally, a perceived difference does not necessarily bring about the response 'not the same'.

On their own the laws of perceptual organisation are, therefore, far from enabling us to predict the response the child will make, because this appears to depend also on the extent of his visual exploration and his criteria for making a decision.

### 3   *The Perception of Differences Caused by the Permutation of Components*

The experiment of Vurpillot and Moal (1970) compares judgments of difference in two situations, one in which the difference between two figures is obtained by substituting one component for another, the other in which there is simply a permutation of two components. One hundred and fifty children from 3 years 9 months to 7 years, divided into three age groups, had to judge twelve pairs of drawings of houses each containing six windows. In six of the pairs the houses were physically identical; the other six differed in two respects. The six windows of each house had different contents: in the identical pairs the windows in the same position in both houses had identical contents (fig. 22a); in the differing pairs the windows in the same position had contents that differed from one another. The differences were introduced either by substitution or by permutation amongst the contents of the windows: in the case of substitution the contents of two of the windows of one house were not repeated in the other house (fig. 22b); in the case of permutation each window of one house corresponded to a window with the same contents in the other house – except that for two of these windows identical contents appeared in different positions (22c). The child was asked to say whether the two houses of a pair were identical or not.

The factors of content and position having been offset, the judgments of difference, when the pairs differed by substitution and when they differed by permutation, could be made. At all age-levels, from 4 to $6\frac{1}{2}$ years, errors were much more numerous when there was a permutation than when there was a substitution. The houses which differed in the content of the windows in the same position (substitution) were judged as different in more than half the cases by the 4-year-olds, and in more than 90 per cent of the cases by the 5-year-olds. But when the difference was one of permutation, the 4-year-olds gave less than 10 per cent correct responses ('not the same') and those of $6\frac{1}{2}$ years still responded incorrectly in almost half the cases.

It seems very clear that young children in making their judgments pay attention, almost exclusively, to the contents of the windows and only begin to see a permutation of the components as a modification of the configuration which the house constitutes, from about the age of 6 years.

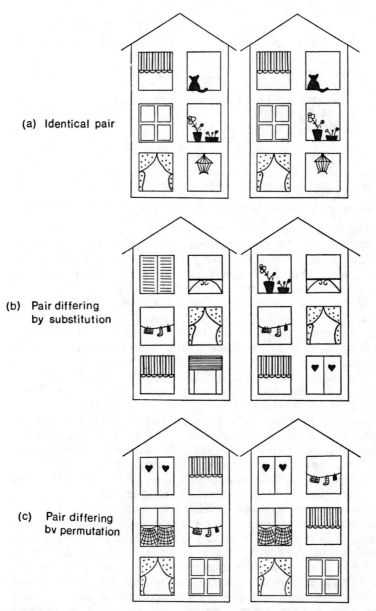

(a) Identical pair

(b) Pair differing by substitution

(c) Pair differing by permutation

Fig. 22. Example of the material used in the permutations experiment (Vurpillot and Moal, 1970).

Table 9   *Percentage of correct responses*

|  | (*Age in years and months*) | | |
|---|---|---|---|
| Types of pairs | 4y. | 5y. | 6y. 6m. |
| Identical pairs ('same' responses) | 96·0 | 97·3 | 97·0 |
| Pairs differing by substitution ('not the same' responses) | 55·3 | 92·0 | 99·3 |
| Pairs differing by permutation ('not the same' responses) | 8·7 | 23·3 | 55·3 |

The results are expressed as percentages of correct responses based on the total number of responses obtained with the pairs in question (after Vurpillot and Moal, 1970).

The results could be interpreted either in terms of perceptual inadequacy or the use of an inadequate criterion for decision-making. It would seem that, lacking a satisfactory system of reference, young children do not differentiate the varying positions of the windows. Such an explanation would suffice if the errors were divided equally amongst all the permutations and if specific investigations of spatial localisation provided supportive data – which is not the case, as we have just seen. The development of the criteria for making a judgment or decision will be examined in detail in Chapter 11.

The analysis of the distribution of correct responses reveals a clear distinction between two categories of permutations. Those where the two windows are in the same horizontal line are the last to give rise to judgments of difference. At $6\frac{1}{2}$ years only 10 per cent of those pairs in which the difference was a horizontal permutation received correct responses, whilst for the other types of permutation 66·7 per cent correct responses were obtained at the same age. Although results of this order would seem to be very definite, the counter-balancing of the factors of content and position does not allow us to draw conclusions other than those relating to a comparison of permutations. In consequence a complementary experiment was carried out, using very similar material. In this (Moal, 1969; Vurpillot, Lécuyer, Moal and Pineau, 1971) each child had to judge as 'same' or 'not the same' twelve pairs of drawings of houses of which three were identical and nine different. Each differing pair differed in two respects, as a result of permutation, and each child saw three horizontal permutations, two permutations of windows some way apart, situated on the top and bottom rows, and four permutations of windows close together and not horizontal, situated on adjoining rows.

Table 10 *Percentage of correct responses according to the localisation of the permutation*

|  | Age (in years and months) | | |
| --- | --- | --- | --- |
| Types of permutation | 4y. | 5y. | 6y. 6m. |
| Non-horizontal permutations | 4·2 | 36·4 | 97·3 |
| Horizontal permutations | 1·1 | 7·3 | 71·8 |

(After Moal, 1969)

Table 10 shows that at 4 years there were practically no correct responses, whatever the permutation. At 5 years correct responses involving horizontal permutations were still rare, whilst correct responses for the other permutations exceeded a third of the total. Finally, at $6\frac{1}{2}$ years perfect performances were achieved for all permutations except the horizontal ones, which still showed an error rate of almost 30 per cent. On the whole the level of performance was higher than in the preceding experiment (Vurpillot and Moal, 1970): it is possible that presenting pairs differing by substitution at the same time as those differing by permutation rendered the task more difficult in the former investigation.

Nonetheless, in both experiments children above the age of 4 years performed differently when presented with pairs involving horizontal permutations than with the others. The former appeared to be more difficult to discern than the latter. If we take account of the results of the investigation of spatial localisation (Vurpillot and Berthoud, 1969), the use of a single axis of reference could be held responsible for the failure to perceive horizontal permutations. But such an explanation can only account for the errors of the youngest children, since from the age of $5\frac{1}{2}$ the great majority of children localise the windows by reference to two rectangular axes (Vurpillot and Berthoud, 1969). A deficiency in terms of the ability to localise spatially is not sufficient to explain the particular difficulty in perceiving horizontal permutations.

We have considered the possibility that the difficulty in detecting a permutation difference might be bound up with the structure of the configuration. The regular arrangement of the windows of a house into rows and columns would make it easier to confuse positions. Indeed, beyond a certain level of complexity the localisation of a unit in a row or column means that you have to count on systematically from the starting point; as every adult has demonstrated to himself at one time or another – and with more reason for localising a particular window – it is impossible to count the storeys of a skyscraper. Visual displacement on its own proves to be an inadequate and unreliable means of localisation. For the young child, whose visuo-motor exploration is less precise than the adult's and who cannot yet count, units that are regularly distributed, even when few in number, can constitute a handicap.

A supplementary experiment (Lécuyer, 1969; Vurpillot, Lécuyer, Moal and Pineau, 1971) verified this hypothesis. Three configurations were constructed using nine components; these components were drawings of familiar objects (toothbrush, comb, cup, umbrella, glove, etc.). The first configuration, A, was a circle in which all the components were equidistant; the second configuration, B, was a circle in which eight components were close together whilst the ninth was distinctly separate; finally, in the third configuration eight components were placed in a circle and the ninth outside the circle (fig. 23). Not all the components have the same status in these configurations; the isolated component in configurations B and C is clearly individualised, or 'singularised', compared with the others. On the other hand the components of circle A and of the arcs of a circle in configurations B and C have uniform status and can be described as 'non-singularised', with one exception: the components situated at the ends of the arcs in B and C can be classed as 'partly singularised' since, although they are less individualised than the 'singularised' components, they still occupy a privileged position amongst those that make up the arc of the circle. Children in the age-range 4 to 6 years had to compare twelve pairs of drawings based on the three configurations – three identical pairs (one for each configuration) and nine differing pairs. The latter each had two differences introduced by the permutation of two components. These permutations involved one of five combinations – either a singularised component and a partly singularised component, or a singularised and a non-singularised one, or two partly singularised ones, or a partly singularised and a non-singularised one, or finally, two non-singularised ones.

The distance between the permutated components was maintained as constant as possible, and the situation of the various components of a configuration, like the order of presentation, was randomised. As in the preceding experiments involving permutations, the child had to decide whether the drawings in a pair were exactly the same or not.

The results clearly demonstrated that the number of correct responses to the different pairs was directly proportional to the degree of singularity of the permutated components (fig. 24). Thus at 4 and 5 years, the pairs in which the permutations included two non-

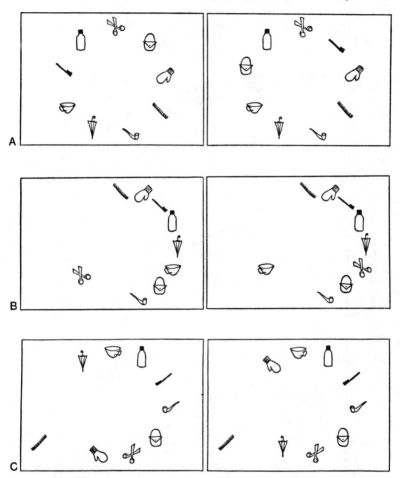

Fig. 23. Example of the configurations used in the investigation of the 'singularity' of a component in the perception of permutations (Lécuyer, 1969).

A: permutation of components, which have not been singularised, in a regular structure. B: permutation of a component which has been singularised and one which has not, in a partially regular structure (configuration B). C: permutation of two components which are partly singularised, in a partially regular structure (configuration C).

singularised components received a proportion of correct responses very close to that obtained for non-horizontal permutations in the second experiment with houses (table 10). By comparison, the percentage of correct responses for those pairs which included a singu-

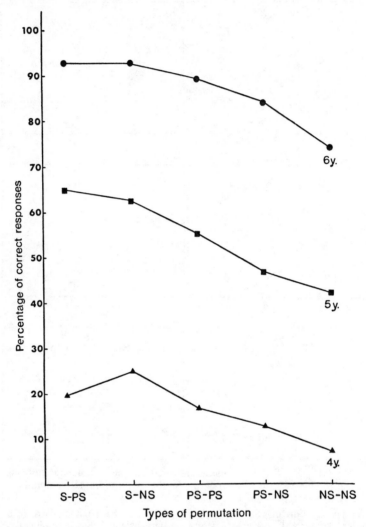

Fig. 24. Distribution of correct responses as a function of age and the degree of singularisation of the permutated component (Lécuyer, 1969).

S=singularised component; PS=partly singularised component; NS= non-singularised component; S-PS=permutation involving a singularised and a partly singularised component, etc.

larised component was significantly higher at all age-levels (fig. 24). However, even in the most favourable example, a permutation difference produced fewer 'not the same' responses than those in-volving a substitution difference (Vurpillot and Moal, 1970).

## CONCLUSION OF CHAPTERS 2, 3 AND 4

All points in the physical world can be localised in terms of a system of reference formed by three axes of orthogonal co-ordinates. It is in this three-dimensional world that the child makes his visual dis-placements. In the course of his first year of life he learns to dis-tinguish between changes of identity and changes of position so that by about 15 months he is in possession of a system of perceptual space, isomorphic to physical space, in which permanent objects, in-variant in terms of size, form, colour, and reflectivity, are integrated in the system of spatial relationships of the set of displacements.

There then follows the superimposition of representational space on to this perceptual space, a much slower development since it is only completed around the ages of 9–10 years.

The development of the capacity for representing the different possible aspects of an object is accompanied by a refinement in the analysis of the sensory tableau in terms of data relative both to various intrinsic properties of the object and its location with reference to the subject, and a progressive accumulation of know-ledge about shape, size, colour, etc. which characterise familiar objects. The conjunction of these various factors means that the comparison between several objects situated in different positions in space is subject to an increasing number of variables. Conflicts become apparent between what one knows – for example, that a man does not change in size as he goes further away, or that a door always remains rectangular – and what one sees: the man looks smaller when he is in the distance and the door may have the appearance of being trapezoidal. The more that is known about an object and its relationship with other objects, the more complex and structured the conceptual system into which it is incorporated, the more diffi-cult judgment becomes – the usual result being a compromise or a choice. Thus, the evolution with age of perceptual constancies seems to take place not so much at the perceptual level as at the level of the interaction between various cognitive processes.

Neither perceptual space nor representational space is completely homogeneous; two directions are privileged, the vertical which coin-cides with the line of terrestrial attraction and the horizontal which is perpendicular to it in the fronto-parallel plane. These two axes divide space into an upper and lower part, a right and a left. Whilst the right and the left parts seem to be visually homogeneous, at least at the age-levels which were studied here, the upper part has privileged status from a very early age. The heterogeneity of space around a vertical axis, as opposed to its homogeneity around a horizontal axis, is very probably at the root of the relatively precocious differentiation between upper and lower as against left and right. The concept of the 'above-below' relationship is acquired earlier than that between right and left (Vereecken, 1961); mirror images are more often confused when they are type H inversions (with reference to a vertical axis) than type V inversions (with reference to a horizontal axis) (Rudel and Teuber, 1963; Huttenlocher, 1967a, b). Geometric forms are perceived as having a top and a bottom, and thus a subjective orientation, by very young children (Ghent, 1956, 1961, etc.). Initially, therefore, objects and forms appear to be situated with reference to the vertical axis.

There is, however, one activity in which the horizontal direction enjoys a privileged role, this being visuo-motor exploration. The anatomical and physiological characteristics of the visual system are such that the visual field is more extensive horizontally and horizontal eye movements easier than vertical ones.

The localisation of a particular point or object is always made within a system of reference. To begin with, this is totally subjective: the vertical coincides with the axis of the body (Wapner, 1968) and the various points of a physical object are situated, like the proximal stimulus to which they give rise, by reference to the vertical and horizontal meridians of the retina.

To the system of reference which his own body constitutes, the child goes on to add a more objective system in the form of an external frame of reference. Initially this frame is limited to one object or a group of objects close together, and it is only when representational space is complete that the child has at his disposal a Euclidean system of reference, with three imaginary orthogonal axes, and where the point of origin is arbitrary.

A distinction is often made between intrafigural and interfigural relationships – the former being those established between the various points of a structure, whilst the latter relate the location of each of these structures (objects or figures) with reference to each other. Such a distinction would seem to be somewhat artificial. It is usable enough when the figures are isolated primary structures; when this is the case, each structure can be defined in terms of a set of intrafigural relationships, whilst the form of the whole configuration – made up of the separate units of these structures – is defined in terms of the interfigural relationships which locate each of these structures by reference to the others. When the primary structures have points of contact and form larger units of overlapping or juxtaposed figures, it is still possible, if a degree of arbitrariness is accepted, to describe them in terms of inter- and intra-figural relationships. But when the whole is perceived as a complex figure made up of simpler figures, every relationship between these is, at the same time, interfigural from the point of view of these simple structures, and intrafigural from the point of view of the whole.

The spatial relationships, intra-or interfigural, can be topological, projective, or metric according to the geometry that is chosen. It appears that topological relationships are used by the child earlier than projective or metric relationships. Piaget and Inhelder (1948) go so far as to postulate that topological relationships are the first to be acquired and that they are organised in topological space which is succeeded by metric space. This transition from a topological to a Euclidean geometry is replicated in the construction of representational space. The development does not in fact appear to be as simple as this, since everything topological does not precede everything metric. The distinction between curvilinearity and rectilinearity, which is Euclidean, occurs as early as the distinction between open and closed, which is topological. In one and the same situation, for example copying drawings, the child is capable of neglecting certain topological relationships whilst respecting metric ones. It seems probable that the child very soon makes use of topological, projective and metric relationships, but that these are not integrated in organised systems; consequently, when the task is difficult and various types of relationships need to be taken into account at the same time, then conflicts arise. Unable to satisfy both metric and topological requirements, the child chooses to respect those which seem to him to be the most important in the circumstances he encounters.

# Chapter 5

# Perceptual Organisation and the Process of Identification and Differentiation: The Child's 'Syncretism'

It has been known for a long time that pre-school children do badly on tasks of perceptual identification and differentiation. The fine discrimination of their absolute and differential thresholds means that their inferiority, compared with their elders, cannot be attributed to a lack of sensitivity in their sensory receptors. Thus, in order to explain this poor performance, one must think in terms of a psychological deficiency rather than some form of biological immaturity.

The behaviour of young children seems to be characterised by an inability to integrate the various units of information they have available into structured wholes within which all the elements are articulated in a network of relationships. From the perceptual point of view, this inability is manifested, in particular, by the failure to relate parts to each other and each part to the whole.

For classic associationism, the repeated appearance of the same parts together is sufficient for associations to be formed and for structured wholes of increasing complexity – and increasingly better organised – to develop. The inferiority of young children would be ascribed to the fact that their relatively short existence had not yet allowed them to acquire sufficient experience. The number of associations between parts being insufficient for these to form larger structures, the child consequently responds only to details. At the end of the last century this simple explanation of the development of children's performances was vigorously challenged and an alternative explanation put forward according to which a general and confused view of the whole would always precede the distinct and analytic view of the parts (Renan, 1890). Thus the behaviour of the very young child, far from being characterised by a sensibility attuned to tiny details, was, on the contrary, syncretic and typified by a predominance of unstructured, unanalysed wholes.

The stimulus given to research into the perception of the child by the controversy which sprang up between the proponents of classic associationism and those of the new theory of 'syncretism', and the place taken by this term in the literature, are such that it seems appropriate to take an historical perspective in order to present the available data in its context.

## I THE PREDOMINANCE OF THE WHOLE OR OF THE PARTS

### 1 *The Concept of Syncretism*

The term 'syncretism' was introduced by Renan, who postulated an analogy between the slow historical evolution of human intelligence and the rapid unfolding of the stages of any and every human behaviour (Renan, 1890; Compayré, in Sully, 1898, p. 12).

'Just as the most ordinary act of human cognition involving a complex object is made up of three phases: (1) a general and confused view of the whole; (2) a distinct and analytic view of the parts; and (3) synthetic reconstitution of the whole from the knowledge of the parts; so does the human mind progress through three stages that can be designated under the three headings of *syncretism*, analysis and synthesis, which correspond to these three phases of knowledge' (Renan, 1890, p. 301).

Sully (1898), followed by Claparède (1909), added a third volet[1] to Renan's dyptich: an individual man's development recapitulated that of the human species, and in the child one saw, successively, a syncretic stage followed by an analytic stage and, finally, a synthetic stage. The description given by Renan of the behaviour of primitive man was compared with the results of observations carried out on children. A striking resemblance was ascertained and subsequently a number of analogies were drawn in various areas: the prelogical thought of the child and uncivilised races (Compayré, 1898; Lévy-Bruhl, 1910), the drawings of children and those of cavemen (Busse, 1914; Kretchmer, 1910; Lamprecht, 1905, 1906, 1914; Van Gennep, 1911; Luquet, 1927a, 1927b, etc.). The development of the child was seen, within the framework of the theory of evolution, as the application to psychology of Haeckel's law of recapitulation.

[1]*Translator's note.* Mlle Vurpillot's very apt image requires the use of this somewhat technical term which may not be familiar to those readers unacquainted with religious art. 'Volet' is the term used to describe one of the (movable) sections of an icon, which is usually in three parts (i.e. a *triptych*).

In fact Renan's three stages aroused a markedly unequal interest: analysis and synthesis were old acquaintances whilst syncretism appeared as a novel and original idea, the key, perhaps, to child behaviour – hence the infatuation which it aroused in psychologists and educationists (Decroly, 1929) during the first quarter of this century. There were very few who interested themselves in the development of the successive stages; in the main, the speculations, the controversies, the researches and the applications were concerned with syncretism alone.

## 2  *Experimental Evidence*

In an initial period, which extended from approximately 1890 to 1925, the perception of the whole was seen as strictly opposed to the perception of the parts: either the young child always perceived the whole more easily than the parts, and the perception of the child was syncretic (Binet, 1890; Claparède, 1909, 1925; Luquet, 1913, 1927; Demoor and Jonckheere, 1920; Volkelt, 1926; Decroly, 1929, etc.), or this same child always perceived the parts more easily than the whole (Compayré, 1898; Cramaussel, 1909, 1924, 1927) and the perception of the child was analytic. Syncretism was given the restricted meaning of globalism, which enforced a choice between two mutually exclusive alternatives. Thus observations and experiments were set up to demonstrate the cogency either of globalism (or syncretism) or of elementarism (or pointillism), the latter seen as the opposite of syncretism.

The most commonly held hypotheses were that the identification of an object would be facilitated by means of a syncretic perception, whilst the perception of differences would be better if details were seen rather than the whole.

The earliest publications reported observations of individual cases. Claparède (1906) reported that his son, aged 4 years, was perfectly capable of identifying in a music album the pages which corresponded to various rondos by Dalcroze, even when the book was given to him upside-down, although he could read neither the words nor the musical notes. Claparède concluded that the identification was made on the basis of the general physiognomy of the page, in other words the *whole*. But nothing in Claparède's account enables one to determine the actual index employed by the child; it could have been the area occupied by the title, or indeed the presence of such a characteristic feature; it could be that the criterion changed from one rondo to another.

Similar observations by Jonckheere (1903, 1908) confirmed Claparède's results and the impossibility of interpreting them in an unequivocal fashion. A backward child was able to recognise, at a glance, the perforated rolls of a pianola (Jonckheere, 1903). A 5-year-old child had a collection of twenty-eight pictures, each one of a postman from a different country. The latter could be identified by the uniform of the postman, by the countryside in which the postman was depicted, by the national flag drawn in the top right-hand corner, by a postage-stamp drawn in the bottom left-hand corner and, finally, by the name of the country.

After a very rapid training session, the child showed himself capable of recognising each of these factors. When questioned, he justified his identification by the shape of the hat in one case, the stamp in another, the flag in a third. Not that this prevented his identifying the postman just as well when the hat, the stamp or the flag were hidden. Does this mean, as Jonckheere supposed, that the child had a picture of the whole and that this was adequate even when one part was blocked out, or is it that he used indiscriminately first one index then another? The absence of a systematic criterion is certainly what shows up most clearly in this particular observation.

Segers (1926a) presented children with drawings of monstrous animals made up of the head of one animal and the body of another, successively, for periods of five seconds each. Before the age of 7 years the children did not seem to be affected by the presence of an anomaly and identified the drawings either by the shape of the body or by the head. The existence of two contradictory possibilities of identification was not perceived, and only troubled those children of around 7–8 years. Segers attributed the behaviour of the younger children to the globalistic nature of their perception.

Whilst Claparède (1907, 1909), Jonckheere (1903, 1908) and Segers (1926b) ascribed the identification of objects to a perception of the whole, other investigators, at the same time, insisted on the attraction for children of tiny details (Cramaussel, 1924, 1927). In the task of describing a picture included in their developmental scale, Binet and Simon (1908) specified three stages: enumeration, description, interpretation. The first of these, attained at the age of 3 years, is not supplanted until the age of 7 years. Before this age, when given a picture, very young children see only a juxtaposition of components between which they establish no connection, neither spatial (description) nor meaningful (interpretation). Each part is perceived individually: there is no conception of the whole. However, it could be that this is due to the size of the pictures concerned. The child, unable to take in the whole at a single glance, would be obliged to explore the picture and would thus have only partial and successive images. Moreover, the pictures contained varied and clearly individualised components such as pots, chairs, people; the child saw these different components successively, in visual exploration, and enumerated them as he progressed. However, when children of 3½ years were shown the postage stamp of the Sower[1] (Simon, 1913; Mosés, 1913), which is an uncomplicated drawing of a woman and small enough to be seen in its entirety at a glance, they enumerated nothing and contented themselves with a global identification. In dealing with the postage stamp used by Simon (1913) and Mosés (1913), as with the large drawings of Binet and Simon (1908), or the reconstructed pictures of Segers (1926a), the youngest children behaved in the same way: they identified what they could see in a single visual fixation. The increase with age of the number of components enumerated stems as much from an improved visual exploration as a larger repertoire of identifiable forms.

Demoor and Jonckheere were of the opinion that if young children were content to enumerate the objects perceived it was because the 'linking together of visual ideas does not take place and is of no interest . . . We see what we are able to see; and we are able to see everything that we can identify, focusing on it, among the other objects perceived, as being meaningful and substantial' (Demoor and Jonckheere, 1920, p. 95).

The influence of motivation had already been emphasised by Claparède who thought that objects were, initially, the goal of activity and the trigger of behavioural response. 'Details can only leave him [the child] indifferent, just as we are indifferent to the details of a car which we have to avoid if we are not to be knocked down' (Claparède, 1909, p. 522).

These various observations agree in showing that, when presented with an object, the young child seeks to identify it, for preference, in terms of his interests, whilst including it in a scheme of action. The methods of identification show themselves to be varied and generally effective, but nothing in the reported observations permits a definite conclusion as to the existence of a globalist rather than a pointillist perception. The conditions under which these early investigations were carried out were either badly controlled or only controlled to a limited extent, and the subjects were few in number; nonetheless the data obtained have provided a powerful stimulus for the execution of better controlled investigations involving respectable numbers of children. The aim of these experiments has been not only the study of the child's capacities for identification but also his ability to make comparisons and detect differences and similarities between objects.

[1]*Translator's note.* The French postage stamp bearing the picture of *La Semeuse* was first issued in 1903, being used for all common denominations. The basic design has continued in use up to recent times, and has been part of the detail of everyday experience for French children.

A technique derived from Heilbronner involves presenting the child with incomplete drawings representing familiar objects; more and more complete drawings of the same object are shown to the subject who must say what it represents (identification) and in what respect each drawing differs from the preceding one (differentiation). Two authors, Van der Torren (1907) and Schober and Schober (1919), carried out investigations using this technique, the only difference between them being that, in the former, isolated details are juxtaposed more or less by chance, whilst in the latter the general outline is present from the first drawing and acts as a frame for the details as they are added (fig. 25). However, at the same age, Van der Torren's subjects reported more differences and identified the drawings at a later stage than the subjects of Schober and Schober. These two investigations have been reported and discussed time and time again in the literature, but they are far from clarifying for us the globalist or pointillist nature of perception in children. Is it possible to say that Schober and Schober's results support globalism? To do so would be to equate global perception with the perception of the contour. The most that can be said is that it appears that easy identification is accompanied by a lack of attention to details. In every respect the task seems to be ill designed for studying the capacity for perceptual differentiation.

The paired comparison tasks involving a model and a number of variables constructed by Segers (1926c) and Cramaussel (1927) led them to completely opposite conclusions, since for the former they confirmed the globalist character of perception, whilst for the latter they proved that syncretism did not exist. The differences in the material and the intervention of multiple and uncontrolled variables renders interpretation very difficult. In Cramaussel's (1927) experiment, the child had to indicate from amongst three or four painted wooden squares the one identical to a model. The squares were painted with coloured stripes, the differences involving either the colour of the stripe, or the colour of the dots painted on one of the stripes, or the relative position of two stripes. The task was in general successfully completed by a substantial proportion of children in the age-range 5–6$\frac{1}{2}$ years. The greatest number of mistakes was made when the difference involved a change in the position of two stripes (the model square had three stripes in the order red, blue, yellow, whilst the stripes of the square that differed were in the order blue, red, yellow). Increasing the number of stripes in the squares to be compared and a rotation through 90°, in relation to the model, increased the degree of difficulty.

Segers (1926c) employed a lotto game technique: on a large card divided up into compartments he drew a series of pictures – one to

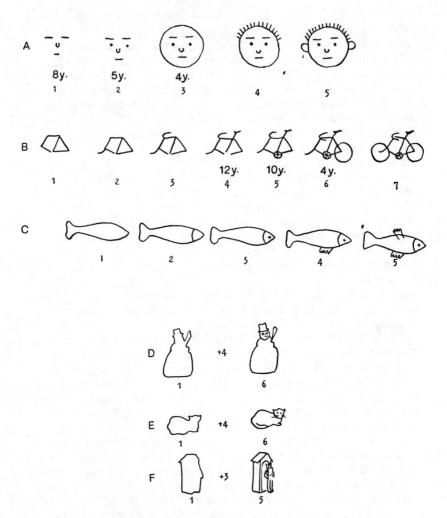

Fig. 25. Examples of incomplete drawings which have to be identified.

Series A, B and C are taken from Van Der Torren (1907). Series D, E and F are from Schober and Schober (1919); only the first and the last drawings are reproduced for series D, E and F.

each compartment – and then gave the child a pack of small cards each bearing one of the pictures on the big card. The child had to place each of the small cards, one by one, on the picture that was identical; after each response the small card was removed so that all the compartments were available for each selection. A first experiment involved lotto cards with four compartments and drawings of the silhouettes of boys and girls in different colours. Segers obtained an error-rate of a little over 50 per cent between 3 and 3½ years and almost perfect performance from the age of 5 years.

A second experiment involved a lotto card with sixteen compartments, each one occupied by a drawing of a house (fig. 26). The

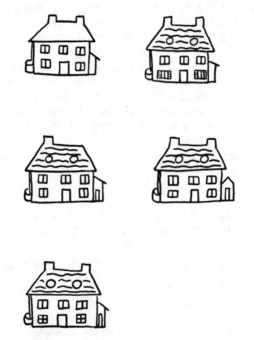

Fig. 26. Examples of the lotto drawings of Segers (1926).

level of performance was not very high, with success rates of only 24 per cent at 4½ years, 60 per cent at 5½ years, 79 per cent at 7½ years, 85 per cent at 9½ years. Segers concluded that perception of differences was poor up to the age of 7 years and attributed it to a globalistic perception. The experiment is well known but several criticisms can be made of it. To begin with, the objective differences between the houses are rather heterogeneous, some involving the presence or absence of a component, others its form or position; even the number of differences varies from one to three depending on which pair is selected. Furthermore, it can be seen that each house must be compared successively with each of the drawings on the lotto card; the possession of a strategy of comparison is indispensable and one is tempted to attribute the poor performance of the youngest children to the absence or poor quality of their strategy rather than their limited perception of differences.

The results of systematic investigations appear to be as contradictory and difficult to interpret as the data obtained from observation. As Cramaussel (1911, 1927) pointed out, this seems to be due largely to a confusion between tasks of specific identification (Claparède, 1908; Jonckheere, 1908; Cramaussel, 1909; Segers, 1926a), categorial identification (Van der Torren, 1907; Schober and Schober, 1919; Cramaussel, 1924), and similarity (Cramaussel, 1911; Van Wayenburg, 1913). As to the actual tests of perceptual differentiation employed, some involve the comparison of an object which is present with one which preceded it but is now absent (Van der Torren, 1907; Schober and Schober, 1919), others present them side by side; the number and kind of physical differences, as well as the number of objects to be compared, vary markedly from author to author.

In short, if any conclusion can be drawn, it relates to the influence on the performance of children in the age-range 3 to 6 years of the objective properties of the experimental setting, and particularly the stimulus. This is the kind of interpretation offered by Meili (1931), who views the 'syncretism' of children in terms of an exaggerated dependence on the characteristics of the stimulus.

## II   THE ABSENCE OF ARTICULATION BETWEEN THE WHOLE AND THE PARTS

### 1   *Part–Whole Confusion*

An error often made by young children is, on the one hand, to identify an object on the basis of a single detail and, on the other hand, to judge two objects as identical because they have a part in common. In both cases there is some form of assimilation between the whole and one of its parts. Cramaussel (1924) insisted on the role of certain distinctive parts, the perceived value of which determined the interpretation of the whole. Thus two 2- to 3-year-old children, turning over the pages of a picture book, called a drawing of a fish a chicken, and a drawing of a sea-gull a fish. 'It is in the sharp curve of the open jaws of the fish that the child sees the menacing beak of the chicken. After that the tail and the fins matter little. In the same way the oblique, tapering shape of the sea-gull immediately suggests a fish. The feet and the folded wings are not seen because they have no reason to be seen' (Cramaussel, 1924, p. 167).

Cramaussel deduced from this that the whole is uncertain, of little interest, whilst the individualised detail is seen and recognised accurately; it is therefore on this that the identification of an object depends. Since details are perceived better and sooner than the whole, then syncretic perception does not exist. Claparède very properly replied to this by saying that 'syncretism does not constitute fidelity to the whole, as is the case with synthesis, but the *confused* perception of it. This confused perception does not exclude details, but these details do not occupy their proper place or take their proper role in the whole' (Claparède, 1938, p. 371).

The inference of the existence of a whole on the basis of the perception of a part is a general and very precocious phenomenon which is related to the amodal perception of Michotte (1946). We hardly ever see an object in its entirety before identifying it, and, as Bruner says (1958), we are always going beyond the information supplied by sensory stimuli. What changes with age is, firstly, the model to which the stimulus information is related, which serves as an index, and secondly, the amount of verification the individual requires.

In *The Construction of Reality* (*La Construction du Réel*), Piaget (1937) cites an example of the inference of the whole from a part. He presented a baby of $8\frac{1}{2}$ months with a familiar toy, a stork, more or less hidden by a cloth. If the head or the tail were visible, the baby pulled out the toy; if only the feet appeared or even if, with the baby watching, the toy was covered completely, there was no search for it. Thus the presence of an object was anticipated only if a part of it were visible and if this part was an interesting one. Piaget concluded that the action could only be released by an identified sensory image and that '. . . the action of grasping released in this fashion confers the quality of a whole on what has been perceived' (Piaget, 1937, p. 15). At this age the model to which the information obtained is referred is a sensori-motor schema. At a later stage this model could be a representational image or a concept.

The process of assimilation between the whole and one of its parts can also take the form of a contamination between the identification of one or the other (Piaget, 1923; Claparède, 1938; Dworetzki, 1939).

The interpretive responses of children, and the mentally ill, to the Rorschach test provide numerous examples of this. A typical example of the confusion between part of a form and the whole is provided by Dworetzki (1939). He presented children in the age-range 3 to 15 years, and also some adults, with pictures that could be identified either as wholes or as a collection of parts. In other words, each picture could be subdivided into a certain number of pieces each one of which had a particular identity. At the same time the juxtaposition of these pieces was organised in such a way that the whole also had a particular identity. For example, bananas, plums, cherries, strawberries and apples made up a cyclist; a cotton reel and the thread unwinding from it, together with a pair of scissors, made up a picture of a face (fig. 27). The experimenter asked each child to report 'everything he saw and what it was'. In many cases the child combined two perceptual organisations. Thus in figure 27c the pair of scissors was perhaps recognised individually or was interpreted as making up the eyes and nose of a comic face. One child identified the figure as 'A man, somebody has thrown some scissors in his face' (Dworetzki, 1939, p. 265).

In *Language and Thought* (*Le Language et la Pensée*, 1923) Piaget had already emphasised the confused interdependence of the whole and its parts, insisting at the same time on their simultaneity. For him the schema of the whole and the individual details are bound up together and have no role except in relation to each other. Without the existence of distinctive details there is no whole, and *vice versa*; if it happens that these details precede the whole, they cannot fail to entail its presence.

Janet (1889) described as one of the characteristics of *somnambulisme monoïdéique* the ability to conserve an earlier experience and to make it return as it had been in the past, the presence of some constituents of the earlier experience being sufficient to reinvoke the whole, unchanged. The idea of the formation of a schema is therefore common to many investigators, this schematisation establishing a tenuous link between isolated parts and an unstructured whole.

## 2   *The Rigidity of Perceptual Organisation: the Exclusive Perception of the Whole or of the Parts*

It was within the framework of Gestalt theory that Meili, in 1931, put forward a new interpretation of the perceptual behaviour of children. Like the advocates of globalism, he believed that children always perceived in terms of wholes but that these could be of variable size and could refer either to the whole of a picture, or object, presented, or to one or other part of these. The structural properties of the physical object determined whether it would be seen as a unitary whole or as an assembly of smaller structures. This organisation of an object or picture into perceptual structures conformed to the same laws in both children and adults, but, as investigations concerning embedded figures have shown (Ghent, 1956a; Vurpillot, 1964a; Vurpillot and Florès, 1964), whilst an adult is able to consider, at the same time, an organisation in terms of small structures as well as their integration into larger structures, the young child is unable to do this. If the objective situation is such that several small structures are easier to organise than a single large one, children perceive isolated features and not the whole; if, on the other hand, the situation favours organisation in terms of a single unit, that is what is perceived and not the parts. Perceptual organisation is thus, for them, rigid and exclusive; the whole and the parts are not articulated.

Syncretism would imply an extreme conformity to the laws of perceptual organisation, and Meili predicted that there would be global perception when the form was simple and the structure a strong one, and analytic perception when the structure was weak and complex. Furthermore, Meili accorded an important role to experience in the determination of relationships between parts, since he predicted that they would be perceived, preferentially, in terms of the forms taken by familiar objects. He suggested that when the whole had no meaning for the child, but certain of the parts had, then these details would be perceived and there would be no perception of the whole.

Like the Gestaltists, Meili saw the whole as the fundamental psychic datum; '. . . the characteristics of the latter [the whole] cannot be deduced from the separate parts, and these parts themselves and their position within the whole are determined by it' (Meili, 1931, pp. 34 and 35). However, unlike those Gestaltists who seemed to use the terms *Gestalt* (form), *Struktur* (structure) and *Ganzheit* (whole) interchangeably, Meili distinguished between form, the conscious, phenomenal aspect of the perception of the whole, and its structure which was not directly accessible but which prescribed the usual fashion in which the different parts were combined.

Form and structure would thus be two attributes of the perceived whole. The problem is that structure and form are terms relating to perceptions and neither of them is measurable independently in an objective manner. Thus, in both cases strength, weakness, simplicity, complexity, are postulated rather than measurably evidenced, and we fear that Meili's explanation is very much a tautology of this type: 'The child perceives the whole rather than the parts when its structure is strong and simple and its form strong; but the form and the structure are supposedly so when this is what is perceived.'

Meili's approach is of interest because of his basic thesis, which is to explain the way in which a child identifies a picture according to the way in which he organises it, perceptually, into units; only those structures with a strong form are taken into account and identified.

Meili attempts, with more or less success, to interpret the results obtained by other authors as a function of his thesis. Thus the predominance of details reported by Cramaussel (1924, 1927) would be due to the complicated nature and the 'weakness' of structure of the wholes which were used, whilst in Segers' (1926b) experiment the

houses were wholes with a 'strong' structure. The experiments of
Van der Torren (1908) and of Schober and Schober (1919) proved,
in both cases, that children perceived wholes well, but that in a
good many cases the identification of these wholes was incorrect.
The child only perceived the small variations from one picture to
another as differences to the extent that they did not fit into his
interpretation; the more incorrect this interpretation was, the greater
the discordance and the greater the chance of differences being perceived. But in general the children displayed a considerable tolerance
in assimilating to the whole parts that were not concordant.

In summary, Meili was able to find, in each case, an explanation
in terms of the strength and complexity of the structures and forms,
but as he put forward no means of measuring one or the other, his
thesis remains in the realm of speculation.

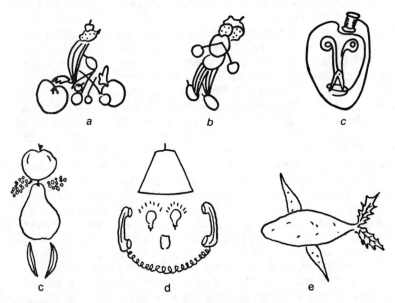

Fig. 27. Examples of ambiguous drawings identifiable in terms of the whole
or of the parts.

(Figures a, b and c after Dworetzki, 1939; figures c, d and e after Elkind,
Koegler and Go, 1964.)

There are a number of experiments which clearly demonstrate
the inability of young children to organise the same set of stimuli
in two different ways. Dworetzki (1939) asked his subjects to identify
some ambiguous figures and reported a very clear developmental
progression. Between the ages of 3 and 6 years only 3 per cent of

the identifications made concerned the whole and the parts of the same figure; this number increased slowly with age, reaching 44·8 per cent in the age-range 10 to 15 years and 80 per cent in adults. In the case of the youngest children identifications were mainly of the whole (80 per cent at 3–5 years); the number of interpretations solely in terms of the parts increased with age without ever exceeding a third of the responses (see table 11). Dworetzki concluded that his experiment verified to a remarkable degree the sequence, in the course of development, of the three stages of syncretism, analysis and synthesis described by Renan (1890) and Claparède (1908). The increase with age of joint interpretations indicated the growing plasticity of the perceptual structures.

Table 11 *Distribution of identifications of ambiguous drawings in terms of the whole (W) or the parts (P), as a percentage.*

| Ages | Dworetzki's results (1939) | | | Elkind, Koegler and Go's results (1964) | | |
|---|---|---|---|---|---|---|
| | *W* | *P* | *W&P* | *W* | *P* | *W&P* |
| 3–5 years | 80 | 10 | 3 | 17 | 71 | 11 |
| 6 years | 47 | 21 | 16 | 27 | 49 | 23 |
| 7 years | 37 | 24 | 19 | 15 | 48 | 37 |
| 8 years | 31 | 28 | 21 | 7 | 32 | 60 |
| 9 years | 16 | 29 | 32 | 0 | 21 | 79 |
| 10–15 years | 10 | 32 | 45 | | | |
| Adults | 2 | 15 | 80 | | | |

The results are expressed as percentages of identifications made. W=identification of whole only. P=identification of parts only. W&P= identification of parts and whole in the same figure. (After Dworetzki, 1939; and Elkind, Koegler and Go, 1964.)

Elkind, Koegler and Go repeated Dworetzki's experiment with material of the same type but differing in two respects. Firstly, the drawings of the component parts of the whole (fruit or objects) were more realistic than those used by Dworetzki. Secondly, several of the drawings were made up of parts that were separate and not joined up (see fig. 27c, d, e). Their results showed the same inability, in children under the age of 6 years, to identify the whole and the parts in the same figure; however, progress in this respect appeared more rapid since at the age of 9 years 78·6 per cent joint interpretations were reported. However, whilst with Dworetzki's material 80 per cent of the interpretations of children from 4 to 5 years were of the whole alone, with Elkind's material 71·42 per cent of the interpretations by children of the same age were only of the parts (see table 11).

Reversible figures which represent familiar objects also make it possible to demonstrate the inability of the young child to identify one figure in two different ways. Elkind (Elkind and Scott, 1962; Elkind, Koegler and Go, 1962; Elkind, 1964; Elkind, Koegler and Van Doorninck, 1965) has devoted a whole series of studies to the

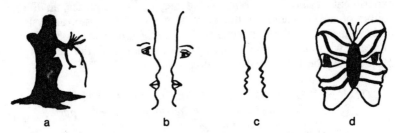

a                          b                          c                          d

Fig. 28. Examples of reversible figures (Elkind, 1964).

developmental evolution of the perception of reversible figures. Each of the figures concerned could be identified in at least two ways; each interpretation would imply one particular organisation of the figure and ground. Thus the drawing *a* in figure 28 (Elkind, 1964) could be identified either as a black tree trunk on a white background, or as a white duck on a black background; drawings *b* and *c* could be seen either as a vase, if the central part took the role of the figure, or as two profiles if the parts to the sides formed the figure and the centre part became the background, etc. Elkind recorded the number of times each of the possible interpretations was given in response to each drawing by children at different age-levels. He observed that the physical properties of each drawing determined which part was most likely to be seen as the figure. At all ages, that part of the drawing which was most 'articulated' – the term by which Elkind (Elkind and Scott, 1962) expressed the degree of resemblance to real objects – was what was most often seen as the figure. It follows from this that the lowest rate of alternation between different interpretations of the same figure was when one of them was very 'articulated' and the other much less so. The alternation was stronger when neither of the possible interpretations was articulated and even more so when both of them were. The influence of the physical properties of a drawing was the same at all age-levels.

As in the experiments concerned with the predominance of the whole or the parts in the identification of ambiguous figures (Dworetzki, 1939; Elkind, Koegler and Go, 1964), the number of separate interpretations given to the same figure increased with age

(Elkind and Scott, 1962); for seven ambiguous figures they went from an average of 7·40 at 6 years to an average of 12·70 at 12 years (Elkind, 1964). Systematic training showed its effects in a substantial increase in the number of interpretations. The training was carried out with a series of six figures and comprised several stages. First of all the experimenter asked the child what he saw, what the drawing might represent, then he added: 'Some children see more than one thing. Do you see anything besides a . . .?' (mentioning the child's first response). During a third stage the experimenter said: 'Sometimes children see a . . . (mentioning an interpretation not given by the child). Did you see a . . .?' Finally, if the child still had not given one or more of the possible identifications, the experimenter, using an appropriate screen, masked all of the figure except for the part which had not yet been identified. For example, in drawing *a* of figure 28 (Elkind, 1964) the screen showed the white duck on a uniform black background. The effect of training was measured by comparing the number of separate identifications made before and after training, using six drawings from a parallel series. There was a definite increase at 6, 7 and 8 years of age (Elkind, Koegler and Go, 1962); it was also apparent in children with brain damage and in retarded children of 8½ years who all had I.Q.s in the range 70–90 (Elkind, Koegler, Go and Van Doornick, 1965).

In the course of training, verbal clues were effective only above 8 years of age; the use of a selector screen proved to be by far the most effective means of teaching a child to reorganise a figure perceptually. The number of instances where the same drawing gave rise to an identification of the whole and more than one partial identification by the same child increased markedly between 4 and 11 years, which confirms the results of the preceding experiments.

The impossibility, for the young child, of employing the same part of a figure in two different perceptual organisations is also apparent in a task involving the reproduction of geometric figures. Geometric figures were presented to children from 4 to 7 years of age (twenty at each age-level), with the instructions to trace in red pencil that part of the figure which resembled one model, and with a blue pencil that part of the same figure which resembled another model (fig. 29).

In order to succeed in such a task the child had to include the same segment successively in two figures, that is, certain lines had to be double traced, a red and a blue one side by side. Below the age of 5 years, fewer than 10 per cent accomplished the task successfully, and even between the ages of 6 and 7 years the proportion of successes did not exceed 50 per cent. In the majority of cases failure occurred, as predicted, where the double-tracing of the line

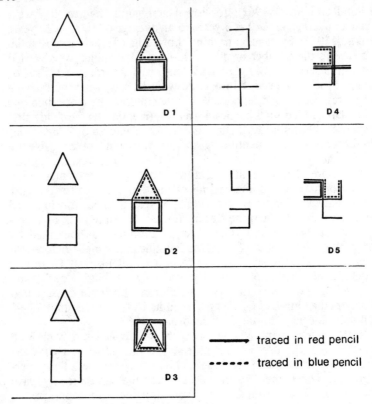

Fig. 29. Material used in the tracing task.

In each case (D1, D2, D3, D4 and D5) the models are on the left, and the complex figure on which they have to be traced is on the right.

in common was involved; the child identified the two figures well enough but, having drawn the first one, he left the second unfinished because the line needed to complete it had already been attributed to the first ('no double line' errors=NDL); sometimes, in his uncertainty, he decided not to use the common line at all rather than select one figure in which to incorporate it (see table 12).

Selinka (1939) studied part-whole integration using material similar to Kohs' blocks. The child was given four blocks which he had to arrange so as to reproduce a design identical to the model. Each block had a quarter of a circle on each of its six sides, but only one of these quarters had a texture identical to that of the model circle. If the child took into consideration only the contour of the design, all he had to do was to position the blocks so as to make up

Table 12   *Development with age of successes in the task involving double lines (percentage).*

| | Age (in years and months) | | | | | |
| | 4y. 6m. | | 5y. 6m. | | 6y. 6m. | |
| Problems | Successes | NDL | Successes | NDL | Successes | NDL |
|---|---|---|---|---|---|---|
| D1 | 12·5 | 52·5 | 32·5 | 55·0 | 40·0 | 57·5 |
| D2 | 7·5 | 15·0 | 30·0 | 35·0 | 52·5 | 30·0 |
| D3 | 2·5 | 52·5 | 27·5 | 52·5 | 42·5 | 32·5 |
| D4 | 5·0 | 20·0 | 55·0 | 17·5 | 57·5 | 20·0 |
| D5 | 10·0 | 12·5 | 37·5 | 15·0 | 55·0 | 27·5 |
| Mean | 7·5 | 30·5 | 36·5 | 35·0 | 49·5 | 33·5 |

The results are expressed as percentages, there being forty subjects at each age-level and for each figure.

NDL=an error in which the two figures are identified but the line in common is absent in one or both cases, that is, one or both figures is incompletely reproduced.

the circle without regard to the interior surface. The care with which he sought to match to the model not only the circular form of the whole, but also the appropriate pattern for each quarter, would show to what extent he took account of details. It appeared that up to the age of 5 years only the form of the whole was correctly reproduced; the maximum degree of progress in the attention given to details occurred between the ages of 7 and 8 years.

Corah and Gospodinoff (1966) used a technique involving a comparison between a model and two other figures from which a choice had to be made; one of these had the same contour as the model but differed in its internal details, whilst the other had the same internal details but differed in its contour. The authors reported that the youngest children, with a mean age-level of 4y. 9m., matched model and variable according to the common contour in ten cases, and according to a common part in another ten cases, whilst the 9-year-olds established identity in terms of the contour in eighteen cases out of twenty. This would suggest that the younger children responded on a chance basis; Corah and Gospodinoff thought that this was not the case, without, however, justifying their conclusion. It is possible that the heterogeneity of the material was also a factor. Ten of the models consisted of overlapping figures, a circle and a triangle for example; one of the figures from which a choice had to be made comprised the two parts (triangle and circle) placed side by side, the other the contour of the whole. The children thus had to choose between forms which reproduced primary contour structures

(Vurpillot and Florès, 1964) of the model and a form which corresponded to a secondary contour structure. If we take into account what we know about the capacities of perceptual organisation of children younger than 5 years (see Chapter 1), it would be expected that they would recognise the primary structures in the model and the variable but would not see the contour as a structured form. In the ten problems of this type, the children probably chose those forms which they recognised, that is, those which Corah and Gospodinoff described as the parts.

The other ten models, however, were made up of irregular, asymmetrical forms, with seven to ten sides and enclosing a small, regular figure: a triangle, a square, or a diamond. The variables comprised either the same contour containing a different small figure, or a different contour containing the same small figure. In this case both the contour and the parts are primary contour structures; in no instance does the passage from the model to the variables modify the nature of the organisation of the structures which make up the whole. The comparison between contours must therefore be an easy one and it could be assumed that choices in terms of the form of the whole (the contour) would be more numerous than with the first series of ten models. Unfortunately, Corah and Gospodinoff (1966) do not give sufficient information, which means that the interpretation which has been proposed remains speculative. Only an analysis of the responses in terms of the contour or of the parts of the different types of models would enable us to say whether the responses of the children at 4y. 9m. were a chance distribution or determined by the perceptual organisation of the material.

In differentiation tasks where the judgments 'same' or 'not the same' have to be made, the differences the experimenter introduces can involve either the form of the whole of the stimulus or small details in it. The manner in which the child organises the stimulus is thus likely to influence the judgments he makes. If each of the figures is perceived as a single structure, they will be judged as 'the same' when the form of the whole is the same, and 'not the same' when it differs; in such cases it will be of little importance whether or not the component parts of the whole differ from one figure to the other. However, if each figure is perceived as a whole made up of small independent structures, the comparison will involve these and, provided that each one has an identical match in the same position in the other figure, the judgment given will be 'the same', even if the configurations of the whole do not have the same form. A recent experiment (Pineau, 1969; Vurpillot, Lécuyer, Moal and Pineau, 1971) seemed to indicate that, in children from $3\frac{1}{2}$ to $5\frac{1}{2}$ years, the response given depended less on the form of the whole of the configurations that were being compared than on an identity of form between the parts of these configurations. The number of 'not the same' responses was, at all the age-levels concerned, greater when the figures to be compared were identical configurations (two circles or two irregular wholes) one of which was made up of nine daisies and the other of nine leaves (pairs *ab* and *cd*), than when a circle and

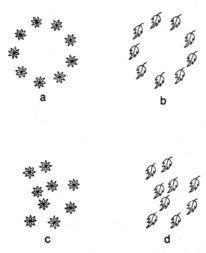

Fig. 30. Material used in making up identical and different pairs (Pineau, 1969).

an irregular configuration were involved, both made up of either daisies or leaves (pairs *ac* and *bd*) (figs 30 and 31). Comments made spontaneously by the children or in response to a question by the experimenter seemed to indicate that in many cases the child perceived the differences in the form of the configuration just as well as the differences in the form of the component parts. But when these were in conflict, the identity of the form of the parts was considered more important than that of the configurations. 'They're the same, that one where they're in a circle [circle made of daisies] and that one where they're muddled up [irregular configuration also made of daisies],' said a child of $3\frac{1}{2}$ years. 'They're the same, that circle's all right, but that one's broken,' said another child of $4\frac{1}{2}$ years about a circle and an irregular configuration, both composed of leaves.

It seems, therefore, that from the age of $3\frac{1}{2}$ years, children are capable of perceiving both small structures and the form of the configurations which they constitute. Incorrect responses would arise then not from an inability to organise the whole and the parts at the same time, but from a failure to relate the existence of differences which involve one of the properties of the objects to a

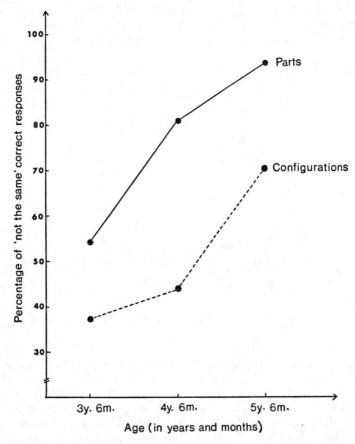

Fig. 31. Evolution with age of the number of 'not the same' correct responses given to figures which differed either in the form of the constituent parts, or by the configurations which these parts constituted.

*Continuous line*: the evolution with age of the number of 'not the same' correct responses to pairs *ab* and *cd*. *Dotted line*: evolution with age of the number of 'not the same' correct responses to pairs *ac* and *bd* (Pineau, 1969).

judgment of identity relative to objects as wholes. The deficiency is therefore at the level of the child's criteria for making decisions; the judgment 'the same' rests on an equivalence and not on an identity. Perceptual organisation is involved only in relation to the choice of the dominant property. The component parts, leaves or daisies, being small, well structured and meaningful, constitute forms stronger than the configuration of the whole, which is large, discontinuous in outline and without representational significance except perhaps in the case of the circle. When the whole is a configuration of separate parts, it is the form of the latter which determines the decision, as in the experiment of Elkind, Koegler and Go (1964) (see pp. 137 and 138).

CONCLUSION

A number of conclusions can be drawn from the research reported in this chapter.

1  The first concerns the relationship between identification and differentiation. In an identification task, attention is drawn to what there is in common between the object to be identified and the various categories the child possesses; in a differentiation task, however, attention is drawn to what two or more objects do not have in common. It is thus a matter of two opposite strategies. However, one of the characteristics of children of pre-school age seems to be a lack of articulation between their various behaviours. When, in one and the same task, the experimenter asks the child both to identify a figure and to say in what respect it differs from the preceding one (Van der Torren, 1907; Schober and Schober, 1919), he introduces a conflict between the two approaches.

However, to be able to identify an object is much more important than differentiating it minutely from another object; the essential requirement for developing economic, adaptive behaviour is to organise information into a limited number of categories before storing it for reference to subsequent experiences. In consequence, the child prefers to use an identification strategy and, in so far as he can place an object he encounters in a familiar category, a few discrepant details are of little significance – and this is even more true when it is just a matter of one detail more or less in an object than in the preceding one. If he can identify an object he pays no attention to differences. However, if an object is not immediately identifiable in terms of the categories the child possesses, then he will carry out a protracted search for a possible cue and will be more likely to see the particular details which make it possible to differentiate it from the preceding object. There is, therefore, an inverse relationship between performances of identification and those of differentiation, but this relationship is not symmetrical since the first of these terms is the determining one: the easier the identification, the less precise the differentiation – but this is not true the other way round.

2   Identification results from the interaction between two processes: the organisation of stimuli into structured perceptual units, and the confrontation of these with the representational or conceptual structures in the child's repertoire. If the physical properties of the stimulus are such that they are organised into unambiguous primary perceptual structures (see Chapter 1), only these will be identified by young children. But if the circumstances are such that the patterns of stimuli are ambiguous and incapable of being organised into structures (if, for example, the stimulus is blurred, poorly illuminated, amorphous) or, on the contrary, so complex that the number of primary structures and the relationships between these structures exceed the child's organisational capacities, then identification will not be determined by the perceptual structures but by the immediate interest of the child.

Moreover, in this sort of situation, a relative order of importance seems to emerge. When the laws of organisation can be applied, they are dominant; the perceptual structure determines the limit of possible identifications, as the Gestaltists would predict (Meili, 1931; Guillaume, 1937). When perceptual organisation becomes difficult or almost impossible, then the laws of category accessibility (Bruner, 1958) constitute better predictors than those of organisation, and only those stimuli which fit the most easily mobilised categories at that point in time are retained.

The child only identifies what he can assimilate to an existing cognitive structure. Between the ages of 3 and 7 years these structures are representational images, akin to the perceptual structures – the communality of the formal properties of the perceptual structure and the categorial model is therefore the determining factor. This model may be crude and inadequate, and identification made on the basis of just a small part of the stimulus, as in the examples provided by Cramaussel and Dworetzki, but without a model there is no identification. In the case of the baby, identification is also made by reference to a model, but this is bound up in his own actions; thus for Piaget (1936, 1937) it is a matter of a sensori-motor schema, for Bruner (1966a, 1966b) one of enactive representation.

3   Identification involves perceptual structures, of greater or lesser size, clearly individualised, which are related in terms of topological characteristics such as contiguity, enclosure, intersection, etc.; these structures cannot be broken up into smaller structures, nor can they be fitted into each other.

The results of the experiments of Dworetzki (1939), Elkind and Scott (1962), Elkind, Koegler and Go (1964), and Vurpillot (1964a) show the influence and interaction of two factors in perceptual identification: on the one hand the determination of the structures to be interpreted by the laws of perceptual organisation, and on the other hand the cognitive possibilities of inserting the same object into two related classes. The preferential discrimination of the whole or the parts would depend on the perceptual organisation, whilst the possibility of switching from the whole to a part, and conversely, would indicate not so much a plasticity of perception, as Dworetzki (1939) suggests, as the application to a perceptual task of a new form of cognitive organisation; such a hypothesis is in accord with the theories of Piaget.

Without entering into interpretations in such terms as strength, weakness, simplicity and complexity in the way that Meili (1931) does, one can describe the results in the following manner. When the physical properties of a figure are such that it is organised preferentially into small independent structures, and these represent objects familiar to the child, he will identify the figure as a collection of objects. If, however, the physical properties of the figure are such that the preferential organisation is that of a single whole, encompassing all the parts, and this whole represents an object the child knows, then *this* will be identified. When the material is such that the whole and each of its parts can be identified without ambiguity it is the objective properties which determine the preferred perceptual organisation and, accordingly, the identification. The possibility of moving from an identification of the parts to an identification of the whole presupposes that the same collection of lines can be seen, for example, either as a banana or as the body of a cyclist. It is this double role of a single unit, a role analogous to that taken by a common element in related classes, that children appear to be incapable of appreciating before the age of about 7 years. Up to that age-level a detail of a figure can constitute either an individualised and identified structure or a part of another structure, also individualised and identified – but it cannot take both roles at the same time. It must be added that this ability to see the same structure both as a whole and as part of another whole is manifested more or less precociously according to whether it involves a task of identification or differentiation, whether the material is meaningful or not, whether it represents very familiar objects or those rarely encountered, whether the contours are continuous or discontinuous, and so on. The age of 7 years is given only as an approximate indication, a mean around which the dispersion is very great.

4   Contrary to what the early proponents of syncretism believed, the notion of three stages corresponding to three successive periods of time is too simple a picture of the child's development. If it were possible, in a sufficiently precise task and during a relatively short period of time, to observe the progress of analysis and synthesis, it is quite certain that the three stages of Renan and Claparède would not always be found at the same ages for all kinds of responses, or for one type of response to all kinds of forms, or, in a particular setting, for all its components. Some examples of globalism and some of pointillism can be observed, simultaneously, with the same child and the same object, from a very young age. As Meili (1931) commented, however young the child may be, he always responds to structured wholes which correspond either to the parts or to the whole of the stimulus or to the total situation. The young child analyses these wholes or units neither into discrete elements nor in terms of dimensional characteristics (colour, brightness, texture, etc.) and so is, from this point of view, globalistic. Nonetheless, these characteristics are perceived from an early age, and on this point the proponents of syncretism deceive themselves when they conclude from an unsuccessful performance on a differentiation task that the child has not perceived the differences, and infer that he sees the object as a confused whole. The available data tend to support the opposite interpretation: the perceived wholes are so strongly organised for the child that it is impossible for him to abstract one feature from them and organise his responses in terms of this alone.

5   It must be noted that by 'part' or 'detail' the authors of the experiments reported in this chapter seem to mean a detachable part and not a characteristic like colour, size, being striped, etc. The impossibility for the very young child of analysing a perceived and identified whole into its parts should manifest itself as much in relation to the abstraction of a property as to the isolation of a particular detail.

Finally, it may be asked whether the claims of the proponents of associationism, like those of syncretism, do not in fact contain the implicit hypothesis that, before being identified, the object must be seen in its entirety. The use of terms such as 'whole', 'global aspect' and 'contour' more or less suggest this. Yet such a hypothesis is far from being supported by the analysis of children's performances and, like Piaget (1961), we think that many of the characteristics of these performances, and, in particular, identification on the basis of a detail or incorrect judgments of identity, are due to insufficient perceptual activity. In the last resort the child identifies a stimulus on the basis of what he has seen and not what he could have seen.

*The figures and tables in Part One have been reproduced with the kind permission of the following authors and publishers:*

Fig. 1     Gottschaldt, K. *Psychologische Forschung*, 1926, **8**, p. 296.

Fig. 2     Vurpillot, E. and Florès, A. *L'Année Psychologique*, 1964, **64**, p. 378.

Fig. 3     Vurpillot, E. and Florès, A. *L'Année Psychologique*, 1964, **64**, p. 380.

Fig. 4A    Piaget, J. and Stettler, B. *Archives de Psychologie*, 1954, **34**, p. 205.

Fig. 4B–C   Ghent, L. 'Perception of overlapping and embedded figures by children of different ages', *American Journal of Psychology*, University of Illinois Press, 1956a, **69**, pp. 575–587.

Fig. 5     Vurpillot, E. and Florès, A. *L'Année Psychologique*, 1964, **64**, p. 385.

Fig. 9     Vurpillot, E. and Florès, A. *L'Année Psychologique*, 1964, **64**, p. 390.

Fig. 10    Gollin, E. S. 'Developmental studies of visual recognition of incomplete objects', *Perceptual and motor skills*, 1960, **11**, pp. 289–298, fig. 1.

Fig. 11    Piaget, J. and Stettler, B. *Archives de Psychologie*, 1954, **34**, p. 216.

Fig. 13    Huttenlocher, J. 'Discrimination of figure orientation: effects of relative position', *Journal of Comparative and Physiological Psychology*, American Psychological Association, 1967b, **63**, pp. 359–361.

Fig. 14    Wohlwill, J. and Wiener, M. 'Discrimination of form orientation in young children', *Child Development*, The Society for Research in Child Development, Inc., 1964, **35**, pp. 81–90, fig. 2, p. 1117.

Fig. 15    Ghent, L. *Canadian Journal of Psychology*, 1960, **14**, pp. 249–256.

Fig. 16    Braine-Ghent, L. 'Age changes in the mode of perceiving geometric forms', *Psychonomic Science*, 1965a, **2**, pp. 155–156.

Fig. 17    Pinard, A. and Laurendeau, M. *International Journal of Psychology*, 1960, **1**, p. 244.

Fig. 18    Piaget, J. and Inhelder, B. *La représentation de l'espace chez l'enfant*, Presses Universitaires de France, 1948, p. 73.

Fig. 19    Vereecken, P. *Spatial development. Constructive praxia from birth to the age of seven*, Groningen, J. B. Wolters, 1961, pp. 58–59.

Fig. 20    Vurpillot, E. and Berthoud, M. *L'Année Psychologique*, 1969, **69**, p. 395.

Fig. 22    Vurpillot, E. and Moal, A. *L'Année Psychologique*, 1970, **70**, p. 395.

Fig. 25    Van der Torren, I. *Zeitschrift für Angewandte Psychologie*, 1907, **1**, pp. 189–232.

Fig. 26    Segers, J. E. *Journal de Psychologie Normale et Pathologique*, 1926a **29**, pp. 608–636.

Fig. 27    Elkind, D., Koegler, R. R. and Go, E. 'Studies in perceptual development: II. Part-whole perception', *Child Development*, The Society for Research in Child Development, Inc., 1964, **35**, pp. 81–90, fig. 1, p. 84.

Fig. 28    Elkind, D. 'Ambiguous pictures for study of perceptual development and learning', *Child Development*, The Society for Research in Child Development, Inc., 1964, **35**, pp. 1391–1396, fig. 1, p. 1392, fig. 2, p. 1393.

Table  6   Vurpillot, E. and Berthoud, M. *L'Année Psychologique*, 1969, **69**, p. 450.

Table  9   Vurpillot, E. and Moal, A. *L'Année Psychologique*, 1970, **70**, p. 398.

Table 11   Elkind, D., Koegler, R. R. and Go, E. 'Studies in perceptual development: II, Part-whole perception', *Child Development*, The Society for Research in Child Development, Inc., 1964, **35**, pp. 81–90, table 1, p. 85.

*PART TWO*

# The Analysis of Visual Structures in Terms of their Properties

# Chapter 6

# The Role of Verbal Mediators in Discrimination Learning

We have put forward the hypothesis (p. 31) that the visual world of the 3- to 4-year-old child is organised into perceptual structures which are indivisible and cannot be analysed or combined. The data obtained in investigations of problems involving embedded figures (Ghent, 1956; Vurpillot, 1964a; Vurpillot and Florès, 1964), reversible figures (Elkind and Scott, 1962; Elkind, Koegler and Go, 1962; Elkind, 1964), or ambiguous figures (Dworetzki, 1939; Elkind, Koegler and Go, 1964) have confirmed, on the one hand, that identification only involves those perceptual structures organised according to the laws of Gestalt, and, on the other hand, that before the age of approximately 6 years a perceptual structure cannot be broken down into its component parts and these related to parts from other structures. It would seem likely that the constraints on the dissociation of structures are valid not only for the parts or detachable pieces just referred to, but also for features which cannot be physically isolated, like the properties of colour, size, texture, etc.

The abstraction of a property from one or more objects involves an isolation of part of the information contained in the sensory stimuli. This part becomes salient for the subject, in a given situation, and it is that which determines the response that is made. One of the properties abstracted from an object can also serve both to categorise it – that is to group it with other objects on the basis of a particular value of this property – and to differentiate it from another object characterised by a different value on this same property. The property abstracted is thus a dimensional variable; this we shall refer to as a 'differentiator' rather than a 'dimension', since it would seem a more appropriate term for the corresponding physical variable. It would then be possible to say that a physical dimension of differentiation, size or brightness for example, is used as a differentiator by a child when ordered variations in the child's responses correspond to ordered variations in this physical dimension. The actual differentiators would constitute scales with a series or ordered values; it is possible that in children these are derived from bipolar differentiators like E. J. Gibson's (1963, 1965, 1969) distinctive features which only present two opposite values: curvilinear-rectilinear, big-small, open-closed, etc.

The existence of a differentiation between different patterns of sensory stimulation – what Piaget calls the 'sensory tableau' (Piaget, 1936) – can be demonstrated at birth (Fantz, 1961, 1963; Hershenson, 1964, etc.). It does not follow from this that the baby already has differentiators available. For example, it would be very imprudent to conclude from the fact that a baby can follow visually the displacement of a coloured point of light on a background of another colour (Chase, 1937) that he has a means of differentiating colour. It is one thing to perceive that two differently coloured objects are not the same; it is quite another thing to judge that these two objects differ in terms of their colour. The former could depend simply on a differential sensibility of the receptors, whilst the latter requires the abstraction of a property of the stimulus.

Within this perspective, the child would pass from a primitive stage during which he would be incapable of abstracting any property of an object, to a final stage where he would be able to classify or differentiate objects according to any of their properties, provided that his sensory receptors were appropriately sensitive. In the course of this process of development certain properties would be abstracted earlier and more easily than others.

Two groups of experimental investigations, unequal in size, are relevant here: one compares the relative facility with which various properties are abstracted, and the other, much more extensive, measures the rapidity of transfer of learning according to whether certain differentiators are or are not used by the subject.

I   THE ROLE OF THE ABSTRACTION OF A DIMENSION OF DIFFERENTATION IN THE TRANSFER OF DISCRIMINATION LEARNING

Discrimination learning can be facilitated or, conversely, impeded by previous learning; the positive or negative effect of the transfer is determined by the nature of what has been learned during the course of the previous task. By comparing what remains constant and what varies from the first to the second learning task, and by relating the factors thus identified and the existence of a positive or negative transfer, it becomes possible to infer the basis of the learning. In consequence, a number of authors have attempted to demonstrate that learning is restricted to the establishment of a simple association between a stimulus object and an instrumental choice response (single-stage learning), whilst others have devoted themselves to proving that it is necessary to infer an unobservable, intermediary process, the supposed nature of which varies according to the author concerned. In this latter instance, the intermediary process means that the final response selected no longer depends on the physical stimulus but on the coding of this stimulus. For one important group of research workers, this coding, whether selective or, on the contrary, elaborative, has the effect of making one particular part of the available information significant, this part relating to a property or dimension of the objects to be discriminated. The concern of the majority of workers is to investigate whether or not the subject makes use of differentiators, and to determine the nature of the influence on his performances, in a transfer task, of maintaining or changing the dimension made relevant in the training session.

1 *Transfer Involving the Conservation of the Relevant Dimension*
As a general rule, a simple learnt discrimination, involving a single dimension of differentiation, is acquired more rapidly when preceded by a training session in which the same dimension is the relevant one, than when the pretraining involves a different dimension, or in the absence of pretraining altogether (Lashley, 1942; Lawrence, 1949, 1950; Mackintosh, 1965a). Lawrence (1949) trained a group of rats in two discrimination tasks in which the same dimension, brightness, was relevant. In the first task the rat learnt to select the black stimulus presented at the same time as the white stimulus (simultaneous discrimination); in the second task it learnt to turn to the right if the black stimulus was presented, to the left if the stimulus was white (successive discrimination). Although the instrumental responses were different, as well as the task, the pretraining facilitated the second learning.

Analogous results can be observed in adults. When a task involving perceptual differentiation between figures precedes an associative learning task involving these same figures and the names of colours, then learning is facilitated when the same dimension of differentiation between the figures is relevant in both tasks; when the reverse is the case, it is hindered (Kurtz, 1955).

2 *Learning Involving Reversal and Non-reversal Shifts*
Experiments involving reversal shifts (or, more simply, reversals) and non-reversal shifts are classed as discrimination, as well as

concept learning. We shall begin by outlining the classic experimental design from which they are all derived, and to which variations have gradually been added.

Using simple material composed of objects which differ along two dimensions, subjects are trained in an initial discrimination in which dimension A is relevant and dimension B is not. A second training involves the same objects; for some subjects the same dimension remains relevant but the positive value changes (reversal shift, R); for other subjects, it is the dimension which was not relevant in the first training session which becomes relevant in the second (non-reversal shift, NR, also called the extra-dimensional shift, ED).

If conserving the same relevant dimension facilitates a second learning, the reversal group (R) should be able to produce a better performance than the non-reversal group (NR). However, the experimental evidence reveals that the relative facility of R and NR learning changes according to the population in question. Thus rats (Kelleher, 1956), monkeys (T. Tighe, 1964), and children of 3 and 4 years (T. Kendler, H. Kendler and Wells, 1960) acquired a second learning more quickly when the dimension was changed (NR) than when the learning involved reversal (R); the two types of learning are of equal difficulty for children from 5 to 7 years of age (T. Kendler and H. Kendler, 1959); learning involving reversal shift is acquired more quickly by adults (Buss, 1953; H. Kendler and d'Amato, 1955; Harrow and Friedman, 1958).

(*a*) *The influence of the status of the non-relevant dimension.* Some investigators (Eimas, 1965, amongst others) have criticised the classic experimental design for ignoring the possibility that the subject may respond in terms of the non-relevant dimension in the second learning (fig. 32); such a procedure, they suggest, facilitates NR learning.

Consequently, several variations have been introduced in order to study the influence of the non-relevant dimension in the second learning task and, particularly, to verify whether, by making it variable instead of keeping it constant, as in the classic procedure, the relative facility of R and NR learning is modified.

T. Tighe and L. Tighe (1967) gave children from $4\frac{1}{2}$ to $10\frac{1}{2}$ years a first discrimination learning task involving two pairs of objects which differed in size and brightness (fig. 32). Then with half the subjects they carried out a training session involving reversal shift learning (R), and with the other half, non-reversal shift learning (NR). Each of these groups was then divided into two sub-groups according to the composition of the stimulus pairs presented in the second learning task. Group 1 saw the same pairs of objects as in the

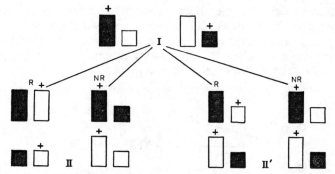

Fig. 32. Schematic representation of the learning experiments involving reversal shift (R) and non-reversal shift (NR).

*Top:* the stimulus-pairs of the first learning task (I). *Bottom:* the stimulus-pairs involved in the second learning task. *On the left:* the non-relevant dimension constant (II); *on the right:* non-relevant dimension variable (II'). In each case the positive stimulus has a + above it.

first learning task, whilst group 2 saw pairs of objects which differed along one dimension only. For group 1 the non-relevant dimension in the second learning task was variable, for group 2 it was constant. Performance, measured in terms of the number of attempts required to attain the criterion, was the same for both groups in children of 4½ years. However, for children of 10 years, maintaining a constant non-relevant dimension made the second learning task much easier, whether this involved a reversal shift or a non-reversal shift. Furthermore, both types of learning, R and NR, were acquired with equal rapidity when the non-relevant dimension was held constant; learning involving reversal shift R was more rapid than non-reversal shift learning NR when the non-relevant dimension varied (group 1). The authors saw in these results confirmation that only the older children in fact used dimensional characteristics for purposes of discrimination; when the objects presented varied conjointly along two dimensions (group 1), they first had to determine which of the two was relevant. Where the non-relevant dimension was kept constant (group 2), however, the composition of the pairs eliminated the possibility of a second choice dimension. The variation of the non-relevant dimension could only affect those who made their selection in terms of dimensional characteristics.

(*b*) *Extra- or intra-dimensional shift.* Other investigators (Furth and Youniss, 1963; Campione, Hyman and Zeaman, 1965; Dickerson, 1966; Mumbauer and Odom, 1967) have compared the relative difficulty of intra-dimensional reversal (R), intra-dimensional change (ID) and extra-dimensional change (ED). Dickerson (1966) used four forms (triangle, circle, square, T-shape) and four colours (red, yellow, green, blue) which could be combined two at a time. In the first phase of his experiment he presented two pairs of objects differing conjointly along two dimensions, a single value being positive in the relevant dimension (classic procedure). For the second

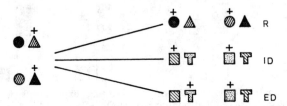

Fig. 33. Example of the design of the learning experiments involving reversal shift (R), intra-dimensional (ID) and extra-dimensional (ED) change (after Dickerson, 1966). *On the left:* the stimulus-figures for the first learning task; *on the right:* those for the second learning task.

phase he divided his subjects into three groups. The first (group R) saw the same pairs as in the first phase, the same dimension remaining relevant but the positive value of this dimension being reversed. The second group (ID) had both pairs of stimulus figures differing in the forms and colours used, but with the same dimension remaining relevant. The third group (ED) had the same stimulus figures as group 2 but with the other dimension as the relevant one. Fig. 33 provides a concrete example. Forty-eight children from 3y. 9m. to 5y. 7m. were involved in the experiment. Their performance, measured by the number of errors in the second learning task, showed that it was the change of both the stimulus and the relevant dimension (colour instead of form) which led to the most errors; second learning was much easier when the same dimension remained relevant, and in this case reversal of the positive and negative values or the choice of other values appeared to be equivalent.

   With older children (aged 7 to 8 years) and an association learning task involving numbers and stimulus figures which varied along two dimensions, Furth and Youniss (1964; Youniss and Furth, 1964) obtained different results. In the first learning task nine stimulus figures made up by combining three forms and three colours were presented one by one to the subject who learnt to respond 1, 2 or 3 to three values of one of the dimensions. During the second training session group R saw the same stimulus figures, the same dimension remained relevant, but the responses 1, 2 and 3 were associated with different values.

   The extra-dimensional shift group (ED) also had the same

stimulus figures but the other dimension became relevant, the responses still being 1, 2 or 3. Finally, group ID saw new stimulus figures composed of three different forms and three different colours, the responses remaining 1, 2 or 3. Without overlearning, the intra-dimensional shift was the easiest, the reversal shift was more difficult, and the extra-dimensional shift was of the same level of difficulty as reversal. With overlearning (eighteen supplementary trials in task 1) the intra-dimensional shift remained the easiest but the extra-dimensional shift showed itself more difficult than reversal.

From the group of investigations which have just been described it emerges that the choice of the experimental setting influences the relative degree of difficulty of transfer tasks involving the maintenance or reversal of the relevant dimension in the first learning task. As a general rule, learning on the second task is more rapid when the same dimension remains relevant (Lawrence, 1949, 1950; Kurtz, 1955; Furth and Youniss, 1964; Youniss and Furth, 1964; Campione, Hyman and Zeaman, 1965; Dickerson, 1966; Mumbauer and Odom, 1967, etc.). However, there are some exceptions to this: when both successive learning trials involve the same stimulus objects, animals and young children learn more rapidly when an extra-dimensional shift is involved (ED or NR) than when it is an intra-dimensional reversal shift (R). (Kelleher, 1955; Kendler, Kendler and Wells, 1960; Tighe, 1964, etc.)

## II THEORETICAL INTERPRETATIONS

All the work reported is derived from the connectionist learning model of Hull (1943, etc.) but it is possible to distinguish several lines of interpretation.

### 1 *The Single-stage Connectionist Model*

Discrimination learning can be defined as the acquisition of different responses to different stimuli due to the differential reinforcement of responses made to these stimuli (Tighe and Tighe, 1966). This sort of learning requires two hierarchical operations: (1) one stimulus must be distinguished from the other; (2) a specific response must be made to each one. These two operations are hierarchical in the sense that the achievement of the second necessarily implies the achievement of the first, without the reverse being true. A successful learning is explained by the fact that the stimuli in question have been both discriminated and identified.

According to Spence (1936) all of the stimuli which actually impinge on the subject, relevant or not, are associated with the response that was reinforced. Thus, when a rat receives a positive reinforcement after having selected the black square situated to the right, each aspect of the stimulus – square, black, to-the-right – is equally reinforced. On the other hand, when no reinforcement follows the choice of a white circle situated to the right, the tendency to approach the characteristics round, white, to-the-right, diminishes. The tendency to approach a composite stimulus (circular/white/to-the-left, or circular/white/to-the-right, or square/black/to-the-left, etc.) is the sum of the tendencies, or forces of habit, to approach each characteristic. Thus the subject selects each time the composite stimulus for which the approach tendency is the strongest. According to Spence's (1936) theory, behaviourally, each attempt corresponds to a single-chain S-R association which is established in terms of the non-selectivity of components.

Spence's single-chain, non-selective model explains the greater rapidity of learning involving an extra-dimensional shift compared with reversal shift learning when the same stimulus objects are used in both tasks. If, in the first learning trial, the positive stimuli are large and small black squares, to the right and to the left, then the characteristics 'black' and 'square' would always be reinforced, 'white' never, whilst 'large', 'small', 'right' and 'left' would have been equally reinforced, that is, in 50 per cent of the cases. In a transfer task involving reversal the positive stimuli are large and small white squares, to the right and to the left; thus white, previously never reinforced, takes the place of black which was always reinforced. If the transfer is extra-dimensional the positive stimuli become, for example, black or white large squares, to the right or the left; these new positive stimuli have thus been reinforced in 50 per cent of cases during the first learning task. It follows that the approach tendency is stronger than in the preceding case (50 per cent as against 0); an extra-dimensional NR second learning must therefore be more rapid than a learning involving reversal shift. This is indeed what one finds in animals and young children but not in adults and older children.

If another experimental setting is selected, that of Dickerson (1966), for example, only the reversal shift situation retains the same stimulus objects, the other two, extra-dimensional and intra-dimensional, involve new objects which differ from the previous ones in both characteristics, colour and form (fig. 33). In this case the Spencian model would predict that the three situations are of equal difficulty. However, although the two situations, R and ID, in which the relevant dimension is maintained, seem to be equivalent, the extra-dimensional situation, ED, although relating to the same stimulus objects as the intra-dimensional situation ID, is clearly more difficult. The predictions from the Spencian model are not realised.

## 2 The Intervention of Language in Discrimination Learning

(a) *Responses involving verbal mediation.* Impressed by the qualitative difference which separates the performances of young children and animals from those of older children and adults, Kendler and Kendler proposed a two-stage model (Kendler and Kendler, 1959, 1962, 1968, 1969) according to which the differences, as much comparative as developmental, can only be interpreted in a satisfactory manner if the existence of two fundamentally different mechanisms is postulated. For these authors, animals and very young children would behave according to the predictions of Spence's single-stage S-R model. But the learning of older children would be in terms of a mediational model. In this model, intermediary responses, acquired before the instrumental choice responses, are intercalated between the stimulus objects and the responses; the stimuli from these mediational responses are added to the external stimuli and can enhance the discriminability of the object (Miller and Dollard, 1941). For Kendler and Kendler the mediating response is representational in nature and constitutes some form of coding of the stimulus; the learning thus occurs in two stages: the subject first learns to code the stimulus and, in particular, to respond to the relevant dimension of differentiation; and only subsequently does he learn which is the positive value on this dimension. Under these conditions a second learning in which the same dimension remains relevant is acquired more quickly than a learning in which another dimension becomes the relevant one, since in the first case only the choice response changes, whilst in the second a new mediating response must be employed as well as a new choice response. Thus, in line with Spence's predictions, a NR learning would be easier than an R learning for very young children, whilst with older children the opposite would be the case since they would conform to the mediational model.

The age at which the transition to mediational learning occurs is not easy to determine. On the basis of the evidence relating to transfer involving reversal and non-reversal shift in the original experimental situation (T. Kendler and H. Kendler, 1959), this transition would take place around the age of 5 to 7 years. Before 5 years of age non-reversal shift learning is clearly easier (T. Kendler, H. Kendler and Wells, 1960); between 5 and 7 years children are divided almost equally into two groups, one behaving like children of 3 to 4 years and the other like older children (T. Kendler and H. Kendler, 1959).

But the relative difficulty of learning involving reversal or non-reversal shift depends not only on age but also on the dimension of differentiation concerned. It would seem that the capacity for responding to a particular dimension is more or less precocious depending on which it is.

Furthermore, it is soon obvious that the simple comparison between reversal shift and non-reversal shift learning, carried out on the same material with different subjects, is a crude method of determining the presence of mediational responses. In consequence, a further refinement – optional shift – was developed.

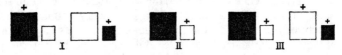

Fig. 34. Optional shift learning.

I, II, III: stimulus figures used in the three successive learning tasks.

The experiment was in three stages. In the first the child learnt to select a stimulus figure as a function of a single value in one dimension. If, for example, the relevant dimension was brightness and the selected value was black, he had to respond positively to the black stimulus figure, whether it was large or small. In the second stage he was presented with a single pair of stimulus figures within which the positive object in the first stage was now negative. However, since a single pair of objects was presented, differing in size as well as contrast, both dimensions were relevant so that a correct response could signify that the child had selected white with reference to black, or small with reference to large, or that he had selected small/white/square. The object of the third stage was to determine the response criterion used in this second stage. Two pairs of objects were presented ten times each, one pair being the same as in stage II, with the same positive and negative stimulus figures, and the other a complementary test pair (fig. 34). On the basis of their responses to these, subjects were classified in three groups: reversal shift R, extra-dimensional ED or NR, and non-selective NS (T. Kendler, H. Kendler and Learnard, 1962).

In the example given (fig. 34) a subject was classed R if, from the test pair, he selected the large white stimulus figure at least eight times out of ten, thus indicating that, during the three stages, he had conserved the dimension of differentiation which was significant in the first learning task, namely contrast; it could be assumed, therefore, that at stage II he had responded to White, thus effecting a reversal shift of the value on one dimension in moving from I to II, hence the classification R (reversal). ·

A subject was classed NR or ED if he selected the small black square at least eight times out of ten, a choice which would indicate that in stage II he had responded in terms of size. In this case, in moving from I to II he had changed the dimension of differentiation, hence the classification NR (non-reversal) or ED (extra-dimensional).

Finally, a subject who in stage III sometimes selected the small black stimulus figure and sometimes the large white one, was classified as non-selective NS and it was hypothesised that his responses were not made as a function of a single dimension.

T. Kendler, H. Kendler and Learnard (1962) postulated that a subject whose responses were classified as R definitely utilised mediational responses; having learnt to respond as a function of a single dimension of differentiation during the first learning task, he retained it for those which followed since it remained relevant. The authors' developmental hypothesis would predict that the number of children utilising mediational responses should increase with age, and this was verified by the results. Thus, whilst at $3\frac{1}{2}$ years less than 40 per cent of the subjects were in group R ('mediating subjects'), this proportion increased to 50 per cent at $4\frac{1}{2}$ years and exceeded 60 per cent at 10 years of age (fig. 35). These results have been confirmed in other experiments where the material involved other dimensions of differentiation (Kendler and Kendler, 1968). It is interesting to note that if one extrapolates the curve relating to the 'mediating' subjects R (H. Kendler and T. Kendler, 1969), the abscissa is reached at the age of 2 years (fig. 35); it must be added that, in an optional shift task, the number of rats in group R was almost nil (T. Kendler, H. Kendler and Silfen, 1964). It is impossible not to relate these results to what we know from other sources about the development of the child. The emergence of mediators or of differentiators, according to the terminology preferred, would coincide with that of representational capacities. Thus rats would behave like 2-year-old children because, like them, they lack the symbolic function.

Kendler and Kendler classed those subjects who made NR responses with those who made non-selective responses on the supposition that they did not employ mediational responses. Such a decision could be seen as arbitrary, and the authors have referred to Spence (1936, 1952) to justify themselves. Within the Spencian perspective, each object is seen as a complex unit formed of two stimulus components each of which could individually acquire a response tendency as a function of reinforcement. At the end of stage I, the response

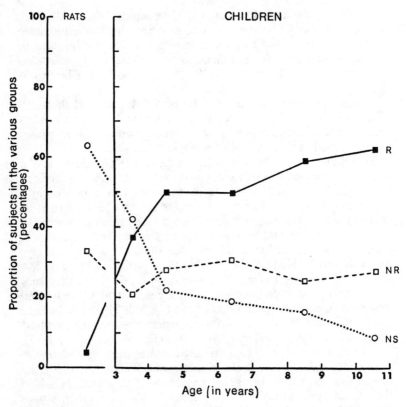

Fig. 35. Changes with age in the proportion of subjects in three groups in an optional shift learning task (Kendler and Kendler, 1969).

Group R=reversal shift; NR=extra-dimensional choice; NS=non-selective.

tendency of the positive component of the relevant dimension (black in the example selected), would be very strong since all the responses which had been made to it had been reinforced; on the other hand the response tendency of the negative component of this same dimension (white) would be slight since no response made to it would have been reinforced. The response tendencies of both components of the non-relevant dimension (small and large) would be equal, of median value, since the corresponding responses had been equally reinforced – that is, 50 per cent of the time. In stage II the child would respond to the compound stimulus which was correct in stage I, for instance the large black square, until the response tendencies established in stage I were sufficiently reduced, due to the non-reinforcement of the response, so that the responses to the other compound stimulus, the small white square, could be established. But, because of the training experienced in stage I, the two components (small and white) of the new positive stimulus would not be equal: 'small' would have a stronger response tendency than 'white', and this inequality would be maintained in stage II. Consequently in stage III, having to choose between 'small' and 'white', it would be 'small' that he would respond to preferentially. However, it must be added that if the number of trials was increased in stage II, the response tendencies of small and white would be simultaneously augmented up to a ceiling level; it would thus come about that 'small' would attain its maximal value and stay at that level whilst the response tendency of 'white' would continue to increase and approach that of 'small' until it was at the same level. If the number of trials was sufficiently large in stage II, the choices at stage III would then be distributed equally between the small black square and the large white one. Amongst the 'non-mediating' subjects those who acquired the second learning rapidly would thus be in group NR, and those who acquired it slowly would be in the non-selective group. The results are in agreement with this latter hypothesis. The NS (non-selective) group needed an average of 17·4 trials to attain the criterion fixed for the second learning task and the NR group only 14·7. The subjects in group R ('mediators') learnt much more quickly than the others, needing 8·4 trials for the second learning task and only 12·3 for the first, as against 31·1 trials for the NR subjects and 45·2 for the non-selective group at this same stage I.

Working on the hypothesis that the mediation process involved was verbal in nature, the investigators, at the end of the experiment, put to the children a certain number of questions designed to elucidate the manner in which they had perceived and resolved the task in series III. A child was classed as verbalising the correct dimension when his justification corresponded to the direction of his responses, for example when having responded in III to the contrast, he said that the correct stimulus was the white one. A child was classed as verbalising the incorrect dimension when his justification did not correspond to the direction of his responses, as when, for example, he said that the correct stimulus was the white one whilst his choices had been made as a function of size. Finally, a subject was classed as not verbalising in a relevant fashion when he did not give a justification or if it was not in terms of a particular dimension.

Table 13 shows that almost half (42 per cent) of the children described as non-selective made no mention of any dimension of differentiation in their verbalisations, whilst the great majority of 'mediating' children (84·8 per cent) cited the dimension which corresponded to their actual response. Group NR is the one which poses the most problems; in their analysis the authors classed these subjects as non-mediators; however, in contrast to the non-selective subjects, these children gave responses consistent with the use of a dimension of differentiation, and in their verbalisations they justified their choice in terms of a value on a single dimension, as often as the 'mediating' subjects. These children therefore showed themselves quite capable of abstracting the dimensions of the objects presented to them.

Table 13    *Proportions of subjects as a function of their behavioural responses and their verbalisations (percentage)*

| Subjects | *Verbalisation of the correct dimension* | *Verbalisation of the incorrect dimension* | *No relevant verbalisation* |
|---|---|---|---|
| R | 84·8 | 7·6 | 7·6 |
| NR | 66·7 | 25·6 | 7·7 |
| NS | | 57·7[1] | 42·3 |

[1]For the non-selective (NS) subjects no dimension can be considered correct (after T. Kendler, 1963).

Some supplementary experiments (H. Kendler and T. Kendler, 1961; T. Kendler, 1963, 1964) have defined the role of language more precisely in reversal shift learning of children from 4 to 7 years of age. In a first stage the child learned to respond positively to one of two objects both of which differed along two dimensions (a large black square and a small white one). Before giving his choice response the child, following the instructions of the experimenter, had to verbalise one of the properties of the positive object. In the second learning task two pairs of objects were presented (a large black square with a small white one, and a small black square with a large white one) and only one dimension was relevant. For half the children the verbalisation learnt in stage I related to the relevant dimension in stage II. If, for example, the large black square was the positive stimulus in I and the child had to say 'black', in II the positive stimulus figures for the same child would be the white squares: the same dimension is relevant but the value within this dimension is reversed. For the other half of the children the verbalisation related to the non-relevant dimension in II; for example, for a child who, in I, had learnt to say 'black' to the large black square, the positive stimulus figures in II would be the large (or the small) squares. A third, control, group did not learn a verbal response.

The results are very straightforward: a verbal response relating to the non-relevant dimension (group II) clearly retarded the learning that followed, particularly in the older children. A verbal response relating to the relevant dimension did not accelerate second learning in the older children, but made it more rapid in the younger ones. Kendler concluded that the older children would use mediators in any case; for them the verbal signalling of the relevant dimension added nothing, whilst to emphasise a dimension they would not need to use in the second learning hindered them to a considerable extent. The act of verbalising had much less effect on the younger children because the verbal responses were much less likely to be transformed into mediators.

Table 14   *Number of trials needed to attain the learning criterion in the second task*

|  | Relevant | Non-relevant | None |
|---|---|---|---|
|  | *Nature of verbalisations in the first task* | | |
|  | *Relevant* | *Non-relevant* | *None* |
| 4 years | 16·1 | 30·4 | 22·2 |
| 7 years | 8·3 | 35·6 | 8·8 |

(After T. Kendler, 1963)

Kendler and Kendler conclude from this important series of investigations that verbalisation can play a role in the mediational process but that the extent of this role depends on the child's level of development. Concurring with the views of Spence (1937) and Kuenne (1946), they are of the opinion that, in the course of development, the relationships between verbal behaviour and discrimination learning pass through three stages which correspond to those described by Luria (1957). At the *preverbal* stage the child does not possess the words corresponding to the relevant dimensions of differentiation. At a later stage of *verbal deficiency*, the child has the words in his vocabulary but does not use them to solve a discrimination problem. At a final, *verbal mediational* stage, discrimination is controlled by linguistic processes (H. Kendler and T. Kendler, 1969). As these authors observe, a child does not attain stages 2 and 3 simultaneously for all words; it could be the case, for example, that he discriminates a fish from a marine mammal at the preverbal stage, furniture from means of transport at the level of verbal deficiency, and chickens and cows at the level of verbal mediation.

Combining the results of two optional shift experiments (H. Kendler and T. Kendler, 1961; T. Kendler, 1964), Kendler and Kendler noted that 48 per cent of the children in control group C made an R selection; thus these subjects possessed implicit representational responses which they utilised spontaneously. The children in group V were given verbal instructions concerning the relevant dimension by the experimenter, and of these 82 per cent made an R selection. If the number of mediating (R) subjects in groups C and V is compared, and if it is assumed that the groups were homogeneous, it can be seen that 34 per cent (82 per cent − 48 per cent) of the children in the second group (V) only gave the representational response because they had been guided by the instructions. For the remaining 18 per cent 'non-mediating' children in group V, language had exercised no control over their choice response. It can be assumed therefore, taking account of their age (mean of 5y. 10m.), that all the children had passed the preverbal stage; that 18 per cent were at the stage of verbal deficiency, whatever instructions they had been given; that 34 per cent had obeyed the instructions given to them and so showed themselves capable of adopting representational responses produced by others and passed on to them; and that 48 per cent were capable of constructing representational responses themselves.

(*b*) *The role of verbal labels.* It is a familiar hypothesis that explicit responses, acquired during the course of a first learning task, remain during a second task as implicit responses. The latter are, according to Hull (1930, 1939), the source of the stimulus *s* which is added to the stimulus-objects *S*; the choice response is then made to a combination of two stimuli: *S*+*s*. According to the degree of similarity or, conversely, of difference, which obtains between the stimuli on the one hand and the responses learnt in the first task on the other, there will be a positive or negative transfer in the second task, during the course of which new responses will become linked to the same stimulus-objects.

Where the stimulus-objects are very similar, a pretraining which associates each of them with very different responses will tend to make them more discriminable. Because of the differential reinforcement provided by these responses, stimulus generalisation will be decreased and a second learning facilitated. This is known as the hypothesis of the *acquired distinctiveness of cues* (Miller and Dollard, 1941).

In the opposite case, where an identical response is associated with quite different stimulus-objects, the characteristics of each stimulus-object and the stimulus arising from this response will be made more similar. The generalisation between stimulus-objects will be increased and a second learning retarded. This is known as the hypothesis of the *acquired equivalence of cues* (N. Miller and Dollard, 1941; N. Miller, 1948), also known as *mediational generalisation.*

Both hypotheses are valid whatever the nature of the responses involved; thus Lawrence (1949, 1950) has shown them to be valid for motor learning tasks with rats. However, the majority of experiments of this type have involved the use of verbal responses in the first learning task and have been concerned to demonstrate the privileged character of the latter.

1 *Verbal labels and the acquired distinctiveness of cues.* The typical experimental design, such as one finds in Spiker (1963) and Cantor (1965) is reproduced in fig. 36. Spiker insists on the fact that certain conditions must be obtained in order for the responses learnt in the first task to result in an acquired distinctiveness of the cues.

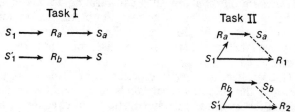

Fig. 36. Schematic representation of the acquired distinctiveness of cues.

In the first task the subject learns to give the responses $R_a$ or $R_b$ to the stimuli $S_1$ and $S'_1$. It is assumed that $R_a$ emanates from stimulus $S_a$ and $R_b$ from stimulus $S_b$. During the second learning task response $R_1$ is associated with the complex $S_1 + S_a$, and $R_2$ with the complex $S'_1 + S_b$.

The stimuli $S_1$ and $S'_1$ must be sufficiently similar for there to be the possibility of confusion between them because of primary generalisation (Spiker, 1963); they must not induce spontaneous naming on the part of the subject; the second task must involve more than a simple psychophysical discrimination; responses $R_1$ and $R_2$ must be distinct and should not demand any special ability on the part of the subject.

A series of experiments by Cantor (1955) presents positive results in favour of the role of verbal labels. Cantor compared the performance of preschool children on a discrimination learning task involving two line-drawings of adult female faces, as a function of three types of pretraining. For a first group of twenty children, described as the *Relevant* group, pretraining involved learning verbal labels attached to the stimuli in the test trial; one of the pictures of a woman was called Jane, the other, Peg. A second group, described as the *Irrelevant* group, learnt during pretraining to put the name Jack to the picture of one boy and Pete to the picture of another boy; thus verbal labels were attached to stimuli which would not appear in the test task. A third group, described as the *Attention* group, received approximately as many presentations of the relevant stimuli, the pictures of the women, as the *Relevant* group; they were instructed to point with their finger to the main features of the drawings but did not learn the verbal label. The discrimination learning test task was the same for the subjects in all three groups; one of the stimuli was positive and each correct choice was rewarded. The comparison between groups was in terms of the number of correct responses in each block of five successive trials, for a total of thirty trials. From the sixth trial the *Relevant* group gave significantly more correct responses than the two other groups, between which there was no statistically significant difference although there appeared to be a slight degree of superiority in favour of the *Irrelevant* group. Factors such as 'warming up' and 'learning to learn' being the same for all groups, the better performance of the *Relevant* group can be attributed to the fact that they had learnt to attach verbal labels to the stimuli to be discriminated in the second learning task.

Kurtz (1955) offers another interpretation of Cantor's results in particular, and the role of verbal labels in general. According to Kurtz, verbal labels would merely constitute an effective means of establishing observing responses[1] to the stimuli. Any other technique which could give rise to these responses should therefore produce the same results as a pretraining involving the learning of verbal labels. In the case of Cantor's (1955) experiment the view could be taken that the *Attention* group had not had the chance to acquire observing responses since they did not have to give discriminative responses in the course of their pretraining.

In order to meet this criticism, Norcross and Spiker (1957; Spiker and Norcross, 1957) repeated Cantor's experiment with slight modifications. Norcross and Spiker (1957) used Cantor's material and a similar population which was divided into three groups: the *Relevant* group and the *Irrelevant* group operated in the same fashion as those in Cantor's experiment; only the third group, called the *Discrimination* group, differed, since for them pretraining involved giving judgments of 'same' or 'not the same' to pairs formed either of the two stimulus-figures of the test task, or one of these and its replica. Discrimination learning was clearly involved since the responses were corrected where necessary. The results confirmed those of Cantor (1955): the *Relevant* group gave significantly more correct responses in the test trial than both the *Irrelevant* and *Discrimination* groups, whose responses were essentially equivalent.

A third experiment (Spiker and Norcross, 1957) involved two *Discrimination* groups; during pretraining, one group compared stimulus-figures presented simultaneously, the other stimulus-figures presented successively. The authors found no difference between the *Discrimination* groups and verified the superiority of the *Relevant* group. They concluded that learning to name the stimuli, in itself, brought about a facilitation of all the subsequent discrimination learning, without there being any need to implicate observing responses.

2 *The influence of the degree of similarity between verbal labels.* The hypothesis of the facilitating role of verbal labels leads to the prediction that the more different the labels are, the greater should be the degree of facilitation (N. Miller, 1948). Indeed, in the theory of the acquired distinctiveness of cues, the final responses are determined by the visible stimuli (the objects to be discriminated) to which are added the implicit responses, acquired in the course of pretraining. The more these implicit responses differ, the more different will be the stimuli to which they give rise and the more distinct will be the objects themselves. The facilitating effect of verbal labels that were similar would, therefore, be considerably inferior to those which were clearly distinguishable.

An experiment by Norcross (1958) verified these predictions. In this experiment 5-year-old children learnt during pretraining to give names to four pictures: two of girls, two of boys. Their names consisted of trigrams, two of which were very similar, Zim and Zam, and two very different, Wug and Kos. For half the children the similar names were given to the pictures of boys, and for the other half to the pictures of girls. The test task involved learning to press

Table 15

| Pretraining | | Transfer task |
| Group 1 | Group 2 | Groups 1 and 2 |
| --- | --- | --- |
| 1st boy — Zim | 1st boy — Wug | 1st boy — 1st button |
| 2nd boy — Zam | 2nd boy — Kos | 2nd boy — 2nd button |
| 1st girl — Wug | 1st girl — Zim | 1st girl — 3rd button |
| 2nd girl — Kos | 2nd girl — Zam | 2nd girl — 4th button |
| | | (After Norcross, 1958) |

a particular button when each of the four stimulus-figures was presented. The subject was instructed to say out loud the name of the picture before pressing the button selected.

Performance was clearly better with the two pictures to which the child had learnt to give very different names – pictures of girls for group 1 and pictures of boys for group 2. Since each child had learnt to respond differentially to each stimulus-figure during pre-training, they had all been given the same chance to establish observing responses. If Kurtz's (1955) hypothesis had been correct, one would have expected these responses to transfer to the second task so that the performances would be the same on all the pictures. Since this was not the case, Spiker (1963) concluded that verbal labels played a privileged role in the discrimination of objects.

An experiment by Katz (1963) employed a design a little more complicated than the preceding one. The stimulus-figures were four irregular polygons constructed according to the principles described by Attneave (1954). The subjects, children from 6 to 8 years, were divided into three groups as a function of the pretraining they received. The first group, described as the different label (DL) group, learnt to associate a different syllable (buz, ric, jan or sol) to each of the four polygons. The second group, described as the common label (CL) group learnt to associate one of the labels to two of the polygons and another label to the other two polygons. The stimulus-figures were presented one by one, for a two-second exposure; the experimenter said whether the response was right or not but did not give a correction. The third group received the same number of presentations of the stimulus-figures as the other groups, that is, 150, but did not learn labels. In order to prevent them from assigning one themselves, they were instructed to count in series whilst the stimulus was presented. Two test tasks followed the pretraining, and were the same for all three groups. In the first test task pairs of polygons were presented for 200 ms each and the subject had to say whether they were identical or different. Within these pairs, 8 were composed of two identical polygons, 10 consisted of two polygons to which group 2 had learnt to give the same name (test pairs) and 10 consisted of two polygons to which this same group had learnt to give different names. The second trial involved a discrimination learning task in which the positive stimulus was always one of those that had received the same name in the group 2 pretraining.

In the test task of judgments of identity or difference, the performances with identical pairs were excellent for all three groups, which is in agreement with numerous other experimental results (Vurpillot and Zoberman, 1965; Vurpillot, 1968, 1969a; Vurpillot and Moal, 1970). On the other hand, for the test pairs, the three groups produced different performances, the number of errors (those judged 'the same') being smallest for group 1, median for group 3 and greatest for group 2. Giving different names to each polygon facilitated their discrimination; giving the same name to two polygons hindered it. The second test task confirmed the results of the first. Katz's results are therefore in support of the hypotheses of the acquired distinctiveness of cues and mediational generalisation: verbal labels can facilitate or hinder later learning by their greater or lesser similarity.

The results of Katz's experiment would therefore seem to be very positive. However, using other syllables with the same polygons and the same experimental technique as that of Katz (1963), Oléron (1967a) did not find any difference between groups DL and CL. With the same exposure time, children of the same age did not differentiate those polygons to which they had learnt to give different names better than those they had learnt to give the same name. The hypothesis of the acquired equivalence of cues would only predict errors of confusion between stimuli affected by the same verbal label; however, in Oléron's experiment (1967a) confusions were as numerous between polygons associated with different verbal labels as between polygons with the same name. Oléron proposed the following interpretation of his results. The act of naming the polygons induced in the subject a categorising set which applied to all the stimulus figures. These would be treated as members of common classes, members between which differences were tolerated to the extent that they would cease to be noticed. To this cognitive set would be added a perceptual set tending towards the search for points of resemblance. Finally it might come about that the subject declares the stimulus-figures to be the same simply because they have the same name, even though he perceives differences between them. Within this perspective, perception is not modified by the addition of labels, but rather by the orientation of attention towards differences or similarities, towards one property rather than another.

The possibility of verbalising and the form that it takes during a discrimination learning task do have an influence on performance and, as Oléron says, '. . . the verbal statement is a stimulus which contributes to the determination of the observed response . . .' (Oléron, 1967b, p. 173). But the mediational schema which sees the word as a simple intermediary between the stimulus and the response is too simple to correspond to reality. The role of language cannot be reduced to the addition of a label because the word is a function of the cognitive activity of whoever employs it. If the level of this activity is high, the word becomes an instrument capable of influencing what is produced: an adequate verbalisation facilitates the processes of differentiation, whilst an inadequate verbalisation hinders them. But if the level of cognitive activity is low, the verbal statement is limited to its articulation, which cannot influence performance.

# Chapter 7

# Selective Attention

In contrast to the theories of verbal mediation, described in the preceding chapter, is another group of theories for which *attention* is the factor involved in discrimination learning in general and the discovery of dimensions of differentiation in particular. As Kendler and Kendler observe (H. Kendler and T. Kendler, 1969), in the literature concerned with discrimination learning the word 'attention' appears to be used in at least three different ways. Attention has been defined as an instrumental orientation response of the receptors (Spence, 1940; Wyckoff, 1952; White and Plum, 1964, etc.). It has also been conceptualised as a filter having the effect of conserving the relevant part of the available information whilst inhibiting the rest (Sutherland, 1959; Mackintosh, 1962, 1965b). Finally, some have seen it as a process of coding sensory stimuli (Lawrence, 1963). Some workers distinguish between these various meanings and grant an essential role to one specific aspect of attention whilst others subsume all three senses of the term under the concept of attention (Kurtz, 1955; Zeaman and House, 1963, etc.).

## I  OBSERVING RESPONSES AND DISCRIMINATION LEARNING

In order to refute the arguments put forward by Lashley (1929) and Krechevski (1932) in support of a discontinuity in learning, Spence added a link to his schema of association between a stimulus and a response (Spence, 1940, 1951).

In a discrimination learning task, the animal would learn a chain of two responses of which the first would be 'to orient and fixate its head and eyes so as to receive the critical stimuli' (Spence, 1940, p. 276), in other words to obtain discriminable retinal stimuli from the objects presented. The observed errors would thus be due to the fact that the animal looked at only one part of the stimulus, one which did not contain the details which were critical for discrimination. Wyckoff (1952) took Spence's idea and, in order to show the importance of observing responses, devised an ingenious piece of experimental apparatus to make it easier to record such responses. · The animal, a pigeon, operated the illumination of the stimulus by pressing on a pedal. This action was called the *observing response.*

The importance, indeed the existence of observing responses has been vigorously debated by learning theorists. Lashley (1942) rejected Spence's explanation, commenting that the value taken by the angle encompassing the various parts of the stimulus is such that all the parts are seen in one visual fixation; the absence of an observing response is thus not adequate as an explanation of the rat's behaviour during the period preceding the solution. Mackintosh (1965b) expresses surprise at the success of Spence's hypothesis in the absence of evidence concerning the role of effective observing responses, manifested in discrimination learning tasks. Wyckoff's experiments, he says, were ingenious but did not involve the orientation of receptors, a justified criticism, to which he adds, aligning himself with Lashley, that, taking into account the experimental conditions, such an orientation was unnecessary (Mackintosh, 1965b).

However, fine visual orienting responses could escape the experimenter. It is possible that in the majority of the experiments cited by Mackintosh, the experimental setting was such that the whole of the stimuli could be included in a single visual field and that gross orienting responses such as observable movements of the head would not be necessary. But, when presented with the same stimulus-figures, for example two rectangles, is it not the case that the subject tends to fixate the centre when he has to discriminate them in terms of contrast, and on the other hand, the contour and the angles when he has to differentiate them in terms of their orientations (H. Kendler and T. Kendler, 1966)?

A number of investigations, using groups of children, have attempted to relate the existence of instrumental observing responses and performance on discrimination learning tasks.

S. White has tried a succession of different techniques in an attempt to evaluate observing responses in children from 3 to 5 years. One involved placing the stimulus-figures to be discriminated at the front and at the back of a revolving door, another made the appearance of the stimulus-figure dependent upon pressing a lever (S. White, 1962). In both cases the task became too complex for such young children. In consequence, White (S. White and Plum, 1964) then decided to measure directly the activity of spontaneous visual exploration in children from $3\frac{1}{2}$ years to 5 years by recording their eye movements during discrimination learning. The distance between the two stimulus-figures was 30 cm, and a camera, situated between the two, recorded the visual fixations at the rate of three frames per second. These were divided into four categories: fixation on the stimulus to the left, on the stimulus to the right, on the centre, and 'unclassifiable'. White treated as an eye movement only the movement from one stimulus to the other, whether or not there had been, between the two, a pause in the centre or an unclassifiable displacement. The number of eye movements provided a measure of the children's observing activity.

The experimenters presented a series of eight discrimination learning problems to each child. There were two series: the 'easy' one involved coloured pictures of birds; the 'difficult' series consisted of figures made up of a vertical line with two small lateral lines coming out of it, the difference between the two figures of a pair relating to the orientation of one of these small lines.

The number of exploratory movements was greater for the 'easy' series than for the 'difficult' one; however, the rate of observing activity was not constant throughout the task (which continued for a number of sessions over two or three days) and reached a maximum point within each problem and within the series of problems. This maximum coincided, in a problem, with the attainment of the criterion; if presentation of the figures was continued, performance remained excellent but the number of eye movements decreased. Within a series of problems the maximum was located at the point where the child had acquired what was for him the best possible strategy and where he was learning each problem relatively quickly. In this case also, the number of eye movements subsequently decreased, but to a lesser extent than in the case of a single problem.

The rate of exploration is thus positively associated with its efficiency. For White this formulation is valid in two senses: the discriminability of the stimuli and the interest they arouse stimulate exploratory activity – this is the case, for example, with the pictures of birds; at the same time the exploration of the pictures facilitates their discrimination.

During the 'pre-solution' period, the child seems at first to respond by chance (40–45 per cent correct responses), then, simultaneously, he displays a more extensive activity of comparison between the stimulus-figures and begins to respond correctly. White compares this with the behaviour of rats, who make numerous side-to-side head movements at a point of choice in the maze, just at the moment when they are about to discover the correct solution. According to Tolman (1939) this maximum of observing activity corresponds to the sudden discovery of the correct hypothesis; only at that moment does the animal know on what cues to rely in order to select the right path and it then starts to seek to discover them in earnest. It is possibly the same for children, and that they also form the hypothesis that there must be something in the figures which will enable them to discover how to give a response which will bring about a favourable result; on the basis of this hypothesis they set about seriously comparing the two objects. It must be observed that the average number of movements observed per trial was very small: 1·48 in the 'easy' series and 0·69 in the 'difficult' series of experiment I, 0·73 and 0·39 for the same series in experiment II of White and Plum (1964). If the curves relating to the level of exploration during trials on a particular problem are examined, it can be seen that it is only at the moment when the subject attains the necessary criterion that the number of movements exceeds 1. This could mean that before the trial where the criterion is attained the child is satisfied with looking at one stimulus-figure for most of the time, and that as soon as he looks at them both, he is able to respond correctly on each occasion.

Using the same technique as White and Plum but applied to even simpler stimulus-figures (a circle and a diamond in different colours), Scott and Christy (1968) found a maximum of exploratory activity during the first presentation of the objects. It would seem that the curiosity aroused by these simple stimulus-figures was exhausted at the first presentation and that the children made hardly any effort to improve performance, as if a partial reinforcement were sufficient for them.

The results of the experiments of White and Plum (1964) and Scott and Christy (1968) show that the first stage in a discrimination learning task, for a very young child, involves the discovery that it is necessary to have looked at both stimulus-objects before giving a response. If the primitive response-style of taking the chance that one of them is the correct one persists for a relatively long time, the responses given in this way are reinforced in a significant number of cases. It is even possible that, for the child, the simple act of giving a response and by this means of playing with the experimental material constitutes a reward as worthwhile – if not more so – as the praise of the experimenter, or a marble or a sweet, or some other small present.

Systematic training in one instrumental comparison activity should transfer to other tasks; the acquisition of observing responses to the cues relating to a dimension of differentiation should facilitate a second learning in which this dimension remains relevant whilst it should be a handicap if this dimension becomes non-relevant. A number of experimental results provide effective support for this assumption.

Wright and Daehler (1966) selected a task involving the discovery of the object which did not belong with the others (oddity problem). Training consisted of sixteen trials with material which comprised blue cubes with yellow discs stuck on them. The control group differentiated cubes with six large discs on them from plain cubes, in the course of sixteen trials. For the experimental group, difficulty increased with each successive trial because the yellow discs became smaller and smaller, forming more and more complex configurations so that gradually it became necessary to manipulate the cubes in order to see the distinctive features. The test task, the same for both groups, comprised ten problems involving the discovery of the 'odd' object amongst three toys which differed in a minor detail. The experiment involved children from 3 to 9 years of age; the number of objects handled provided a measure of observing activity during the training periods and in the test problems. The results obtained showed that the experimental group achieved a higher level of performance than the other, at all age-levels, and that the observing activity in that group was more intense. It is thus possible to train a child, from the age of 3 years, to make observing responses – or, if another terminology is preferred, to increase his perceptual, manipulatory activity. From the same age of 3 years, the responses thus acquired are transferred to tasks of the same order carried out with the same material. The rate of perceptual activity observed in the second task remained almost constant up to 5 years and then after 6 years of age, but there was a rapid and quite definite increase between 5 and 6 years. Performances on the test task evolved in a parallel fashion to perceptual activity, indicating a significant move forward between 5 and 6 years; the correlation between the number of observing responses and performance was positive.

The results from the control group showed that the observing responses appeared spontaneously and increased in number with age. As in the case of the experimental group, the progression was not regular and the maximum increase was between 7 and 8 years, that is, at a later age. The improvement in performance was regular from age-level to age-level. The differences between the experimental group and the control group were not simply quantitative, and the training given to the children did not just have the effect of speeding up the acquisition and transfer of observing activity; it also induced a systematised approach to the experimental task, which manifested itself in a certain rigidity of behaviour. If the performances of the experimental and the control group at 8 and 9 years are compared, they can be seen to be equal; however, the number of manipulations of the objects remains distinctly higher for the experimental group. It is possible that, due to the formation of a set during pretraining, these children continued to explore the objects more than was necessary in order to differentiate them.

Another experiment (Wright and Gliner, 1967) provides more precise information on the role of observing responses. They studied the conjoint action of two factors – the discovery of the relevant dimension, and the discriminability of the values on this dimension – in the performance of 10-year-old children. The experiment was designed in such a way that the relevant and non-relevant cues were situated in different parts of the stimulus. It was thus possible, during the first phase, to train (or not to train) the children to explore systematically one area of the objects and then to measure to what degree the observing responses thus acquired were transferred to a second learning task. Wright and Gliner decided to use tactile perception, the sequential nature of which would make it easier to isolate the areas which were explored from those that were not. During pretraining, the stimulus-objects were four amoeboid forms which differed along two dimensions, the contour (two different forms) and the texture (fur or rough sponge). The textured part was confined to one small area of each object. In order to differentiate the objects in terms of their form the subject had to follow the contour with a finger; to differentiate them in terms of their texture he had to explore the central part of their surface area. The children were divided into four experimental groups. Group T learned to explore the textured part; group S learned to explore the contour; in group B exploration involved the contour and the textured part alternately; group N received no pretraining. In groups T, S and B the child explored one object after another, without seeing them and using his preferred hand, and received reinforcement in the sound of a bell when he followed the instructions correctly. Once the criterion was attained, that is, the exploration of the correct area only, the subject proceeded to the test task – half the children being given an easy discrimination task, the other half a difficult one.

Knowing that the form dimension is spontaneously preferred, the experimenters used only texture as the relevant dimension in the test task. The objects presented at this stage were two pentagons and two octogons, on each of which was a small disc of glass-paper differing in the coarseness of the grain. This difference in coarseness was slight for the 'difficult discrimination' group and marked for the other. The objects were presented in pairs, handled one after the other, following which the child identified one of them and received a positive or negative reinforcement. For each response the exploratory activity was recorded on a 5-point scale: 5 corresponded to exploration involving texture only, 4 indicated exploration mainly involving texture, 3 represented equal exploration of contour and texture, and so on. This activity was recorded during pretraining and during the test task.

As in the preceding experiment (Wright and Daehler, 1966), it was confirmed that it is possible to acquire training in exploration and that this transfers to other materials. When the same dimension was relevant in both tasks (group T) the effect was facilitating; however, when the relevant dimension in the first group became non-relevant in the second learning task (group S), the effect was inhibitory. The amount of perceptual activity manifested was independent of the degree of discriminability of the objects; the authors concluded that this second factor was only relevant in the second stage (choice-response) of the learning task.

This series of investigations demonstrates, as one might have expected, that the exploration of the stimulus-objects to be differentiated is a necessary condition for the acquisition of appropriate choice-responses. The results which have been obtained[1] are very interesting from the point of view of the development of spontaneous exploratory activity and the possibilities of its training and transfer. As to the relationship between observing responses and the abstraction of the relevant dimension for differentiation, this only seems to be in evidence in those special cases where the information relating to the competing dimensions is situated at points some way apart in the stimulus-object, so that changes in visual fixation must accompany the attention directed to one as against the other. It is quite certain that a possible discontinuity in discrimination learning cannot be interpreted simply in terms of the orientation of the receptors. Experimental settings are usually such that the stimulus-objects to be compared can be included entirely and simultaneously within one visual field (Mackintosh, 1965b). Finally, as has been demonstrated many times, it is important not to confuse looking and seeing, receiving sensory stimuli and perceiving them; an article by Horn (1965) provides important data on this point. To cite just one example: in a tachistoscopic presentation involving a fixation point, perception can differ according to whether attention is drawn to one aspect or another of the stimulus, although the patterns of sensory stimulation remain the same (Fraisse, Ehrlich and Vurpillot, 1956; Fraisse and Vurpillot, 1956).

## II SELECTIVE ATTENTION

The great disproportion between the mass of information contained

---

[1]It might seem more appropriate to describe these in the chapters devoted to perceptual activity (chapters 9 and 10). However, the theoretical framework in which the experiments were conceived seemed to indicate that they should be included here.

in the sensory stimulation provided by objects to be discriminated, and the limited capacity of the nervous system to process and store the information, means that the organism is obliged to make a choice (G. Miller, 1956; Broadbent, 1958). This selection can take place at two levels: at the receptor level and at the level of the integration of neural excitation by the central nervous system. Presented with a stimulus-object the subject can orient his receptors and so obtain only a part of the information available; this type of selection has been discussed in the preceding pages. Furthermore, the subject is able to retain only part of the information he has gathered – that which he judges to be significant – this selection taking place at the moment when the information is processed.

Some investigators see the first level as being of negligible importance and give it no place in their theoretical model (Goodwin and Lawrence, 1955; Sutherland, 1959; Mackintosh, 1962; House and Zeaman, 1960; Zeaman and House, 1963). Others take into account both the orientation of the receptors and the selection of a property of the stimulus-objects (Lawrence, 1963; Polidora and Fletcher, 1964; Wright, 1964, etc.).

All of these models, which L. Tighe and T. Tighe (1966) describe as subtractive mediation theories, have in common, after the sensory reception of stimuli, the intervention of a transformational process. This transformation mainly consists of a filtering process which retains only that part of the sensory stimulation relative to a particular property of the stimulus-objects; the hypothetical filtering mechanisms differ according to the investigator concerned.

### 1   *Mackintosh's Hypothesis.*

Sutherland and Mackintosh (Sutherland, 1959, 1963; Mackintosh, 1962, 1963, etc.) have proposed the hypothesis that all animals possess a set of analysers corresponding to particular dimensions of differentiation of objects they encounter. The first stage of learning consists therefore of engaging the appropriate analyser. For these authors no response is necessary prior to the orientation of the receptors, and their model postulates that the subject receives all the stimuli emitted by the objects to be compared. The analyser is a neurological mechanism which acts on the sensory excitation resulting from receptor stimulation in such a way as to produce different messages for the objects which differ along the dimension to which the analyser in question corresponds. For example, Sutherland (1957a and b, 1960b) postulates the existence of an analyser which would measure the horizonal extension of a form for each point on its vertical axis, and its vertical extension for each point on its horizontal axis. This analyser would make possible the discrimination of forms which differed in terms of the values of either the vertical or horizontal extension (Sutherland, 1957a, 1957b). The model postulates that two analysers cannot function simultaneously. Thus, without any training, an animal would be able to respond to all of those dimensions of differentiation – but only those – for which it possessed a corresponding analyser. The distribution of the responses as a function of one dimension rather than another would not be the product of cognitive abstraction or of the acquisition of an implicit response, but would follow from a simple orientation of attention.

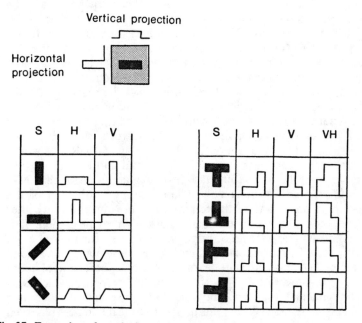

Fig. 37. Examples of vertical and horizontal projections of rectangles and T shapes after Sutherland's (1960b) model.

$S$=stimulus; $H$=horizontal projection; $V$=vertical projection.

Although the animal may be capable of responding to all the dimensions for which it has an analyser, Mackintosh (1965b) states that it does not follow that at the beginning of a task the animal's attention is divided equally between all these dimensions, nor that, in the course of learning, it learns the same amount concerning all the properties of a stimulus-object.

A rat was trained to jump towards a simple stimulus-figure identified in terms of its values along two dimensions – for example, a vertical black rectangle. The degree of generalisation of the acquired response was then measured in situations where the stimulus-figure retained the same value as the initial stimulus on one dimension and varied on the other (Mackintosh, 1965c). The author found that there was generalisation on both dimensions and that, in consequence, the rat had learnt something relating to both the contrast and the orientation of the rectangle.

However, the more it learnt on one dimension, the less it learnt on the other. When, initially, a rat learnt to discriminate objects – for example, a vertical black triangle and a horizontal white triangle – with the aid of the two relevant indices, and subsequently was subjected to two transfer tasks where first one and then the other of the initial dimensions was relevant, a negative correlation was found between the performance of the same subject on the two transfer tasks. If it learnt to respond to contrast rapidly, then it was very slow to acquire a discrimination on the basis of orientation alone, and vice versa (Sutherland and Mackintosh, 1964). Mackintosh (1965b) raises a number of objections to the interpretation given by Kendler and Kendler to the evolution with age of children's performances on transfer tasks involving reversal and non-reversal shift. He argues that it is not evident that a model of the two-stage S-r-s-R type would predict that a second learning involving reversal shift R would always be more rapid than a learning task involving non-reversal shift NR, since this would depend on the relative rate of extinction of the choice response R and of the response r to the dimension, whether this response was one of orientation, attention, or mediation. If it was predicted that the choice response would be extinguished more quickly than the mediation (or attention) response during the second learning, then reversal shift learning R would be acquired more rapidly; if, however, it was the mediation response which was extinguished first, then a non-reversal shift NR second stage learning would be more rapid. Within this perspective the differences observed between animals and young children on the one hand, and older children and adults on the other, could be interpreted within the framework of the same two-stage model and not in terms of transition from a single-stage S-R learning to a two-stage S-r-s-R learning as Kendler and Kendler postulated (H. Kendler and T. Kendler, 1959, 1962; T. Kendler, 1963). As Mackintosh (1965b) observes, overlearning could influence the second learning in two ways, either by accelerating the rate of extinction of choice responses acquired during the first task, or by slowing down the extinction of the response of orientation or discrimination of the relevant dimension. However, numerous experimental results seem to show that one of the most distinct effects of overlearning is to slow down the rate of extinction of choice responses, at least in animals (Komaki, 1961; Mackintosh, 1962, 1963a and b, 1964, 1965a). But the second interpretation seems to be confirmed by complementary experiments. Two groups of rats accomplished an initial discrimination learning task. For the first group, as soon as the chosen criterion was attained, reinforcement ceased and presentation of the stimulus-objects continued until the choice responses were extinguished, that is, when responses were equally divided between the positive stimulus and the negative stimulus. For the second group a certain number of reinforced overlearning trials were inserted between the point where learning was established and the period of extinction. Both groups were then put through a second, reversal shift, learning task. A distinct difference in the behaviour of the two groups was noted. Those in group 1, for whom the intercalated trials had not been reinforced, showed increasingly regular choices in favour of the new positive stimulus, whilst the others began to respond preferentially to the former positive stimulus (d'Amato and Jagoda, 1960; Mackintosh, 1963b, 1965a). Mackintosh (1965b) concluded that the overtrained subjects had indeed extinguished their choice responses but not those of attention to the relevant dimension.

The influence of overlearning can also be explained in terms of a greater slowness in acquiring orienting responses than choice responses. Only a large enough number of supplementary trials would allow the former to establish themselves firmly enough to be effective in the second learning task (Oléron, 1967a, b). For Mackintosh (1965c), as for Oléron (1967a, b), overtraining could have the vital role of reinforcing the probability of paying attention to the relevant dimension and, therefore, of responding to it. Mackintosh's thesis is based on the fact that various experiments have effectively demonstrated that if the number of trials is increased after attaining the required criterion in the first learning task, the rate of acquisition of a second learning involving reversal shift is proportional to the number of overlearning trials (Reid, 1953; Pubols, 1956; Capaldi and Stevenson, 1957). It does not follow that reversal shift learning then becomes, in all subjects, more rapid than non-reversal shift learning. Some investigators have reported that 200 overlearning trials did not bring about any modification of the relative difficulty of R and NR learning in the rat (T. Tighe, Brown and Youngs, 1965). However, in pre-school children, a number of overlearning trials facilitate reversal shift learning (R) to the extent of making it more rapid than non-reversal shift learning (NR). (Marsh, 1964; L. Tighe and T. Tighe, 1966.)

If we have understood Mackintosh correctly, he disagrees with Kendler and Kendler on at least two points. Firstly, an explanation of learning in terms of selective attention is seen by him as clearly superior to an explanation in terms of mediational responses because it accounts for results obtained with animals as well as with humans; it is thus unnecessary to think in terms of two types of learning, S-R for one, S-r-s-R for the other, the former constituting a satisfactory interpretation of the data for neither population. Instead a two-stage learning model is valid, for both; this model brings in the operation of selective attention rather than the addition of an implicit mediational response. Furthermore, Mackintosh postulates that any living organism is capable of responding effectively to one or other variable dimension of the stimulus, provided that he possesses the appropriate analyser. The capacity for responding to a dimension being innate, learning has the effect of focusing attention on one dimension rather than another. However, results obtained in optional shift experiments would seem to contradict this.

The experiment of T. Kendler, H. Kendler and Learnard (1962) had shown that the number of children who chose to respond, in the second learning, as a function of the relevant dimension in the first one (*Reversal* subjects) increased very clearly with age; the same experiment carried out with albino rats showed that practically none of them could behave in this way, some choosing to respond to the dimension which had not been relevant in the first learning (*Non Reversal* subjects), and the majority responding to specific properties of the objects ('non-selective' subjects). (T. Kendler, H. Kendler and Silfen, 1964.) Using different material, L. Tighe and T. Tighe (1965) obtained results very similar to those of Kendler *et al.* (1962, 1964).

Children of 3 and 4 years responded more often than the rats as a function of the dimensions of differentiation of the stimuli, but they preferred to change the dimension (NR) rather than retain the same one by reversing the positive value (R). Overlearning involving two or three hundred supplementary trials in the rat, after having attained the criterion during the first learning, or one-hundred supplementary trials in the case of children, had opposite effects on the two populations. Overlearning increased the number of children who conserved the same dimension (group R), but had the opposite effect on rats (L. Tighe and T. Tighe, 1965).

## 2  Transfer Along a Continuum

As early as 1890, James suggested that a difficult discrimination learning task, impossible when first presented, could be accomplished when it was preceded by several learning episodes graduated from the easiest to the most difficult, provided that the same dimension of discrimination remained relevant throughout. In general the validity of James's predictions has been confirmed, but the available data do not make it possible to decide between the varying interpretations offered.

Mackintosh (1965b) points out that in order to succeed in a discrimination learning task the subject must be in a situation where there is a heightened probability of his attending to the relevant dimension and selecting the positive stimulus. An unsuccessful performance could be due to the fact that either one, or both of these probabilities are too low. A discrimination learning task could be difficult because the two stimulus-objects to be discriminated are too similar. In this case, Mackintosh states, the central representations of $S+$ and $S-$ are partially obscured in such a way that, even when the subject attends appropriately to the relevant dimension during each trial, it is impossible for him always to give the correct response; in certain instances the two stimuli will appear indistinguishable. Since he will make errors even when he takes the relevant dimension into account, the likelihood is that he will not attend to the latter in a consistent manner. Consequently one of the remedies would involve inducing the subject always to respond as a function of the relevant dimension. An easy initial learning achieves this by making it possible for the subject to firmly establish the use of the relevant dimension; by subsequently presenting more and more difficult discriminations in which the stimuli are more and more similar, whilst still being discriminable in the same dimension, the correct orientation is achieved, resulting in satisfactory performances (Pavlov, 1927; Sutherland, Mackintosh and Mackintosh, 1963; House and Zeaman, 1960).

A number of authors have reported that retarded children are particularly slow in the acquisition of a simple discrimination learning, compared with other children of the same mental age (Stevenson and Iscoe, 1955; House and Zeaman, 1958, 1960). However, in analysing individual learning curves, Zeaman and House (1963) noted that the initial plateau was particularly long in retardates; from the point where the curve started to move upwards as a result of other than chance successes, the gradient was the same for all children of the same mental age, retarded or not. The more the child was retarded, the longer the plateau in the learning curve. The authors concluded that this initial part of the curve corresponded to a period during which the subject was not responding to the relevant dimension. It was sufficient to orient the attention of the child towards this dimension, by means of an easy discrimination task, to bring about a significant reduction of the plateau section of the curve and, consequently, an acceleration in the rate of learning in a difficult discrimination task. Thus preliminary training in the discrimination of cut-out forms produced a success-rate of 68 per cent in a discrimination learning task involving the same forms, but as drawings, whilst a success-rate of only 10 per cent was achieved in a group which had not been given pretraining (House and Zeaman, 1960).

Some investigators have thought that by raising the general level of arousal they would be able to increase the amount of selective attention given to one dimension; thus they have introduced novel stimuli, positive or negative, in the middle of a learning series, the novelty being seen as a factor in the alerting of attention (Berlyne, 1960). The results are not very convincing. Zeaman, House and Orlando (1958) report having obtained a sudden elevation of performance in imbeciles by this means; but with normal subjects from 4 to 9 years S. White (1964) found no change with the older children whilst the 4-year-olds were confused and hindered in their learning. It is likely that the appearance of this unexpected stimulus did indeed attract their attention but that this was drawn to the non-relevant rather than to the relevant aspects of the stimuli.

It is by no means evident that, during a learning task, attention is focused preferentially on the relevant dimension. When a first learning is difficult, the subject's attention tends to take in all the properties of the object, including those not relevant in that particular task. It can be seen, therefore, that a second learning in which one of these dimensions became relevant would be facilitated (MacCaslin, Wodinsky and Bitterman, 1952; Perkins, Hersberger and Weyant, 1959; Mackintosh, 1965a).

III   GIBSON AND GIBSON'S THEORY OF PERCEPTUAL DIFFERENTIATION

With the exception of the one- or two-stage Spencian models, which deal with the association between stimuli and instrumental responses, all of the models described in Chapter 6 and at the beginning of Chapter 7 can be classed under the general heading of mediational theories of learning. Against these, Tighe and Tighe (1966) contrast the Gibsons' theory of perceptual differentiation (J. J. Gibson, 1950, 1959, 1960, 1963; E. J. Gibson, 1963, 1965, 1969; Gibson and Gibson, 1955). For both types of theory, discrimination learning consists of passing from the non-utilisation to the utilisation of stimulus variables corresponding to properties of the stimulus-object, present from the beginning of the task, and which the subject's nervous system is sensitive to. For S-R theorists, the properties of the stimulus-objects simply act as possible signals for mediational responses which become the primary determinants of discrimination behaviour – consequently it is the acquisition of mediating responses that has to be studied and interpreted. For the Gibsons, the characteristics of the patterns of stimulation constitute the primary determinants of discrimination responses, and so their interest is focused mainly on the subject's sensitivity to the variety of stimulus variables during the course of learning.

## 1  Outline of the Theory

Perceptual learning in children is seen as obeying the same laws as in adults and is defined as an increase in the ability of the organism to obtain information from his environment, this progress resulting from repeated encounters with the patterns of stimulation which this environment affords. It is postulated that all the information picked up by the receptors is transmitted to the central nervous system, that the degree of maturation of the receptors determines the amount of information collected, but that perceptual learning relates only to the selection made from the mass of information received.

When the perception of a particular stimulus pattern is modified, it does not mean that a new response has been acquired or substituted for another but that one or several higher-order variables have been abstracted, which was not the case before. The change involves the relationship between an organism and its environment and it consists of an increasing specification of the correspondence between percepts and stimulus variables.

E. J. Gibson (1969) distinguishes two main areas of study in perceptual learning, on the one hand those supervening changes that clarify what has been learnt, and on the other the mechanisms which bring about these changes. Reading E. J. Gibson's work, it is immediately apparent that her research activity has been mainly concerned with the first of these.

Development takes place in terms of an increasing refinement of perceptual differentiation; the result of perceptual learning is that the organism now responds in a differential manner to stimulus-patterns to which, formerly, it responded in an undifferentiated manner. Perfect learning would enable the organism to distinguish all possible variables and to respond specifically to each of them. But this increasing specificity, which consists of the establishment of a more and more extensive repertoire of differentiators corresponding to the various stimulus variables, is accompanied by the extraction of relational invariants. A primary generalisation in terms of which an identical response is given to several objects because their differences are not perceived, is succeeded by a secondary generalisation within which a selection takes place in terms of critical and non-critical variables; the variations of the latter, although perceived, are ignored and the identity of the response is related to the value, or the relationship, or the set of values or relationships which remain invariant from one object to another.

The discovery and utilisation of dimensions of differentiation such as size, colour, number of points of inflexion, etc. can be sufficient to judge whether two objects are identical or not, but not to identify them. In order to regroup objects into categories, in order to recognise that a particular object is the one which has been seen before or that it belongs to a specific category of objects – chairs or letter A's, for example – it is necessary to establish what it is that remains invariant in all chairs or all letter A's and which, at the same time, is quite distinct from what characterises an armchair or a letter B.

Complex objects are identified by means of the presence of critical differences. Within a particular set of objects, the letters of the alphabet for example, it is possible to establish a list of distinctive features such that each object within the set can be distinguished from the others without ambiguity, because of the unique set of values which characterise it on the list. The concept of the distinctive feature is borrowed from Jakobson and Halle (1956), who had applied it to speech phonemes. A distinctive feature is a bipolar dimension on which each object of the set in question is affected by one or the other value. The list of distinctive features is built up in such a way that their number is the smallest possible and so that none of the objects in the set has the same values as another on *all* dimensions; particular values on particular dimensions are common to several objects. The bipolarity of a distinctive feature is determined by the presence or absence of a quality or even by opposite values on a single dimension. The description of an object in terms of distinctive features is a kind of coding of the object which is used not to describe its objective properties in terms of the absolute value of each of them, but to define it on the basis of what permits it to be differentiated from the others. A distinctive feature is thus, above all, relational – furthermore it remains invariant across certain transformations such as the stress or tone of voice in the case of phonemes, the size or the style of type-face in the case of printed letters.

The succession of processes which lead to the identification of an object, letter A for example, is as follows. In the first stage there is the learning of the set of letters of the alphabet, the discovery of the dimensions of differentiation, and the determination of those that are critical and those that are not (distortions due to perspective or size, for example). Then a list of distinctive features is established and an invariant corresponding to each one of the letters made up from this list. This list depends on the composition of the set involved during the learning stage; there will not be as many critical dimensions if the set is restricted to six letters as if it comprises all twenty-six letters of the alphabet; if, however, these twenty-six letters have to be learnt at the same time as other forms presented conjointly, then probably other distinctive features would have to be added to the list.

Once learning is finished, the identification of an object constitutes an ordered set of operations (Gibson and Yonas, 1966). To begin with, it is necessary to determine to which set or category the object to be identified belongs, and then to explore sequentially the list of distinctive features relating to this set. This exploration involves a series of ratings made on the basis of a set of standards; when a single object has to be identified, the entire list of features must be checked because only the composite formula of the invariant permits a specific response. But when it is simply a matter of finding, amongst others, the object identical to a model, for example a letter A in a list of letters, each object does not have to be checked against the entire list of features, since it is sufficient to discover a single difference between this object and the model in order to eliminate it and pass on to the next one. The order in which a list of features is scanned is of some importance since, for a given set of objects and in a specific task, certain features are more critical than others. Consequently there are optimal strategies which vary according to the task, the pattern that is being looked for, and the objects amongst which the search must take place.

E. J. Gibson is of the opinion that in the course of learning, the list of distinctive features relative to a particular set develops in a hierarchical fashion by an ordered differentiation and division into stratified categories. An initial critical dimension is abstracted which permits the division of the set into two sub-sets, then another, and so on; at each stage the differentiation becomes finer but only the possession of the complete list of distinctive features and the establishment of the appropriate invariants for each object removes all confusion between the members of the set.

One could reply to Gibson that the identification of an object on the basis of a list of distinctive features assumes a previous decision as to which category the object belongs and, consequently, which list is appropriate; how is the identification of this category made? Although the author does not deal with this problem explicitly, there seems to be no fundamental difference between the identification of objects of a particular category and the identification of several categories of objects. The same principle of ordered differentiation could operate at all levels and the categories of objects be isolated by a succession of hierarchical divisions, proceeding from an initial single category. There is nothing to prevent our assuming that in the visual domain, for example, all perceptual categories are derived from an initial segregation between homogeneous and heterogeneous stimulus-groupings. Research on the neonate (Fantz, 1963, etc.) has demonstrated that they respond to such a dimension of differentiation. For E. J. Gibson, the discovery of a critical dimension is accompanied by an orientation of attention; that is, it makes for a more effective exploration of the environment and is, by this means, conducive to the discovery of other dimensions.

The Gibsons' theory of differentiation predicts that in the course of his development the child is, essentially, going to learn to discover more and more information in his environment and to retain what seems to him most appropriate to the problem he proposes to tackle. The progress observed will thus depend both on a refinement of his ability to differentiate between the stimulus-variables and on a selection of the variables to which he will respond. The specificity of his responses will increase with the number of variables which he is capable of detecting in the flux of stimulation. At the same time he will learn to distinguish, in each situation, those variables which are critical from those which are not, and to respond only to the former.

There is no lack in the literature of examples of the refining of perceptual discrimination by simple repetition of the same task or the same type of task although the responses made are not progressively corrected. Only those investigations carried out by E. J. Gibson and her students will be reported here.

## 2　*The Influence of Repetition on Performance in a Differentiation Task*

Gibson and Gibson (1955) gave children in the age-range 6 to 11 years, as well as adults, thirty non-representational scribbles to identify. The experiment was organised in the following way: one of the figures was presented on its own for a period of five seconds, then removed; the subject was then given a pack of 34 figures containing 4 reproductions of the standard and 30 other scribbles; he looked at each one of them for three seconds and said whether or not it was identical to the standard. When the 34 cards had been scrutinised in this fashion, the standard was re-presented and a new series of 34 figures examined, and so on. Amongst the figures, 12 differed from the standard on a number of dimensions and so were easy, 17 others closely resembled the standard from which they could differ along three dimensions: the number of whirls (3 values), the degree of horizontal compression (3 values), and the orientation (2 values). (Fig. 38.)

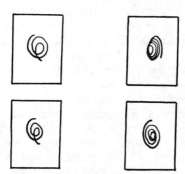

Fig. 38. Examples of the forms which had to be discriminated (Gibson and Gibson, 1955).

At the beginning of the task the youngest children identified 13 of the 17 difficult scribbles as being the same as the standard, whilst in the adults' case there was an average of only three confusions on these same figures. With all the subjects, and despite the fact that their responses were not corrected, the number of confusions diminished from series to series, and the older the subject the quicker this was. Thus learning took place together with a refinement in discrimination. However, this was limited and slow in the youngest subjects, only two out of ten attaining a perfect criterion of identification; after seven series of presentations there were still almost four confusions in one series for the other eight children of the same age. Errors were far from being equally distributed between all the variables; the fewer the number of dimensions on which the variable and the standard differed, the greater the number of errors. Thus, at 8 years, 53 incorrect identifications were recorded when the model and the variable differed on one dimension, 35 when it differed on two dimensions, and 28 when it differed on three.

Gibson and Gibson concluded from this experiment that the repeated perception of a set of figures brings about a refinement of perceptual differentiation and the progressive isolation of the relevant dimensions of differentiation.

### 3 *The Effects of Perceptual Pretraining on Learning Involving Reversal Shift*

The numerous experiments on the effects of overlearning have shown that, as a general rule, it improves the performance of children in a new learning task involving reversal shift (Furth and Youniss, 1964; Youniss and Furth, 1964; L. Tighe and T. Tighe, 1965, 1966). An experiment by L. Tighe (1965) showed that pretraining of a perceptual kind produced the same effect, in an even more distinct fashion. According to Gibson and Gibson's theory of perceptual differentiation (Gibson and Gibson, 1955) the relative facility of learning involving reversal shift or non-reversal shift is determined by the level of perceptual learning attained in the first task. Attainment of a fixed criterion by a subject can correspond to two possible levels of perceptual learning. Either the subject has isolated the relevant dimension of differentiation and discriminates the two objects on the basis of differences on this dimension, independently of the differences they present on other dimensions, or he has not isolated the dimensions of differentiation and discriminates the objects in terms of the combined values of their properties, choosing the 'big white one' as against the 'small black one', for example. Thus the level of perceptual learning determines which property of the stimulus-objects is going to be linked to the reinforcement of the choice response. Consequently, a subject who has isolated the relevant dimension discovers an invariant relationship between one value of this dimension and the reinforcement, whilst a subject who has not abstracted this dimension must learn two relationships, one between each of the objects and the reinforcement. The relative facility of learning tasks involving reversal shift or non-reversal shift, depends therefore on what, for the subject, constitutes the real stimulus, the stimulus-pattern provided by each of the objects or the values on a higher-order variable, the relevant dimension.

Like the mediational theories, the Gibsons' theory of differentiation predicts that everything which reinforces the use of dimensions of differentiation facilitates reversal shift learning. However, whilst the first group of theories relies upon classic concepts of reinforcement, the second assumes that it is sufficient to orient the attention of the subject to the variable dimensions of the stimulus without its being necessary to reward preferentially those responses made as a function of the relevant dimension.

L. Tighe (1965) took a group of a hundred 5- to 6-year-old children, the age-level at which reversal shift and non-reversal shift learning present about equal difficulty (T. Kendler and H. Kendler, 1959). During pretraining each child was asked to give a series of non-reinforced judgments of identity or difference between a standard beaker of a particular brightness and a particular height and beakers of varying height and brightness. Each child compared, successively, four standard beakers with others, some of which were the same height but different brightness (4 values), and some the same brightness but differing in height (4 values), and, finally, some differing in both height and brightness. Pretraining of this kind puts the accent on the independence of the properties of the stimulus-objects and their dimensional character, since the series of variables demonstrates that each property can remain constant whilst the other varies. The author insists on the fact that this pretraining is essentially perceptual, that the responses are not reinforced and so cannot be transformed into mediational responses according to learning theory. A second group of children (the control group) carried out, at the same time, tasks which bore no relation to the test tasks. The latter consisted of an initial discrimination learning task followed by a learning task involving reversal of the criterion for half the subjects and a change of criterion for the other half; the material and the experimental design were analogous to those in the first investigations of Kendler and Kendler (T. Kendler and H. Kendler, 1959). Whilst the subjects in the control group had the same level of performance in both transfer tasks, the children who had had pretraining with the beakers did better on the reversal shift learning task than on the non-reversal shift one. In other words, a relatively brief perceptual pretraining session, of twenty minutes' duration, without verbalisation of the properties – relevant or not – of the objects, was sufficient to induce in children of 5–6 years behaviour which appeared to be characteristic of older children. The discovery and subsequent use of a critical dimension of discrimination can thus be explained other than in terms of the intervention of verbal mediators, that is, simply by means of perceptual training which focuses attention on the independence of the variations of the properties of the material concerned.

## IV  LEARNING A DIMENSION OR LEARNING A PROTOTYPE

Almost all of the theoretical models mentioned so far have postulated that the discovery of the relevant dimension facilitates discrimination learning. However, other models postulate that in the course of discrimination learning the organism constructs increasingly refined categories which ultimately make possible the matching of a given pattern of sensory stimulation with the appropriate category (Bruner, 1958). The immediately perceived differences between the objects to be discriminated serve to construct appropriate categories. A category is always representational by nature and three levels of representation can be distinguished: *enactive, iconic* and *symbolic* (Bruner, 1966a). In enactive representation, a pattern of activity is organised sequentially in terms of a schema, the unfolding of which is controlled by sensori-motor feedback; at this level the object is recognised by the activity it invokes. The orientation reflex of Sokolov (1963) could be an enactive representation (Bruner 1966a). This form of representation would be based on the learning of responses and the formation of habits (Bruner, 1966b). Iconic representation would not mirror reality, but would be selective, although not in an arbitrary fashion; it would be regulated principally by the laws of perceptual organisation such as those expounded by the Gestalt theorists and interpreted by Attneave (1954) within the framework of information theory. Symbolic representation would always result from a coding process which would transform the object (in the widest sense of that term) to be represented. In its three forms, the purpose of representation is always to conserve past experience by means of a model; the formation of categories conforms to the laws of information storage, and the act of identification depends on the information stored within this model. A category is thus always the result of the individual operating on the information which his environment has made available to him through sensory channels; it is not discovered but invented, and if the categories employed differ very little from one individual to another of the same species, the same age and the same period in history, it is because these individuals possess the same sensory receptor system and live within the same physical and cultural environment.

The process of discrimination itself does not appear to interest Bruner; it would seem that, for him, discriminability stems from a difference between patterns of sensory excitation and that, apart from exceptional cases, these patterns always differ in one way or another. Every perceptual judgment, whether it is a matter of deciding if two objects are identical or different, or if one is an apple and the other a square, is based on a selection between those variations which are relevant and those which are not. Furthermore, to perceive an object is above all to identify it, to place it in a category. Even a process as simple as the segregation between figure and ground can be considered as the separation of the effective stimuli into two perceptual categories, figure and ground; the existence of events, objects and sensations which are totally unclassifiable is considered by Bruner to be extremely doubtful.

It is to other investigators that we owe an experimental confrontation between both types of models: that is, the abstraction of the relevant dimension or the construction of prototypes. An experiment involving learning transfer (A. Pick, 1965, experiment I) was carried out with 5-year-old children and using forms resembling letters of the alphabet. The set of forms comprised six standards and their six transformations; these transformations involved the alteration of one or two straight lines into curved ones, a change in size, a mirror-image reversal, a 45° rotation, and a transformation of perspective (fig. 39). In a first task, all the children learnt by reinforced trial and error to match three standards perfectly with their replicas, presented at the same time as three of their transformations. The transfer task was analogous to the initial learning task, but the drawings presented were different and no correction of responses

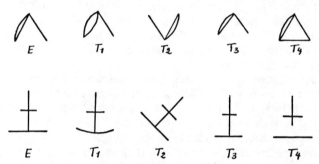

Fig. 39. Examples of letter-like forms (Gibson, Gibson, Pick and Osser, 1962).

E=standard; $T_1$=transformation of a straight line into a curved one; $T_2$=rotation; $T_3$=transformation of perspective: in space or through a plane; $T_4$=topological transformation: closed, broken.

was given. In this transfer task, the children were divided into three groups. Group $E_1$ received the same standards as during initial learning but the variables involved other transformations (for example, reversal, rotation and perspective if the initial learning task had involved a change from a straight to a curved line and a change in size). Group $E_2$ had three standards other than those used in initial learning but the variables involved the same transformations. Control group C had three standards and variables constructed according to three transformations, both differing from those which had been seen during learning.

If, during the first stage, the child had learnt to identify the standards and to recognise them amongst the variables because he had progressively constructed a representative schema for each of the standards, then group $E_1$ should have had a superior performance in the second task to group $E_2$. Furthermore, since the standards in group $E_1$ were the same in the transfer task, the same schemas could be utilised, whilst group $E_2$, who had different standards, would have to construct new schemas.

However, if the child learnt to discriminate objects by discovering which dimensions of differentiation were relevant, transfer would be easier for group $E_2$, for whom the same transformations were applied to the new standards, than for group $E_1$, who had to discover the new transformations applied to the same standards.

The results showed a definite superiority for group $E_2$ with only 39 errors, as against 69 in group $E_1$. But both experimental groups were superior to the control group, who made a total of 101 errors.

Thus familiarity with objects helps in their discrimination from other objects, but it is even more useful to know which dimensions are relevant for discrimination. This superiority of the dimensions of differentiation over the image, the schema, of an object, seems quite clear, particularly when the objects to be discriminated or recognised are presented simultaneously.

Subsequent investigations have shown that the role of the schema is greater to the extent that there is more reliance on memory. In a further experiment, A. Pick used the same material of letter-like forms and brought in the tactile modality.

This experiment (A. Pick, 1965, experiment II) replicated the preceding one as far as possible but with reference to tactile-kinaesthetic perception. The material consisted of forms made of metal, resembling letters of the alphabet; it was composed of four standard forms and their ten transformations (three changes from a straight to a curved line, two topological transformations, one change in size, one right-left reversal, two rotations of 45° and 90°, and one transformation of perspective). During pretraining the child, his eyes covered, felt one of the standard forms with his preferred hand and then, with the same hand, one of its transformations, following which he had to say whether the two objects were the same or different; then he compared a second pair of forms and so on. In this way one standard was presented successively with five of its transformations and two replicas, the responses were corrected, and the series of seven comparisons repeated until the criterion of perfect learning was attained with the exception that an error on the transformations of perspective or size was allowed. Each standard was learnt in turn, by this procedure.

The transfer tasks were the same as in the preceding experiment (A. Pick, 1965, experiment I) and the subjects were divided into three groups according to whether they were given the same standards with different transformations (group $E_1$), different standards with the same transformations (group $E_2$), or different standards and different transformations (group C). The children concerned were from 6 to 7 years old.

Group C had, as in the visual condition, an inferior performance to those of groups $E_1$ and $E_2$, but the performances of these two groups were equivalent. The results of the two experiments are thus not in perfect agreement. However, in going from one to the other it was not only the sensory modality that was changed, but also the experimental procedure itself. In the visual condition (experiment I), the forms to be compared were presented simultaneously; in the tactile condition (experiment II), the comparison between a standard and a variable was always successive. In order to decide whether the change in performance was due to the use of another sensory modality or to the change from a simultaneous to a successive comparison, A. Pick repeated experiment II, asking the child to feel the standard in one hand and the variable in the other; in this condition group $E_2$ produced better results in the test task than $E_1$ and C groups. A. Pick concluded that the discovery of the relevant dimension of differentiation was only more effective than learning a schema, model or prototype in the case where the objects were seen or felt simultaneously. The efficacy of the schema compared with the dimensions of differentiation would thus be greater when there was more reliance on memory.

Still with the same material, A. Pick (A. Pick, H. Pick and Thomas, 1966) compared the capacity for intermodal transfer in the various experimental groups $E_1$, $E_2$ and C. Some results were clear; thus the visual perceptual learning of the test task was more rapid for the two groups $E_1$ and $E_2$ when it had been preceded by an initial learning in terms of tactile perception, than when there had been no pretraining; however, only group $E_2$ learnt a tactile discrimination more easily when they had had visual perceptual pretraining. In other words, there was intermodal transfer in both directions for those subjects who had learnt the relevant dimensions of differentiation in the first task. There was intermodal transfer from the tactile to the visual for those subjects who had learnt the schema of the standard objects. Since we know that tactile learning is slow and difficult to acquire, it is permissible to hypothesise that a longer time is necessary in order to construct a schema than to discover the dimensions of differentiation, at least with this material and with these dimensions of differentiation; the schema would not have long enough to develop during a rapid visual pretraining as it would have in the course of a long tactile pretraining.

Some of the data from transfer tasks involving extra- or intradimensional shift can be understood in this way. Thus, in the experiment by Dickerson (1966), the objects used in the initial learning appeared again in the reversal shift task (R), whilst new objects were presented in the tasks involving intra-dimensional (ID) or extra-dimensional (ED) shift (see pp. 156–158). If the degree of familiarity with the objects to be discriminated was relevant, one would expect that the second learning would be acquired more quickly by group R than by group ID, but in fact the difference in performance between the two groups was not significant.

In a more complex association learning experiment, it was groups R and ED which had the same objects in the two successive learning tasks, whilst group ID saw different objects in the second learning task (Furth and Youniss, 1964; Youniss and Furth, 1964). On this occasion the performance of this last group was superior to that of the other two, which were equivalent. Here, too, a previous familiarisation with the stimulus-objects did not facilitate discrimination learning.

However, it must be pointed out that, in the two examples given, either the same choice-responses had to be given successively to different objects (group ED of Furth and Youniss) or different choice-responses given to the same objects (groups R of Dickerson and of Furth and Youniss). The difficulty introduced by modifying the relationship between the stimulus and the choice response could thus be sufficient to compensate, or even exceed, the facilitation provided by experience of the objects.

# Chapter 8

# The Emergence of Differentiators

The experimental data provided by studies of discrimination learning in children have shown that, whatever the theoretical model to which such studies refer in order to account for the process of acquisition, all research workers agree in recognising that the abstraction of the dimensions of differentiation and the selection of these as organisational elements of the system of choice responses are the major factors in the process. From the developmental point of view, it is evident that the older the child the greater the use of differentiators, and that the point at which a differentiator corresponding to a physical dimension of differentiation makes its appearance is far from being the same for all of these dimensions.

## I DATA CONCERNING THE ORDER OF APPEARANCE OF DIFFERENTIATORS

### 1 Data from Discrimination Learning Experiments

Two-stage models, such as that of Kendler and Kendler (1959, 1963, 1969) or that of E. J. Gibson (1963, 1969), postulate that discrimination learning consists, above all, of learning which dimension of differentiation is relevant, and only then which value on this dimension is the positive one. In terms of these models, the maintenance of the same relevant dimension from one learning to another must advantage this second learning. On this basis it is assumed that when a subject acquires a learning involving an intra-dimensional shift (R or ID) more rapidly than an analogous learning involving an extra-dimensional shift (NR or ED), it is because this subject has organised his responses as a function of the dimensions of differentiation entailed in the experimental task and thus possesses corresponding differentiators. On the other hand, when a second learning involving extra-dimensional shift (NR or ED) is acquired equally, or more rapidly than one involving intra-dimensional shift

(R or ID), it is assumed either that he has learnt in a non-selective fashion forming simple S-R associations (Spence, 1936; Kendler and Kendler, 1959, 1962, 1969) or that he does not yet possess a differentiator corresponding to the physical dimension of differentiation concerned.

The precise determination of an age-level below which one could demonstrate that children do not learn by initially abstracting dimensions of differentiation would seem to be impossible in practice, whether this be with the classic learning technique of extra- or intra-dimensional shift or with that of optional shift. The youngest children examined have been at least three years old and it was by extrapolating the curve of development, constructed on the basis of results obtained with older children, that Kendler and Kendler (1969) placed the beginning of the capacity to respond in terms of dimensions of differentiation at 2 years.

In the first investigations the dividing line appeared to be situated between 5 and 7 years; before 5 years of age reversal learning was slower than non-reversal learning; after the age of 7 years it was more rapid, indicating the utilisation of dimensions of differentiation (T. Kendler and H. Kendler, 1959; T. Kendler, H. Kendler and Wells, 1960; L. Tighe, 1965, etc.). All of these investigators have in common the use of such dimensions as size (big or small) and brightness (black or white) and the cessation of the first learning as soon as the criterion is attained. However, it is only necessary to use other dimensions, to increase overlearning trials, or to introduce perceptual pretraining, in order to lower the age at which reversal shift learning (R) becomes more rapid than extra-dimensional shift learning (NR). Thus, using the dimensions of size and brightness, the superiority of R over NR appears between 6 and 7 years following overlearning (L. Tighe and T. Tighe, 1965), and as early as the age of 5 years following perceptual pretraining (L. Tighe, 1965). Although in the experiment of T. Kendler and H. Kendler (1959) the performances obtained on the dimensions of brightness and size were not different in terms of statistical significance, an examination of the results (T. Kendler and H. Kendler, 1959, table 1, p. 58) seems to suggest that reversal shift learning was more difficult – and thus more slowly acquired – for size than for brightness. For the dimensions of form and colour, reversal shift learning is easier than that involving extra-dimensional shift as early as the age of 5 years, without overlearning (Dickerson, 1966). In an optional shift experiment children of 3 years all selected the reversal R, without overlearning, when the relevant dimension was the thickness of the stimulus objects; when the relevant dimension was the orientation (vertical or horizontal) of stripes, the preference for an R response was shown only in 4-year-old children, and then only following overlearning (L. Tighe and T. Tighe, 1965).

## 2 Data from Comparison Experiments: Detection and Differentiation

A personal investigation (Vurpillot, 1969b), involving children from $4\frac{1}{2}$ to $7\frac{1}{2}$ years, compared differences of four types from the point of view of their relative difficulty of detection. The task was not one of identification, nor one of differentiation by judgment of identity or difference, but of detection: the child was told that there were differences between two objects and was simply asked to indicate them. The experimental task was derived from the seven errors puzzle, well known to readers of a certain daily newspaper;[1] it involved presenting the child with a pair of drawings, one of which was a modified version of the other in certain details. Most of the details in this modified version remained invariant but four of them were altered. The four types of transformation studied were the following: *presence-absence* – a detail present in one drawing was suppressed or absent in the other; *size transformation* – one detail half the size it was in the other; *displacement* or *change of position* – one part was displaced, either by a 45° rotation or by being moved a few centimetres. In the transformations of size and position the form of the part concerned remained invariant. The fourth type of transformation did involve a change of form although the modified part retained a broad categorial identity: the full moon became a crescent moon, a steam-ship a sailing-ship, a round balloon an oval balloon, etc. Experiment I was designed in such a way that each particular model gave rise to four derived versions, each variable part demonstrating the four transformations so that the four types of difference (one for each variable part) were simultaneously present in one pair of pictures (fig. 40). The requirements of the design made it necessary to divide the subjects into four sub-groups in order that each child saw each model only once. The relative difficulty of detecting the various transformations was measured by the number of omissions (differences not reported) and by the order in which the differences were mentioned. As early as $4\frac{1}{2}$ years, suppressions and changes of form were almost all detected and were also the first to be mentioned; it was only at $7\frac{1}{2}$ years that the differences in size were discovered as often as the suppressions and changes in form, but even then they were detected after the latter. Finally, at all ages, differences of displacement took the longest to detect and this category also gave rise to the largest number of omissions (fig. 41). The ascending order

---

[1]*Translator's note.* The newspaper in question is the popular *France Soir.*

of difficulty was thus established as follows: the easiest transformations to detect were the suppressions and changes of form, next came differences of size, and finally those of position.

A second experiment of the same type (Vurpillot, 1969b) seems to indicate that the localisation of the transformed parts – on the contour or in the interior of the picture – interacts with the type

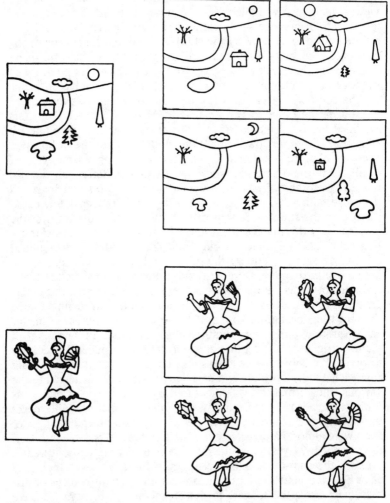

Fig. 40. Examples of the material used in experiment I (Vurpillot, 1969b).

Two models and the four drawings derived from them. The actual size of the cards on which the pictures were drawn was 10cm×10cm.

of transformation in determining the relative difficulty of detecting the differences. On all occasions the comparison involved two pictures, one of which differed from the other on four points; in any given pair the four differences were of the same type and of the transformed parts two were on the contour and the other two in the interior (fig. 42). In the case of any one model, a particular variable part – with the same transformation – appeared on the contour of

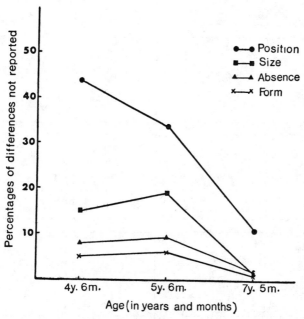

Fig. 41. Number of omissions as a function of the type of differences and the age of the children. Experiment I (Vurpillot, 1969b).

one derived picture and in the interior of another. As in the preceding experiment, the division of the children into four sub-groups meant that each of them only compared one model with one of its derived versions and had to detect the same number of differences of each type. It seemed that situating the variable part on the contour made its discovery more likely and that this effect, very slight at $4\frac{1}{2}$ years, was increasingly manifest with age. But the interaction of type of transformation and the internal or external location of the part concerned was not equivalent. A 'suppression' difference was always detected sooner when it was situated on the contour than when it was in the interior of the picture, and this effect manifested itself as early as $4\frac{1}{2}$ years. The facilitating effect of localisation on the contour was only apparent at $5\frac{1}{2}$ years for changes of form and not until $7\frac{1}{2}$ years for changes in size and position.

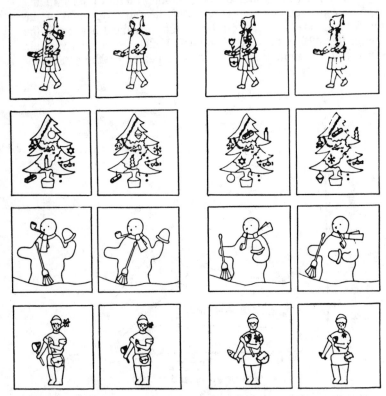

Fig. 42. Examples of material used in experiment II (Vurpillot, 1969b).

In each row there are two models together with one of their derivations. The transformations involved in going from a model to its derivative are: suppressions (row 1); changes of form (row 2); displacements (row 3); or changes in size (row 4). Each card was 10cm×10cm.

The nature of the differences introduced into the material produced a similar effect in the tasks of simple perceptual differentiation as in the tasks involving the detection of differences. In a third experiment (Vurpillot, 1969a) pairs of pictures were made up from the material in experiment II, either a model and its replica (identical pairs), or a model and one of its transformations (differing pairs). The pairs were presented one at a time to children from $3\frac{1}{2}$ to $6\frac{1}{2}$ years of age, who had to judge whether the two pictures were identical or different. The number of correct judgments involving differing pairs was always less when the differences were the consequence of a displacement or a change in size of a part than when they were a result of a suppression or change in form. Since the different types of transformation were applied to different parts of different models, the results of this last experiment – which was designed to verify other hypotheses – are only quoted as tentative evidence.

Table 16    *Number of differences detected early (1 and 2), late (3 and 4), and not detected (Om) as a function of age and situation in relation to the contour*

| | Age (in years and months) | | | | | | | | |
|---|---|---|---|---|---|---|---|---|---|
| | 4y. 6m. | | | 5y. 6m. | | | 7y. 5m. | | |
| Order of detection | 1 and 2 | 3 and 4 | Om | 1 and 2 | 3 and 4 | Om | 1 and 2 | 3 and 4 | Om |
| On the contour | 169 | 109 | 42 | 174 | 110 | 36 | 178 | 139 | 3 |
| In the interior | 145 | 125 | 50 | 144 | 138 | 38 | 142 | 171 | 7 |

The results are expressed in raw figures, based on 640 differences per age-level (320 on the contour, 320 in the interior). Each child had to find the differences in four pairs of pictures; in each pair there were four differences, two situated on the contour, two in the interior of the picture (after Vurpillot, 1969b).

All we need note is that although there were always four trans-formed parts in moving from a model to its derivative, the youngest children judged these as being the same in 80 per cent of cases when the differences were those of size or position, in 60 per cent of cases when they involved changes of form, and in 40 per cent of cases when suppressions were involved. At the same age-level, per-formances involving differentiation were much inferior to those of detection. In experiment III, once the differentiation task was finished, we asked the children to have another look for differences in the differing pairs; at 3 years 8 months the children showed them-selves capable of indicating at least one difference in 85 per cent of cases. It would seem, therefore, that in a differentiation task the poor performance observed cannot be ascribed solely to the absence of adequate differentiators.

A well-known study by Gibson, Gibson, Pick and Osser (1962) provides precise information on the relative difficulty of perception of different spatial transformations applied to geometric forms. Each model was somewhat similar to a capital letter and gave rise to twelve derived forms of which three showed different degrees of transformation from rectilinear to curvilinear, five transformations by rotation or mirror-image reproduction. two transformations of

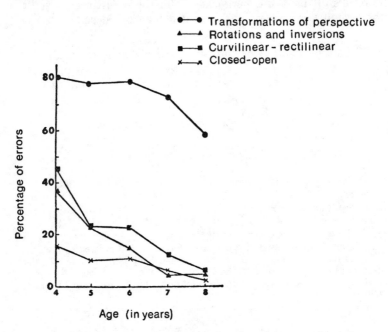

Fig. 43. Evolution with age of errors as a function of the type of transformation (Gibson, Gibson, Pick and Osser, 1962).

perspective, and two topological transformations – open and closed (see fig. 39). The task consisted of finding the forms identical to the model from amongst its twelve transformations. The transformations of perspective were, at all ages, by far the most difficult to detect; even at 8 years, 60 per cent of errors resulted from a confusion between the model and one of its transformations of perspective, whilst at the same age there were fewer than 10 per cent confusions with each of the other types of transformation. At 4 years topological transformations were quite clearly the most easily perceived (only 15 per cent confusions); from 4 to 7 years confusions between a model and its transformations from straight to curved remained distinctly more frequent than those between a model and its open/closed transformation (fig. 43). However, it must be added that in the case of transformations of the curvilinear-rectilinear type, the number of parts transformed, which varied from 1 to 3, played a very important role. The number of confusions was much less when three rather than one of the lines was changed from straight to curved.

## 3 Data from Choice-preference Investigations

The measurement of children's preferences at different ages for particular dimensions of differentiation in a simple categorisation task is a long-established experimental technique. In the classic procedure, a model drawing is presented at the same time as two other drawings, each one of which differs from the model on one dimension whilst retaining the same value on another. For example, variable A might have the same form but another colour, while variable B might have the same colour but a different form from the model. Asked to indicate which of these is most like the model, the child is obliged to abstract the dimensions of differentiation of the objects, and to make a match as a function of one of them.

Various dimensions have been opposed in this fashion: form, colour and number (Descoeudres, 1914); form, colour and size (Kagan and Lemkin, 1961); and, above all, colour and form (Katz, 1913; Tobie, 1926; Volkelt, 1926; Brian and Goodenough, 1929; Colby and Robertson, 1942; Honkavaara, 1958; Gaines, 1964; Corah, 1964, 1966a, 1966b; Corah and Gross, 1967, etc.). For fifty years or so it has been conventional to say that between 3 and 6 years children are more likely to match the stimulus-objects as a function of their colour, whilst those above 6 years of age prefer to classify them in terms of their form. In fact, even the results of the earliest investigations are much less clear-cut than this generally accepted conclusion would lead one to believe. One point on which almost all the investigations are in agreement is that the number of choices made on the basis of form increases with age, whilst those based on colour diminish. Only Kagan and Lemkin (1961) have failed to find this developmental evolution.

If the number of colour-choices is fewer in older than younger children, it does not follow that the latter systematically use colour in preference to form as a matching principle. When the figures were simple geometric forms such as a square, a triangle, a circle, a diamond, the 3- to 6-year-old children seen by Descoeudres (1914) responded as a function of their colour in 70 per cent of cases, but when representations of familiar objects were involved, then, in 60 per cent of cases choices were made as a function of form. In the experiment by Tobie (1926) the children younger than 3 years 8 months responded randomly, whilst those from 3 years 9 months to 5 years 1 month made their choices on the basis of colour; however, the older the children involved in the experiment, the greater the number of choices based on form. This predominance of choices based on colour has not been replicated in more recent investigations (Corah, 1964, 1966a, b, etc.) where the forms were irregular poly- gons with from five to seven sides, differing from each other only in a small portion of the contour. It must be observed that, with such material, if the child did not explore the whole of the contour, he might perceive the three figures as identical in form so that only the colour would allow him to differentiate them; it would no longer be a matter of a choice between two dimensions, the performance being determined by the extent of perceptual activity and not by a prefer- ence for one dimension over another. With simple geometric forms such as those used by Descoeudres, children younger than 6 years showed a massive preference for matching by form. These results indirectly confirm the view of Descoeudres and Tobie, for whom form could only be predominant in the case of familiar, meaningful objects. If, as these authors thought, simple geometric forms lacked meaning for the children of their generation, it is far from being the case today when educational toys familiarise children with geometric forms almost from the cradle.

If form appears as the preferred dimension as early as 4 years, it is nonetheless possible to increase the number of responses in favour of colour either by increasing the extent of the coloured surface (Corah, 1966a) or by providing a pretraining session before the actual choice problem, in which colour is the only relevant dimension (Corah, 1966b). An analogous pretraining in which form was the relevant dimension did not affect the proportion of form- choices. These results link up with those from learning tasks in- volving intra- or extra-dimensional shift. When a dimension has been utilised by a child for some time and is firmly established, verbalisa- tion and overlearning are without effect (T. Kendler, 1963; Mum- bauer and Odom, 1967), this being the case with form. If, on the other hand, the child can abstract the dimension but has not been able to do so for very long, as in the case of colour (Corah, 1966b; Mumbauer and Odom, 1967), then all the techniques for focusing attention and pretraining favour its utilisation. Finally, when a dimension has not been abstracted, no instruction or pretraining can make it emerge. The random responses of children younger than 3 years 8 months, reported by Tobie (1926), the number of children eliminated in Corah's experiments because they responded to the position of the stimulus-object (in one of the experiments 30 per cent of the subjects) lead one to think that a number of children in the age-range from 3 to 4 years are not yet able to abstract even such fundamental dimensions of differentiation as form or colour.

## II THE INTERPRETATION OF THESE RESULTS

**1** *In Terms of a Relative Dominance of Dimensions of Differentiation*

Some authors do not seem to distinguish between the sensitivity of sensory receptors to particular stimulus variables and the capacity to respond electively to variations of these whilst disregarding the other properties of the stimuli. Thus for Sutherland (1959, 1960b) and Mackintosh (1965b) a subject would possess specialised analysers which would allow him to respond to a certain number of dimensions of the stimulus. In other words, the capacity to respond to certain stimulus variables, or dimensions, is built into the central nervous system.

In order to explain why, within the same individual, performance varies according to the dimension of differentiation involved in a task, this group of researchers employ the concept of *dominance*. Certain dimensions would be preferred to others, attention would be drawn more easily to a preferred or dominant dimension than to another, and the duration of the focusing of attention would be proportional to the degree of dominance (Zeaman and House, 1962; Mackintosh, 1965a).

For others (T. Kendler, Basden and Bruckner, 1970) a single-stage learning model could account for the phenomenon of the relative dominance of dimensions without its being necessary to involve selective attention. The dominance of one dimension would be a function of the psychophysical difference between the values on this dimension taken by the objects which have to be discriminated. For example, in a task where the values of the objects (a circle and a square) are kept constant on the form dimension, the other dimension, brightness, could be dominant when its two values are black and white, but non-dominant when it is a matter of two shades of grey (H. Kendler and T. Kendler, 1969).

Both interpretations predict that a problem will be solved more rapidly when the preferred dimension is also the relevant dimension of differentiation (Zeaman and House, 1962; H. Kendler and T. Kendler, 1969). In the case of transfer tasks, if the dominant dimension is the relevant one in the first learning, a second intra-dimensional learning will be acquired more rapidly than an extra-dimensional one, the opposite being the case if the dominant dimension is not relevant in the first learning. These predictions have been confirmed experimentally (T. Kendler, Basden and Bruckner), which supports one interpretation as much as the other.

**2** *In Terms of the Acquisition of Cognitive Structures*

The experimental evidence shows that before 7 years of age children apparently have available only a limited number of differentiators, and that the younger the child the fewer these are. It does not seem possible to explain this fact in terms of insufficient sensory sensitivity or the absence of adequate nervous structures, such as the analysers of Sutherland (1959). Indeed, well before three years, the age of the youngest subjects employed in reversal or non-reversal shift learning tasks, children are aware of differences in brightness, colour, form, size and orientation (at least between vertical and horizontal). We shall quote just two examples. The first concerns the perception of colours. From birth the child shows a differential behavioural response as a function of the wave-length of light emanating from illuminated screens (Staples, 1932; Chase, 1937); from the age of 2 years he is capable of matching them as a function of their shade (Cook, 1931), but he is manifestly unable (for there are tests that could demonstrate his ability, if it existed) to abstract the property of colour before the age of 3 or 4 years. One has here a very clear example of a physical dimension of differentiation, the variations of which a child is sensitive to at an early age but which he does not use as a differentiator until the end of the third or fourth year. The knowledge of colour names and their employment in composite terms such as 'the red ring' or 'the blue dress' comes long before the capacity for abstracting a colour and responding solely as a function of that. Thus it is a matter neither of sensory incapacity nor of inadequate vocabulary.

The second example is drawn from experiments concerned with the displacement of parts of a figure (Vurpillot and Moal, 1970; Vurpillot, Lécuyer, Moal and Pineau, 1971). In these experiments, 5-year-old children were quite able to see permutations involving two of the windows of a house or two parts of a configuration, comment on them, and at the same time conclude that, nonetheless, the house or the configuration had not been changed. The difference of localisation was perceived but not utilised in making the judgment of identity. All this occurs as if, on the basis of differences which have been perceived for a long time, the child only slowly constructs a repertoire of differentiators – and, furthermore, only beyond a certain age. Although the majority of the differences may be perceptible from earliest infancy, some of these become differentiators much earlier than others. The use of terms such as 'preference' or 'dominance' is limited to the descriptive level. E. J. Gibson (1965) offers an explanation which appears to account for the greater part of the available data.

All the variations of stimulation to which the sensory receptors are sensitive can give rise to the construction of differentiators. The order in which they emerge is not so much a function of the greater or lesser sensitivity of the receptors to the physical variables of stimulation as a selection from amongst the information available. Even more limited than the adult in his capacities for processing this information (Santa Barbara and Paré, 1965), the child retains as differentiators only those transformations which are critical for what interests him. At 4 years his interest centres on objects; transformations of perspective, rotations and inversions do not modify the object but only its spatial relationships vis-à-vis the subject or other objects, and so are tolerated. Only the change from open to closed, from unity to incompleteness, affects the integrity of the object itself and is thus, even at this age, treated as a differentiator. As the child grows older and receives formal education, adaptation to the demands of the environment leads him to take account of more subtle modifications, such as the change from a rectilinear to a curvilinear contour. Only transformations of perspective are still tolerated since these do not conflict with the differentiation of objects, and are the only ones compatible with maintaining the invariance of a rigid object in Euclidean space (J. Gibson, 1966). The progress observed with age is not due to the appearance of a capacity to discriminate, but rather to an evolution of the decision criteria and of the capacities for abstraction.

CONCLUSION OF CHAPTERS 6, 7 AND 8

The results obtained in discrimination learning tasks with children seem to show remarkable agreement with results from classic perceptual identification tasks, such as those described in Chapter 5. Just as the very young child shows himself extremely inept at analysing a perceptual structure into separate parts and establishing a network of relationships between a whole and its parts, so too he shows himself incapable of extracting one property from several objects and of responding exclusively in terms of values on it. Before the age of 2 years the child possesses rigid perceptual structures which cannot be analysed in terms of their properties. After this age he has the capacity to take account of a property common to several objects and to judge these on the basis of its values. But this capacity, very limited at the beginning, is only gradually applied to the multiple dimensions of variation to which the nervous system is sensitive. A number of factors would be likely to bring about the behavioural expression of the operation of differentiators; these are, for example, the repetition of the task (overlearning), the verbalisation of the relevant dimension, and so on. It is clear that the outcome of the responses is a determining factor in the acquisition of choice-responses, whatever the age of the subject or the species to which he belongs. However, this outcome is not indispensable, since repeated presentations of objects to a subject, without reinforcement, bring about the same effect (J. Gibson and E. Gibson, 1955; L. Tighe, 1965). The repetition of the trials, the rewards given during the course of the learning tasks only facilitate the mobilisation of those differentiators which the child already possesses. But only a new, poorly-consolidated differentiator appears to be susceptible to overlearning and to verbalisation (H. Kendler and T. Kendler, 1961; T. Kendler, H. Kendler and Learnard, 1962; Mumbauer and Odom, 1967). In the case where a differentiator is not yet part of the child's repertoire, no purpose is served by increasing the number of trials; in this instance learning shows itself to be incapable of bringing about the emergence of a new differentiator, at least in the laboratory. Finally, overlearning is also without effect when the differentiator corresponding to the relevant dimension is firmly established.

Attaching a response to that part of a stimulus which alone provides the critical information for the differentiation in question is universally recognised as a determinant of discrimination learning. There is continuing controversy in the opposition of additive theories which establish a link between a choice-response and a stimulus enricher by the addition of an implicit response, and subtractive theories for which the link is between a stimulus reduced to the relevant information alone and the choice-response. If we take account of the fact that both lead to almost the same predictions, it would seem impossible to decide which one is right.

The role of language has been emphasised by T. Kendler and Spiker. For the former implicit verbal responses play a mediational role and entail the utilisation of dimensions of differentiation; for the latter they increase or diminish the discriminability of the stimulus. There is a significant amount of data in support of the influence of language, but some of the results obtained resist explanation in such terms.

First of all, it must not be forgotten that, even if language can facilitate learning, it is far from being indispensable, since very young children and animals also learn to identify objects and to make appropriate responses to them.

One fact, which is borne out by many observations that have been made relating to tasks of perceptual differentiation, appears to be even more significant – namely, that the child possesses a rich and varied language long before he utilises verbal mediators. T. S. Kendler herself draws attention to this (Kendler, 1963) when she postulates the existence of three levels of language interaction in R and NR learning: a first level before the age of $4\frac{1}{2}$ years where the child does not utilise implicit verbal responses; a second level at which, whilst possessing implicit verbal responses, the child does not use them for the mediation of his responses; and, finally, a level at which verbal mediation plays an essential role.

As for verbal labels, Cantor (1965) comments that it is hardly ever possible, in experiments concerned with the acquired distinctiveness of cues, to attribute the observed effects to the intervention of language alone. By giving the same name to a number of objects, attention is drawn to what they have in common· equally, by giving them different names one invites the child to look for the way in which they differ. A relevant verbalisation would seem to be a particularly powerful factor in mobilising attention as well as a means of coding the information contained in the stimulus. The capacity for coding would appear to depend above all on the level of the child's development, whilst the focusing of attention is more sensitive to factors in the learning situation itself. The way in which the learning is acquired (number of attempts, value of the reward, etc.) determines what receives attention and the intensity of this attention. The focusing of attention at the end of an initial learning phase determines an attitude, or 'set', in the subject, and in consequence facilitates the acquisition of a second learning to a greater or lesser extent.

*The figures and tables in Part Two have been reproduced with the kind permission of the following authors and publishers:*

Fig. 33      Dickerson, D. J. *Psychonomic Science*, 1966, **4**, pp. 417–418.

Fig. 37      Sutherland, N. S. 'Theories of shape discrimination in *Octopus*', *Nature*, London, 1960b, **186**, pp. 840–844.

Fig. 38      Gibson, J. J. and Gibson, E. J. 'Perceptual learning: differentiation or enrichment?', *Psychological Review*, American Psychological Association, 1955, **62**, pp. 32–41, fig. 1.

Figs 39 and 43      Gibson, E. J., Gibson, J. J., Pick, A. D. and Osser, H. 'A developmental study of the discrimination of letter-like forms', *Journal of Comparative and Physiological Psychology*, American Psychological Association, 1962, **55**, pp. 887–906, figs 1 and 4.

Figs 40, 41 and 42      Vurpillot, E. *Enfance*, 1969, **22**, pp. 152, 159.

Tables 13 and 14      Kendler, T. S. 'Development of mediating responses in children', in: J. C. Wright and J. Kagan (eds), 'Basic cognitive processes in children', *Monographs of the Society* for Research in Child Development, 1963, **28**, Ser. 86, Table 1, p. 39, table 2, p. 43.

Table 15   Norcross, K. J. *Journal of Experimental Psychology*, 1958, **56**, p. 305.

Table 16   Vurpillot, E. *Enfance*, 1969, **22**, p. 160.

# PART THREE

## Strategies of Exploration and Criteria of Judgment

# Chapter 9

# An Examination of Some Parameters of Visuo-Motor Exploration

The superabundance of the physical world and the limited capacity of our sensory receptors continually impose on us the need to make a choice from amongst all the information available. We can take in no more than a modest proportion of this information and it is only by the displacement of our receptors that we can compensate, to a certain extent, for these limits. Consequently, exploratory activity would appear to be one of the essential factors in an individual's getting to know his environment. This exploration has two main functions, firstly, to gather information and secondly, to establish relationships between the units of information obtained. Because of this, many authors have seen perceptual activity as crucial in the ontogenesis of perceptual and representational structures (Hebb, 1949; Piaget, 1961; Wekker, 1966; Zaporozhets and Zinchenko, 1966; Leontiev and Gippenreiter, 1966; etc.).

Perceptual exploration takes place in all the sensory modalities, although its extent and plasticity vary enormously from one modality to another. In the areas of olfaction and audition, exploration is limited in man to an orientation of the head to the stimulus source. In the tactile and visual modalities, a developmental evolution can be seen. By taking all objects to his mouth the baby shows that oral exploration in the form of sucking, licking, biting and even eating is his first way of getting to know things around him. This stage is succeeded by a tactile-kinaesthetic type of exploration: objects are then felt, squeezed, banged, put into piles, placed one inside the other, and so on; this new mode of cognition favours the establishment of topological relationships between objects. Finally, visual exploration, present from birth, becomes predominant. The primacy of the tactile-kinaesthetic over the visual modality is postulated by a number of authors (Renshaw, 1930; Birch, 1962; Birch and Lefford, 1963; Hermelin and O'Connor, 1961, 1964; S. White, 1964, 1965) for whom the behaviour of children is organised initially around proximal receptors (tactile, kinaesthetic, proprioceptive, visceral), then, between 5 and 7 years, becomes more dependent on distal receptors (visual and auditory). The arguments put forward by these and others in support of this hypothesis are very limited. We know from the study of surviving premature babies (Hooker, 1936, 1954; Thompson, 1952), that the response to tactile stimulation is clearly manifested earlier than the response to visual or auditory stimulation. Wolff (1963) has demonstrated that the smiling response can be activated by touching the baby's cheek, before the sight of a person or an object has this effect. It also seems to be the case that, when placed in a play situation, the child from 2 to 4 years devotes more of his time to manipulating objects than to looking at them (Zaporozhets, 1961; Schopler, 1964). The tactile-kinaesthetic modality thus appears to mature earlier and to be utilised preferentially by very young children.

The predominant role played by the visual modality in the adult's and the older child's apprehension of the physical world, largely explains the abundance of experimental data relating to visual perceptual exploratory activity, the relative poverty of data relating to tactile, manual exploration, and the absence of studies on oral or auditory exploration. However, the small number of investigations which have been undertaken in the tactile-kinaesthetic area demonstrate the common character of tactile and visual exploration, from the point of view of their developmental evolution. Furthermore, on the basis of investigations carried out in the area of visual perception, it is possible to describe certain characteristics of perceptual exploration independent of the modality involved, and to relate these to the development of the child.

It would seem likely that the perceptual exploratory activity of an individual would reveal what information had been considered sufficiently important to be retained from amongst the mass of potential information, in preference to the rest. The selection from this potential information is both quantitative and qualitative. The number of displacements of the sensory receptor and the surface area of the part explored, provide an estimate of the amount of information obtained. The selection of those parts which are fixated shows the preference in qualitative terms. The sequence of the points explored reflects, in general terms, a strategy of information-search and makes it possible to determine which parts of the stimulus the individual has selected to structure, and according to what plans, what programme of action, he has ordered his exploration. Finally, the duration of a fixation on a point in space corresponds to the time the observer needs to register the information contained in the area fixated.

In visual terms, visuo-motor activity is made up of a succession of eye-movements and pauses or visual fixations. Although it is open to question (Uttal and Smith, 1968), it is usually assumed that afferent messages are inhibited during the displacement of the eye and that perception only takes place during visual fixations. Consequently, the investigations which have been carried out concern themselves only with the information obtained from the localisation of visual fixations; the information which could have been registered visually in the course of displacement is considered as nil or at least negligible.

## I THE EXTENT OF THE EXPLORATION

During the visual scanning of an object, the stimuli issuing from a more or less extensive area of this object excite the subject's receptors and we can say that the object has been partially or completely seen. Because of the heterogeneity of the retina, inspection has extracted from the points fixated – and thus seen in foveal vision – information that is richer and more precise than would have been encountered by peripheral vision alone. As a general rule the extent of visuo-motor exploration is measured by the number of separate fixations and the surface-area in which they are located. But the calculation of the number and location of visual fixations are the only objective data available, and the estimates drawn from these as to the amount of information obtained remain very approximate, insofar as the contribution of peripheral vision to this information-collection is ignored.

The recording of the visuo-motor activity of children is a fairly recent innovation, and the amount of data is as yet rather limited. However, all studies show that this activity becomes, with age, more extensive, more precise and more systematic.

## 1 *Spontaneous Visual Exploration in Familiarisation and Recognition Tasks*

It is to Russian psychologists (Zinchenko, Van Chizi-Tsin and Tarakanov, 1962; Zaporozhets and Zinchenko, 1966) that we owe the first attempts at recording eye movements in children from 3 to 6 years. The children's visuo-motor activity was measured on two tasks, one involving familiarisation, the other recognition of the same objects; systematic differences emerged in the performance of both tasks. The material presented to the children consisted of large line-drawings, asymmetrical and non-representational, 30 cm by 40 cm, adapted from those of Gaydos (1956). For half the subjects, called the 'familiarisation group', the eye-movements were filmed for 20 seconds, at the beginning of the initial presentation of each figure. For the other half, called the 'recognition group', the figures were presented for an initial period but eye-movements were only recorded during the second trial when they were asked to recognise the figure they were shown.

The number of eye-movements and the distribution of the

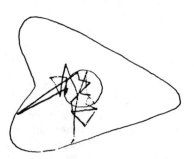

Familiarisation – 3 years

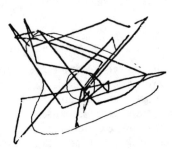

Recognition – 3 years

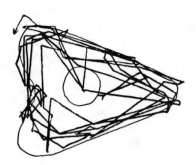

Familiarisation – 6 years

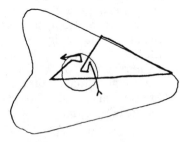

Recognition – 6 years

Fig. 44. Examples of visuo-motor exploration (Zinchenko, Van Chizi-Tsin and Tarakanov, 1962).

The stimulus is drawn in thin lines, the path of visual inspection in thick lines.

The circle in the centre of the stimulus is a hole with the camera lens behind it.

fixations varied with the age of the subject and the task (fig. 44). In the familiarisation task, the 3-year-old children manifested very little activity, visual fixations being in general clustered together in the centre of the figure around the hole which was filled by the lens of the camera. At 4 years of age two sorts of eye-movements were observed: the first, restricted in kind, linked up the fixations which were clustered around the characteristic features of the stimulus such as the centre and the inflexions in the contour; the second, more extensive, went from one extremity to the other and seemed to gauge the surface-area taken up by the figure (Zaporozhets and Zinchenko, 1966). The 5-year-old children performed like the 4-year-olds, except that their examination of the characteristic features was more complete and more systematic. Finally, at 6 years, the path of the eye-movements followed the entire contour in an exhaustive exploration. At the same time as the number of movements increased, so the duration of each visual fixation decreased with age.

On the other hand, in the recognition task, the duration of fixation remained constant from one age-level to another, but the time taken to examine the figure before responding decreased, going from an average of 8 seconds at 3 years, between 4 and 5 seconds at 4 years, and less again at 6 years. The form of the exploration also changed. In the main, the 3-year-old children made large scanning movements which led them outside the contour; those of 4, 5 and 6 years were content to fixate only a certain number of features of the figure, progress being a matter of the more or less adequate choice of the parts fixated.

To summarise: in a familarisation task, exploration is almost nil, or very erratic, in 3-year-olds; 4 years marks the beginning of exploration limited to a few features of the figure, and only after the age of 6 years does the child study the object exhaustively, using a systematic strategy.

## 2   *The Investigation of the Extent of Visual Exploration in a Task of Perceptual Differentiation*

The visuo-motor activity of children has been recorded[1] whilst

[1]The technique of cine-recording the corneal reflection of the stimulus has been described in detail in an article (Vurpillot, 1968); only the essentials are given here. The child is seated on a chair, the height of which can be adjusted, with his head supported on a head-rest, and he is instructed not to move it. Facing him, about 30 cm away, is the stimulus, with a circular hole in the centre and behind this the lens of a television camera. The stimulus is reflected on the subject's cornea in such a way that the part fixated by the eye falls exactly on the centre of the pupil; when the eye is displaced, so also is the centre of the pupil, and thus coincides with a new point of reflection of

comparisons were being made between pictures of houses (Vurpillot, 1968). The stimulus-objects were pairs of houses each of which had six windows; there were three identical pairs of houses and three pairs differing in one, three or five respects (fig. 45). These differences were of the type that we have called 'substitution' (p. 114), that is to say, the contents of a window in one house were absent in the other, their place being taken by different items. The stimulus-objects were distinctly bigger than in the other experiments in which we had used pictures of houses (Vurpillot, 1969a: Vurpillot and Moal, 1970) and the drawings were in white on a black background; the purpose of these characteristics was simply to facilitate the localisation of gaze on the recordings. The instructions were to look at the houses to see if they were exactly the same or not and to give a response immediately a decision was made.

The number of different windows fixated at least once during the exploration of a pair of houses proved to be a good estimate of the amount of information abstracted by the child[1]. The children in the two youngest age-groups, ranging from 3 to 5½ years, looked at essentially the same number of windows, whether identical or differing pairs were involved and whether there were one, three of five differences. Of the twelve windows (six per house), they inspected only six or seven before giving their judgment, whatever this might be. It is thus evident that they made the decision that two houses were the same when they had only looked at half of the windows in them. From the age of 6½ years, the extent of

the stimulus, the one which the subject is now fixating. The TV camera is directed at the left eye of the subject and the picture of this appears on the screen of the monitor; the experimenter can thus constantly regulate the camera so as to keep the eye within the field and within focus despite the slight displacements of the child's head. An ordinary camera situated opposite the monitor screen films the picture at the rate of 7·25 frames per second. The path of inspection during the exploration of a stimulus is reconstructed with the aid of the set of pictures on the film. On each of these the localisation of the visual fixation point is given by the coincidence of the centre of the pupil with a point of reflection of the stimulus. In our investigation we considered it sufficient to record, for each frame, which window was reflected in the centre of the pupil, without taking account of the visual displacements possible within this window. The duration of a fixation was measured by the number of successive frames on which the same window was reflected in the centre of the pupil. The method of recording thus permits the measurement of the number, the duration, the localisation and the sequence of visual fixations.

---

[1]In this experiment, as in the following one, the results were subjected to an analysis of variance, and only those for which Snedecor's F reached a level of at least ·05 are given as significant.

the area explored varied according to the properties of the stimulus; the number of windows fixated was greater for identical pairs than for differing pairs and for pairs with one difference than

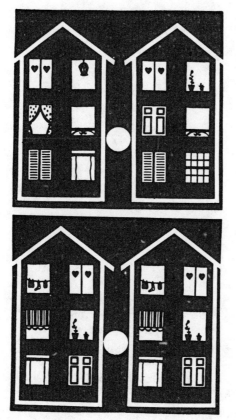

Fig. 45. Examples of the material used in the recording of visuo-motor activity.

*At the top:* pair P3 with three differences. *At the bottom:* an identical pair. The white disc between the two houses represents the hole behind which the lens of the television camera was situated.

for those with three or five differences (fig. 46). The extent of exploration, as far as the last two kinds of pairs were concerned, was essentially the same since, in the case of the pair with three differences, one was located in each row of windows so that the probability of seeing one quickly was almost the same as when the pair differed in five details.

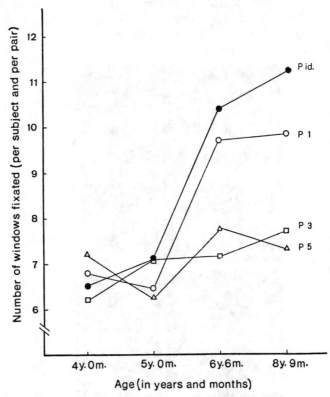

Fig. 46. Evolution with age of the number of windows fixated as a function of the nature of the stimulus.

   P id.=identical pairs; P1=pair with one difference; P3=pair with three differences; P5=pair with five differences.

## 3   *Task Adaptation*

As soon as a task is in progress, even during a short space of time, visual exploration undergoes slight modifications. In the experiment concerned with the recording of eye-movements, the experiment proper was preceded by a short period of familiarisation with both the material and the situation, in the hope that this would overcome any misunderstanding of instructions and reduce the warming-up period. To this end the children were shown, for a fairly long period of time, both a differing and an identical pair – other than the test pairs. No judgment was asked for but the experimenter told the child when the houses were 'exactly the same' and when they were 'not the same'. Despite this preliminary

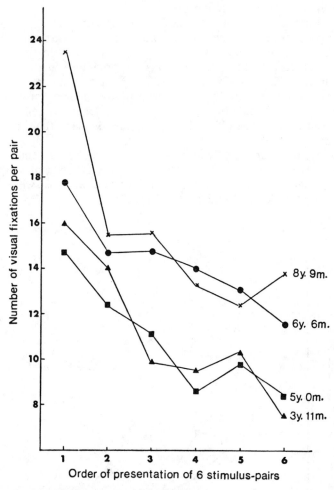

Fig. 47. Evolution, during the course of the experiment, of the number of visual fixations per stimulus-pair.

Each curve corresponds to one age-group; each point on a curve was established on the basis of fifteen measurements, one for each child in the age-group concerned.

familiarisation, at all age-levels it was observed that the time devoted by the child to the examination of a single pair was clearly longer for the first test pair than for those that followed. The order of presentation being random, we then regrouped the data not as a function of the kind of pair involved but simply in terms of its order of presentation.

The duration of exploration of a single pair decreased progressively throughout the experiment, for all age-groups. The analysis of the evolution of various parameters showed that the time taken to explore a stimulus was not employed in the same fashion by children of different ages. The reduction in exploration time was accompanied by a decrease in the number of visual fixations (fig. 47), but throughout the experiment they remained more numerous in the older children, aged 6–9 years, than in the younger ones.

Finally, the number of windows fixated in each pair remained constant from the beginning to the end of the experiment in the children aged 6 years 6 months and 8 years 9 months, while it decreased in those of 4 and 5 years (fig. 48).

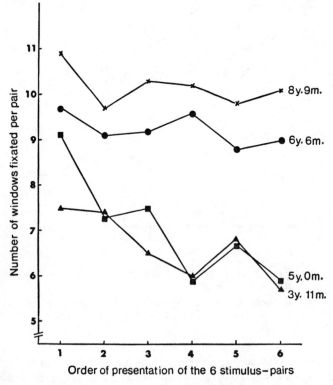

Fig. 48. Evolution, during the course of the experiment, of the number of windows fixated per stimulus-pair. (See fig. 47 for the key.)

From a comparison of these various results we are able to make certain observations.

In the older children the extent of the area explored, measured by the number of windows fixated, is determined only by what is necessary in order to make the judgment of identity or non-identity, and is thus independent of the order of appearance of a pair. In the younger children, however, as we have already seen, the size of the information sample depends neither on the nature (same or different) of the objects compared nor on the type of judgment concerned (same or not the same), whilst it can vary as a function of the child's interest. At the beginning the material used appears novel and interesting and it would take at least the first three or four pairs – bearing in mind the more or less complete character of the exploration and the existence of eleven possible contents for one window – in order that all of these should have been seen at least once. It would seem reasonable to assume that, to the extent that the contents of a window appear novel, the information which it contains will need a longer time to be absorbed than at the end of the experiment where all the various contents have acquired a certain degree of familiarity.

The decrease in the time taken by the exploration before a judgment is made stems from two different causes, according to whether the child is older or younger. In 4- and 5-year-old children the economy is in terms of the number of windows and fixations. The more familiar the material becomes, the more the child loses interest, and the fewer windows he looks at. The amount of useful information abstracted decreases.

In children aged 6–9 years, however, the amount of useful information abstracted remains the same but it is obtained in less time. The same number of windows is inspected, varying only as a function of the judgment to be made, but each one receives on average fewer fixations at the sixth than at the first presentation.

In summary, in the course of the experiment the older children gradually eliminated redundant information arising from multiple fixations of the same windows, whilst the younger ones eliminated useful information.

## 4 *The Effects of Insufficient Exploratory Activity on Performances of Identification and Differentiation*

In recognition tasks (Zinchenko, Van Chizi-Tsin and Tarakanov, 1962) as well as those of differentiation (Vurpillot, 1968, 1969a), the increase in exploratory activity is accompanied by an improvement in performance. Failing to explore the stimulus sufficiently either during the period of familiarisation, or during the comparison period, the young child gains only a part of the information available and, in consequence, his judgment is usually based on incomplete data. This is why, having looked at only a part of the object, he identifies it on the basis of one feature only; the identification of the whole from one part, reported time and again in investigations of children's perception, is certainly due largely to the restricted extent of the area explored on the stimulus. In judgments of differentiation the significant number of 'same' responses given to objects whose differences are clearly supraliminal must be attributed at least in part to the sampling behaviour of young children; when the difference or differences are situated outside the zone explored, the child cannot take them into account and his response is incorrect.

A second experiment (Vurpillot, 1969a) of the same type as the preceding one (Vurpillot, 1968), but without the recording of eye-movements, verified a number of operational hypotheses which were related to the inadequate visual exploration of children under the age of 6 years.

The first hypothesis concerned the number of correct responses. When a pair of houses was physically different, a 'not the same' response – the only correct one – could only be given if at least one of the homologous pairs of windows with different contents was in the area explored visually. The more numerous the differences, the greater the probability that at least one of them would be seen. This hypothesis was verified for 5-year-old children, for whom the number of correct responses increased with the number of differences present. At 6½ years performance was practically perfect whatever number of differences was involved, a result which is in accord with the prediction that after the age of 6 years children no longer sample just a part of the surface-area of the stimulus.

In the case of physically identical pairs, a correct judgment is compatible with a partial exploration, which is supported by the near absence of errors on these pairs even with the youngest subjects.

The second hypothesis concerns the time taken by the child to reach a decision. If we assume that the time necessary for gathering information provided by one window is essentially the same for all, whatever the content, it follows that, for each subject, the time which separates the presentation of a pair from the related judgment is proportional to the number of windows inspected. From this the following hypothesis can be formulated: if the decision criterion rests on the elimination of every possible difference in order to judge two houses as 'the same', whilst they can

be judged 'not the same' if only one difference has been discovered, then a longer time will be needed in order to respond 'the
same' than 'not the same'; the more differences that are present
the less this time will be. However, if the child judges the whole on
the basis of a sample only, exploration will be incomplete for all
the pairs involved and will not depend on their objective characteristics; when this is the case the time taken to formulate a judgment
will be essentially the same for all pairs.

This second hypothesis was confirmed: below the age of 6
years the duration of inspection did not differ systematically from
one pair to another, whilst at the 6½-year level, an age at which
there were practically no errors, the identical pairs were inspected
for a longer time than those that differed, and within this group
the more differences there were, the shorter the length of time
taken by the inspection (fig. 49).

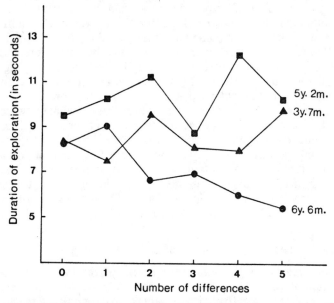

Fig. 49. Duration of exploration of a stimulus-pair as a function of the
number of differences in the pair.

Each curve corresponds to one age-group; each point on a curve is based
on eighteen responses, one for each child of the age-group concerned.

The third hypothesis was that if the poor performance observed
with the differing pairs was a consequence of insufficient explora-

tion, an instruction to look for differences should bring about a more complete exploration and the discovery of these differences. In order to verify this hypothesis, at the end of the experiment all the differing pairs were presented to the child again and he was asked to indicate in what respects the pairs differed, which means that the pairs were described as different by the experimenter. As early as 3½ years at least one difference per pair was indicated in 80 per cent of cases.

The results of this experiment meet criticisms that could be made of the conclusions drawn from the experiment involving the recording of eye-movements.

Although the results of the investigation in question (Vurpillot, 1968) were particularly clear, one could make the objection that the experimental setting selected was very far from the conditions under which the behaviour of children normally occurs, and that this would affect the performance of very young children. It is true that the number of errors made was slightly greater than in the second experiment (Vurpillot, 1969a), in which the comparisons were not accompanied by the recording of eye-movements. However, in both experiments the number of differences present was inversely related to the number of incorrect judgments of 'the same' in the youngest children and to the duration of exploration in the older ones. The inferior performance of those children, at the same age-level, whose eye-movements were recorded, would seem to be of a sensori-motor order, in that children under the age of 7 years, as we shall show later on, experience difficulty in fixating, and maintaining their fixation, on a precise point. In a task involving exploration or free comparison the child guides himself by using his finger, pointing in turn to the parts he intends to examine. He was deprived of this support in the task where eye-movements were recorded.

## II   THE DISTRIBUTION OF VISUAL FIXATIONS

The more restricted the exploration, the more important the localisation of visual fixations would seem to be, since in this case the choice of the area fixated determines what sample of the information is abstracted. However, in children, as in adults, it seems that visual fixations are not distributed in a random manner but are preferentially concentrated in certain areas, determined either by their information value (Mackworth and Bruner, 1966; Mackworth and Morandi, 1967) or by their spatial situation in the visual field (Brandt, 1945; Piaget and Vinh-Bang, 1961a, b; Gould and Schaffer, 1965, etc.).

## 1 *The Concentration of Fixations and Information Value*

An investigation by Mackworth and Bruner (1966) compared the performances of 6-year-old children with those of adults in a task of identifying photographs which were either blurred or clearly focused. In the case of the adults, fixations were grouped systematically in a few areas judged to be the most rich in information; the more blurred the photograph the more definite were these concentrations. The same phenomenon was apparent with the children, but it was less systematic and inter-individual differences were more marked. The location of a concentration was not determined by the physical properties of the stimulus alone, because with one very blurred picture it was the same whether this picture was seen before the clearly focused version – and so without having been identified – or after the clearly focused version, that is, when it *had* been identified.

Not all the points of a stimulus (object, drawing, or photograph) have the same value of visual attraction – some attracting and retaining attention more than others. This is the case, for example, with the angles of a polygon (Zusne and Michels, 1964), or the contour of non-representational forms such as those in the Rorschach test (Thomas, 1963), or in X-ray pictures of lungs (Thomas and Landsdown, 1963). Some investigators (Mackworth and Bruner, 1966) think that in these circumstances the concentration of visual fixations is also determined by the information value of the different parts of the stimulus; those areas markedly contrasting in brightness, the contour, the points of inflexion are in fact the most rich in information (Attneave, 1954). However, visual fixation of these areas cannot be due to deliberate search and orientation for information because the same phenomenon is observed in the neonate. Indeed, the latter preferentially concentrates his fixations on the angles of a triangle (Kessen, 1967). It is therefore necessary to think in terms of an almost reflex, innate, visual attraction, which is, of course, susceptible to subsequent development and integration within a strategy of exploration. The data at present available concerning what one might call the structural poles of visual attraction are very limited – this being as true for adults as for children (Kessen, 1967; Salapatek, 1968; Lévy-Schoen, 1969).

## 2 *The Heterogeneity of the Concentrations of Fixations as a Function of the Spatial Areas of the Stimulus*

It is conventional to say that, as a general rule, the top left-hand quadrant of the visual field attracts more fixations than the others; however, the available evidence is very contradictory and the demands of the task, the subject's hypotheses, and the physical properties of the stimulus have such an influence that it is usually impossible to demonstrate the action of a topographical factor. In a setting sufficiently controlled for the factors we have just mentioned to have a minimum of influence, Piaget and Vinh-Bang (1961a, b) have been able to demonstrate a clear heterogeneity, increasing with age, in the distribution of points of visual fixation on two segments placed end to end in the vertical direction. From the age of 7 years, the upper segment was fixated more often and

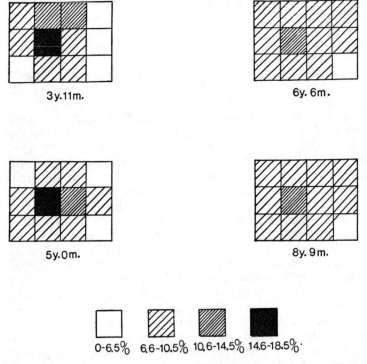

Fig. 50. Topographical distribution of visual fixations on identical stimulus-pairs.

Each diagram relates to the visual fixations of eighteen or twenty children in one age-group on the three identical stimulus-pairs.

The two left-hand columns refer to the house on the left of a stimulus-pair, the two right-hand columns to the house on the right.

Each square corresponds to one window. The degree of shading in a square is proportional to the density of visual fixations in the window situated in that position. This density is expressed in percentages relative to the total number of visual fixations.

for longer periods of time than the lower segment, in the same way that, in a single vertical segment, the upper third was fixated more often than the lower third. The pre-eminence of the upper part of the visual field results in a 'polarisation of explorations' (Piaget, 1961) which is manifested both at the level of the unequal duration of visual fixations and of the 'irreciprocity of movements' (Piaget, 1961, p. 210). During the comparison of the two vertical segments placed one above the other, an unequal duration of fixations in favour of the upper part was indeed observed, but also a privileged direction for eye-movements: 53·3 per cent of the latter going from bottom to top, as against 46·7 per cent from top to bottom (Piaget, 1961, p. 201).

Piaget and Vinh-Bang (1961b) did not find any polarisation of exploration until the age of 7 years, and this polarisation only relates to the vertical axis. During the comparison of the horizontal segments, fixations were divided equally between the one on the right and the one on the left. However, the authors' conclusion as to the homogeneity of the upper and lower parts in space before the age of 7 years is debatable. Piaget and Vinh-Bang present supporting evidence relating to just two children below the age of 7 years, which would seem insufficient. Personally, relying on previous research (Fraisse, 1968) and on data from a spatial localisation task (Vurpillot and Berthoud, 1969) reported earlier (pp. 107 et seq.), we are rather of the opinion that a heterogeneity between the upper and lower parts of perceptual space is manifested much earlier, and that a preference for the upper rather than the lower part can be demonstrated in children relatively early.

In an experiment involving the recording of eye-movements (Vurpillot, 1968), we measured the distribution of visual fixations relating to three pairs of identical houses, in each age-group. Fig. 50 shows, for each age-level, the relative density of fixations on each of twelve windows. It is apparent from the examination of this figure and the statistical analysis (by Chi squares) of the results, that the younger children inspect one area preferentially – left centre. With the older children a degree of preference for the centre remains, but left and right become equivalent. One can see in these results the signs of an improvement in the strategies of comparison, both houses being inspected equally by the older children and the distribution of fixations being homogeneous.

## III STRATEGIES OF EXPLORATION

The strategy of exploration selected by a child shows itself above all in the sequence of points fixated. In the very young child the fixations, which are not very numerous, are concentrated in a few areas which correspond to particular structural properties of the stimulus, and attention seems to go simply from one point of attraction to another. Whilst remaining aware of these points of attraction, the older child gradually frees himself from their influence; from the point of departure the trajectory of his inspection follows a fixed programme of action selected so that the requirements of the task are best met. Those fixations which provide no information are progressively eliminated; at the same time the 'spatial movements' (Piaget, 1961) between proximal stimuli (or the field of centration) increase in number and amplitude.

1   *Strategies of Comparison in Relation to Judgments of 'Same' or 'Not the Same'*
(a) *Size comparison.* The visuo-motor activity of children from 6 to 11 years and adults was recorded during judgments of equivalence or non-equivalence of oblique segments. These were vertical or horizontal, and presented two at a time, either as an extended line separated by a small gap, or joined up to make a right-angle figure (Piaget and Vinh-Bang, 1961a, b).

In general the distribution of fixation points and eye-movements was roughly similar from 6 years to the adult level; however, a developmental evolution can be seen particularly between the ages of 6 and 7 years. Thus the total amount of time devoted to examining the rows before making a judgment decreased with age, and within this period the proportion devoted to fixation became increasingly important. At 6 years the time was divided equally between displacements and pauses; from the age of 7 years only a quarter of the time was given to displacements. Amongst these displacements it was possible to distinguish inter-segmental or comparison movements and movements of inspection from one point to another in the same segment. The former increased in number with age at the same time as the latter decreased, so that at 6 years there was one comparison for three inspections whilst in the adult there were more comparisons than inspections (2·7 as against 2·0).

Piaget and Vinh-Bang see in this development the effects of an increase in the number of spatial movements to the detriment of centration on the parts to be compared. The influence of this increasing decentration on the perceived size of the segments being compared is extremely complex because, on the one hand, the multiplication of fixations compensates for the effects of centration and brings about a decrease in errors due to the unequal fixation of different parts of the figure, but, on the other hand, secondary errors of overestimation arise from the heterogeneity of movements which do not occur equally in all directions.

(b) *The systematisation of the movements between the stimulus-objects being compared.* In several of our experiments (Vurpillot and Zoberman, 1965; Vurpillot, 1968, 1969a, b; Vurpillot and Moal, 1970; Vurpillot, Lécuyer, Moal and Pineau, 1971; etc.), the child had to compare two figures, one beside the other, on a horizontal axis. An economical visuo-motor exploration involved the successive establishment of a correspondence between each part of one figure and its homologue in the other, according to an optimal sequence. The analysis of recordings of eye-movements (fig. 51) has made it possible to examine the improvement with age of the strategies of comparison in one of these experiments (Vurpillot, 1968). As Zinchenko found (Zinchenko, Van Chizi-Tsin and Tarakanov, 1962), the hole between the two houses behind which the camera lens was located constituted a point of visual attraction for the very youngest children. These non-informative fixations were rapidly eliminated between 3 and 6 years. At the same time the movements which linked the two figures being compared became more systematic.

1 *The increase in the number of movements between houses.* Amongst the eye-movements which transferred attention from one window to the other, there were grounds for distinguishing the movements between houses which linked a window in one house with a window in the other house, and the movements within the houses which linked two windows in the same house. In a task involving comparison of two houses only, movements of the first type provided useful information; the second type of movements should only have appeared to the extent that they constituted an economy in exploration.

Figure 52 depicts two theoretical explorations both involving fixations on the twelve windows by means of eleven movements, six of which link homologous windows (homologous comparison movements). Both explorations gather the same information by the same number of movements, but in the first case 100 per cent of the movements are between the houses, in the second only 54·5 per cent. This second form of exploration involves the eye in less total movement than the former, and comprises only seven changes of direction as against ten in the first; it can therefore be considered as more economical. The results in table 17 show that the proportion of movements between houses increases with age, reaching at 9 years the value predicted as a function of an optimal

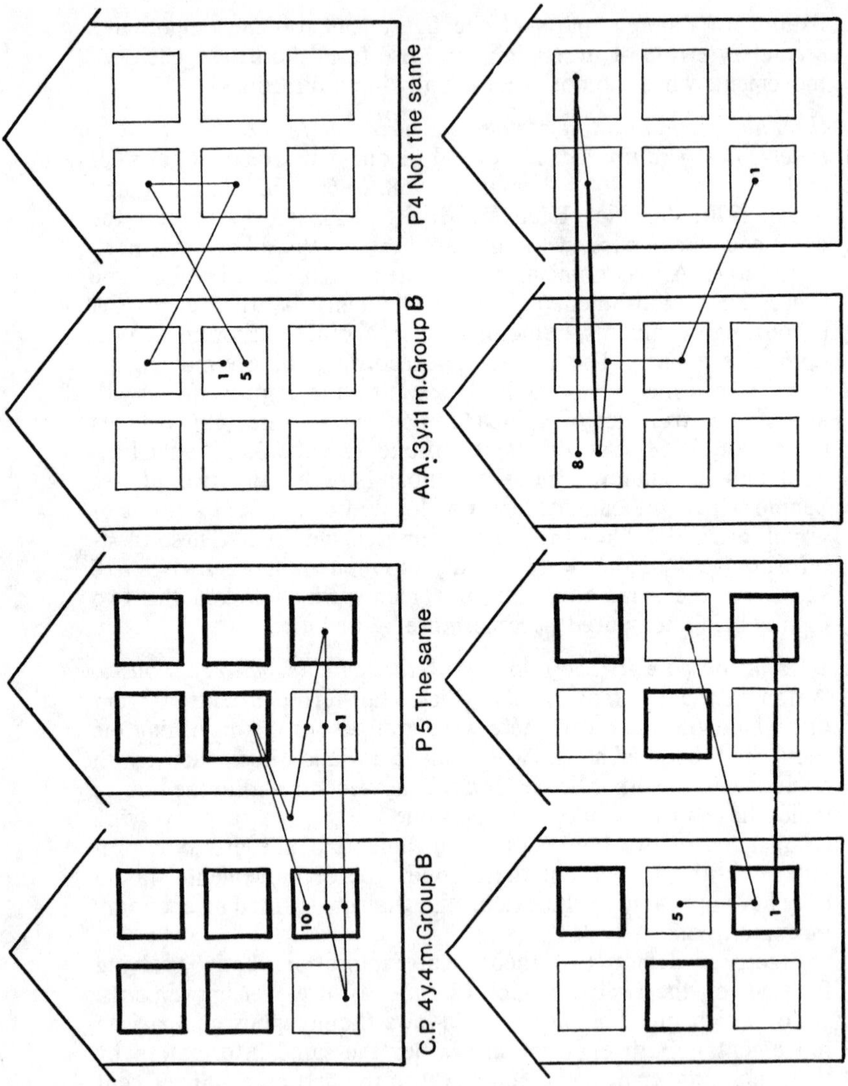

Fig. 51. Examples of visuo-motor explorations (Vurpillot, 1968)
The windows with a thick frame-line are those which differ from one
house to the other. Beneath each pair is given: the initials of the subject, his

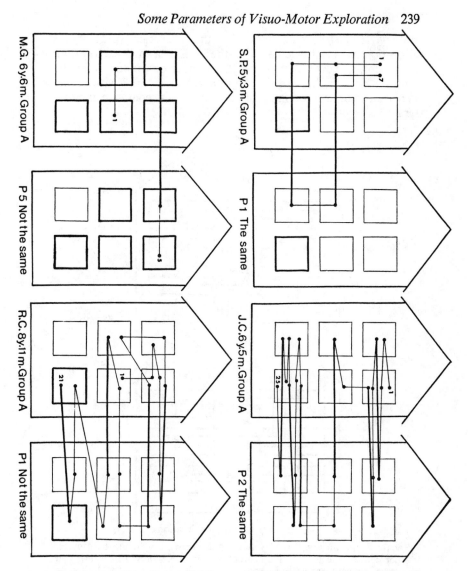

age, the group (A or B) in which he was classified according to his judgment criteria (see ch. 11), the number of the stimulus-pair and his response ('same' or 'not the same').

strategy. It must be made clear that the theoretical value of this proportion has been calculated on the basis of a total exploration; it does not, however, depend on the number of windows actually inspected. It can therefore be legitimately compared with actual percentages obtained on the basis of more or less complete explorations.

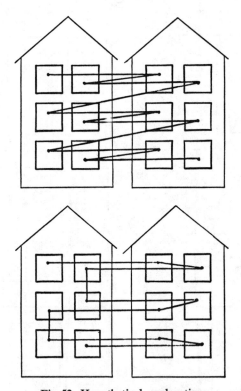

Fig. 52. Hypothetical explorations.

Each exploration involves eleven eye-movements, but in the bottom pair 100 per cent of the movements are between houses, whilst in the top pair, only 54.5 per cent are of this type.

2 *Relative increase in the number of horizontal movements.* Since the two houses are drawn side by side, horizontal movements provide more useful information than oblique or vertical movements. Table 18 shows that the proportion of horizontal movements is already more than 50 per cent at 4 years, and increases with age.

Table 17  *Evolution of comparison movements between houses (percentages)*

| Age (in years and months) | 3y. 11m. | 5y. 0m. | 6y. 6m. | 8y. 9m. |
|---|---|---|---|---|
| $\dfrac{\text{n movements between houses}}{\text{N total number of movements}} \times 100$ | 31·8 | 39·2 | 44·5 | 52·2 |

The results are averages calculated on the basis of individual percentages.

3  *The existence of homologous comparisons.* If horizontal movements between the windows belonging to two houses are those best suited to their comparison, within this group there is a privileged category. The comparison between homologous windows – that is to say, those occupying the identical position in each

Table 18  *Evolution of horizontal movements (percentages)*

| Age (in years and months) | 3y. 11m. | 5y. 0m. | 6y. 6m. | 8y. 9m. |
|---|---|---|---|---|
| $\dfrac{\text{n horizontal movements}}{\text{N total number of movements}} \times 100$ | 55·6 | 64·0 | 69·2 | 74·8 |

The results are averages calculated on the basis of individual percentages.

of the houses – is the sole basis of an effective strategy adapted to the tasks of identification and differentiation.

We shall describe as a homologous comparison an eye-movement which goes directly from window *a* in one house to its homologue *a'* in the other house, without any intermediary fixation. Such movements are apparent in the exploration of the great majority of subjects, and increase with age (fig. 53). One might consider in which cases such movements are due to chance and when they are the result of deliberate action.

Indeed, when a certain number of movements are involved, the probability of a chance homologous comparison occurring is by no means negligible. In consequence, a hypothetical number of comparison movements was calculated for each subject, predictable on the basis of chance from the total number of movements made. This hypothetical value was compared with the actual number of homologous comparison movements, and a subject was considered as having deliberately made homologous com-

parisons only when there was a statistically significant difference
between observed and hypothetical values.

One can see from table 19 that no 4-year-old children made

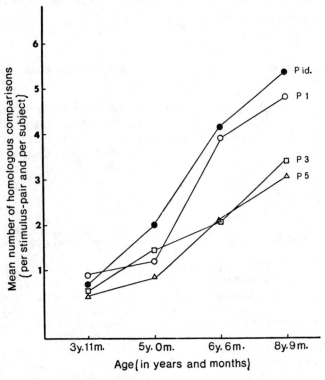

Fig. 53. Evolution with age of the average number of homologous comparisons. (Vurpillot, 1968).

P id.=identical pairs (mean of the results from three pairs); $P_1$=pair with
one difference; $P_3$=pair with three differences; $P_5$=pair with five differences.

Table 19  *Number of subjects making homologous comparisons*

| Age *(in years and months)* | 3y. 11m. | 5y. 0m. | 6y. 6m. | 8y. 9m. |
|---|---|---|---|---|
| *Number of subjects* | 0/18 | 7/20 | 16/20 | 18/20 |

On the bottom line, the figure on the left relates to the subjects who made
homologous comparisons, the figure on the right gives the total number of
subjects in the group (after Vurpillot, 1968).

deliberate homologous comparisons, whilst above the age of 6 years almost all of them employed this strategy.

## 2 *The Influence of Reading on Strategies of Exploration*

The presumed privileged status of the upper left part of the visual field is attributed to the experience of reading which, in our culture, is carried out from left to right and from top to bottom. The large number of studies carried out in this area show that the intensive practice which all adults have of this activity has a certain influence on visuo-motor exploration. Visuo-motor reaction time is more rapid from left to right than from right to left in the adult and the older child (Lesèvre, 1964); left-to-right movements are more regular and more precise than those from right to left (Gassel and Williams, 1963). A left-to-right exploration would thus appear to be favoured.

There are not many studies involving children but they all agree in showing that the direction of exploration becomes more systematic with age. Thus Teegarden (1933) asked children from 4 to 5 years and from 6 to 7 years to name drawings of familiar objects arranged in rows and columns; he found that the order in which they enumerated them was from top to bottom and from left to right in all cases, but more systematically in the older than in the younger children. Gottschalk, Bryden and Rabinovitch (1964) found the same evolution in children from 3 to 6 years. Debot-Sevrin (1962) presented, in a brief exposure, five drawings aligned either vertically or horizontally and asked children to name them; no fixation point was imposed. The tendency to name first the drawing situated at the top and to the left increased with age at the same time as the fixation point selected by the child before the appearance of the stimulus was displaced towards the left.

An enumeration task was also presented by Elkind and Weiss (1967) to children of 5, 6, 7 and 8 years. The children were given two cards one after the other; on the first card twenty-four figures were situated randomly (unstructured stimulus); on the second, eighteen figures were set out in a triangular configuration (structured stimulus) as in fig. 54. The authors recorded the order of the exploration as well as the omissions and repetitions. They distinguished four exploration strategies. The strategy was described as unsystematic when at least five of the pictures named were not adjacent. A left-right strategy corresponded to the naming of pictures, line by line, beginning at the top left and proceeding towards the right. In the top-to-bottom strategy naming also began with the pictures situated in the top left-hand quarter, but

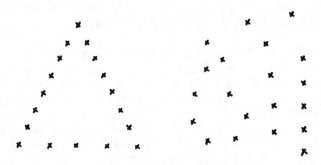

Fig. 54. Distribution of the parts to be named.

The positions occupied by the figures are indicated by crosses; the drawings themselves are not reproduced – pictures of a ship, a chicken, an elephant, a violin, a beetle, a rabbit, etc.

*On the left:* the structured stimulus; *on the right:* the unstructured stimulus.

continued in a vertical direction following the columns. Finally a complex strategy combined the two preceding ones. All four of these strategies were in evidence in the exploration of the unstructured stimulus, the top-to-bottom strategy was relatively rare whilst the left-right strategy was used in half the cases up to 7 years. The complex strategies appeared gradually but became the most frequent by 8 years; random explorations decreased gradually with age, as did the number of errors.

With the structured stimulus only two strategies were observed, that of left-to-right exploration, systematic but uneconomic considering the lay-out of the figures, and a strategy described as triangular in which the naming was step by step, following the configuration. This latter strategy, the most suitable, was always the main one; one interesting point is that the left-right strategy was most apparent at 6 years, the age when children are learning to read (table 20).

One can see from Elkind and Weiss's (1967) experiment that the left-right strategy is already employed by half the 5-year-old children with an unstructured stimulus. Learning to read does not cause it to appear but encourages its more systematic employment, since it is most frequent at 6 years. But later, once reading habits are well established, the child is less bound by this rigid method and seems to feel free to combine more complex strategies.

In a second stage of the analysis of the topographical distribution of fixations during the comparison of the two houses (Vurpillot, 1968), we recorded the localisation of the first three and the last three

Table 20 *Distribution of exploration strategies (percentages)*

| | Age (in years) | | | |
|---|---|---|---|---|
| STRATEGY | 5 | 6 | 7 | 8 |
| *Unstructured card:* | | | | |
| Chance | 50 | 39 | 23 | 5 |
| Left-right | 45 | 52 | 41 | 10 |
| Top-bottom | 5 | 0 | 23 | 30 |
| Complex | 0 | 9 | 13 | 55 |
| *Structured card:* | | | | |
| Left-right | 25 | 48 | 14 | 10 |
| Triangular | 75 | 52 | 86 | 90 |

(After Elkind and Weiss, 1967)

fixations, to determine whether the exploration tended to begin and end in preferred areas[1] (fig. 55).

The comparison, at each age level, of the localisation of the fixations at the beginning and the end reveals a clear developmental sequence. The youngest, the 4-year-olds, began their exploration in the central area of the stimulus, near the initial fixation point and hardly moved from it, although tending to finish up at the top left. The 5-year-olds did not perform very differently, although the area inspected increased.

By far the most systematic strategy was that of the 6½-year-old children who began their exploration at the top left and terminated it at the bottom. Those from 8 to 9 years of age showed a little more imagination since, although the majority performed like the 6-year-olds, some of them began in the middle or at the bottom of the stimulus, which led them to terminate their exhaustive exploration either at the top or at the bottom.

The over-all picture presented by these results might suggest that the tendency to look at the top left-hand part of a stimulus is prior to any learning to read. But we should not overlook the fact that the children concerned all attended nursery schools (*écoles maternelles*) and that it is quite possible that their teachers had already begun to teach them to choose a starting point and a direction of exploration. However, it is at the stage where learning to read proper inculcates a systematic strategy that the child applies it in a rigid and sometimes ill-adapted manner (Elkind and

[1] Chi square comparisons were made between the densities of fixations by row and by column. A difference is reported in the text when the corresponding Chi square was significant at the ·01 level.

Weiss, 1967) to all explorations. Around the age of 8 years, and once he has a firm grasp of reading, the child introduces some variety, whether in his choice of a starting point, or in the organisation of the sequence of fixations, whilst taking care to be thorough and methodical.

## 3 *The Influence of Sensori-motor Variables*

The relative slowness and lack of precision of the sensori-motor activities of young children seem to have their origin in a certain immaturity of the nervous system. At the level of visuo-motor exploration the inferiority manifests itself particularly in the duration of the visuo-motor reaction time and by the difficulty, indeed the impossibility, of maintaining a fixation point and following a set sequence of fixations. These limitations are not without their effects on the child's strategies, and it is often difficult to say to what extent the small number of homologous comparisons in evidence before the age of 6 years is due to the absence of an appropriate programme of action, and to what extent to inadequate visuo-motor control.

(a) *The measurement of visuo-motor reaction time.* Piaget and Vinh-Bang (1961b) measured the time which elapsed between the moment when the subject opened his eyes and his fixation of the figure presented. This latency of the first fixation markedly decreased with age, the greatest progress taking place between 6 and 7 years.

Lesèvre (1964) had subjects fixate a cross situated to one side of the visual field, then caused another cross to appear in another part of the field, and recorded the time which elapsed between the appearance of the new element and its fixation. The subject had been instructed at the beginning to look at the new figure as soon as it was perceived; a displacement of 20° was involved and it could occur in various directions, to the top, to the bottom, to the right and to the left, the possible positions of the figure being 3 o'clock, 6 o'clock, 9 o'clock and 12 o'clock. The figures obtained by Lesèvre are very close to those of Vinh-Bang. As soon as the child was able to read, a lateralisation of inspection was noted, displacements to the right being systematically more rapid than displacements to the left.

To the best of our knowledge there are no data on the visuo-motor reaction time of younger children.

(b) *Maintaining gaze on a fixation point.* All the experimental findings agree in showing that, during the free exploration of a

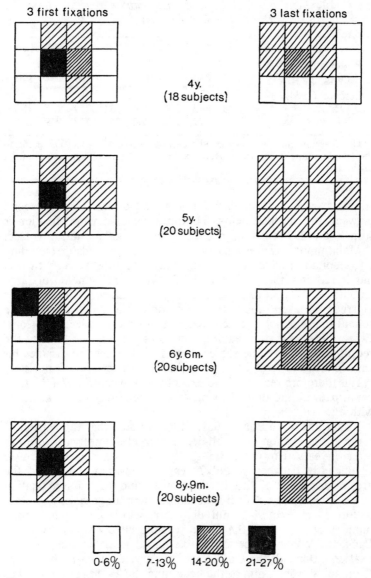

Fig. 55. Topographical distribution of the first 3 and the last 3 visual fixations on the identical stimulus-pairs.

The diagrams are constructed in an analogous fashion to those in fig. 50.

Table 21   *The evolution of visuo-motor reaction time with age (in milliseconds)*

| Age (in years) | 6 | 7 | 8 | 9 | 10 | 11 | 12 | Adult |
|---|---|---|---|---|---|---|---|---|
| Piaget and Vinh-Bang (1961) | 380 | 230 | | 230 | | 210 | | 170 |
| Lesèvre (1964) | | | | | | | | |
| LR | 378 | 302 | 270 | 234 | 231 | 229 | 195 | 188 |
| RL | 379 | 311 | 287 | 260 | 259 | 257 | 229 | 226 |

The reaction-times are expressed in milliseconds. LR = fixation point to the left, stimulus to the right; RL = fixation point to the right and stimulus to the left.

stimulus, gaze is stationary for a period of less than a second between two displacements. The duration of a visual fixation is from about 250 to 800 ms according to the age and task involved.

Maintaining gaze on a particular point for periods greater than one second is a difficult and painful task. To be effectively carried out it requires the subject to inhibit micro-movements of large amplitude. When a fixation is strictly maintained, vision becomes blurred and, even though the condition of the stabilisation of the retinal image is not attained (Riggs, Ratliff, Cornsweet and Cornsweet, 1953), a certain habituation takes place at the level of the receptor neurones. The subject then feels the need to displace his gaze in order to establish the conditions necessary for clear vision.

It is therefore reasonable to expect that the control of a fixation, being painful and difficult, would be increasingly better achieved with age.

Piaget and Vinh-Bang (1961a, 1961b) noted that the margin of error in the fixation of a well-defined target did not vary with age after 7 years. However, the ability to maintain gaze improved significantly between 6 and 7 years. Vinh-Bang calculated the area of dispersion of visual centration around the required fixation point. The adult was capable of maintaining his gaze for 2 seconds within a circle of 4–5 mm diameter, which corresponds to 3 minutes of arc. With the two 6-year-old children seen by Vinh-Bang, the longer the period of fixation, the further the points of fixation extended, the diameter of the circle which encompassed them going from 4 mm at the beginning to 12 mm at 1·18 seconds and to 19 mm (an angle of about 14 minutes) at 1·87 seconds. Stabilisation of gaze fixation began at 7 years, the diameter of the spread then being 5 mm after one second, 8 mm after 2 seconds.

Lesèvre (1964, 1968) observed in some 6- to 7-year-old children small to-and-fro movements around a target. These oscillations indicated a very real difficulty in fixating a particular point in a continuous fashion; they were only observed in the youngest subjects and were rather exceptional even in that group.

However, it must be borne in mind that Vinh-Bang, like Lesèvre, was only able to examine a small number of 6-year-old children, the only ones capable of adapting to the experimental task and setting, a very restricting factor in Vinh-Bang's study. These children were therefore not representative of their age-group, and one might expect that the difficulty in maintaining a fixation would be even more apparent in an unselected population. In any case the study of the capacity for voluntary fixation in children of preschool age has yet to be carried out.

(c) *The voluntary displacement of gaze according to a pre-determined sequence.* As early as the age of 4 weeks the child is able to fixate several points in succession, passing rapidly from one to another (Gesell, Thompson and Amatruda, 1934). However, these fixations are not yet directed in any precise fashion and it is not until the age of 7 years that a child is capable of visually tracking from one point to another along a specified trajectory. Lesèvre reports the results from an investigation of directed exploration involving children from 5 to 12 years, where their eye-movements were recorded (Lesèvre, 1964, pp. 142 et seq.). The figure which had to be explored was made up of fifty-one St Andrew's crosses, each 5 mm by 5 mm, set out in seven lines 22 cm in length, a different number on each line and spaced irregularly. The three crosses on the last line served only as final reference points, so the results relate to forty-eight target-figures only. The subjects were instructed to fixate each cross in succession, as quickly as possible, but without missing any out. The 5-year-olds were incapable of doing the task and simply looked at some of the crosses, while exploring the field on a chance basis, and then stopped.

The ability to direct visual exploration voluntarily and to stop at determined points appeared at 6 years. Of eight subjects, six were able to fixate forty-two crosses out of forty-eight; two could not fixate more than twenty and were eliminated. Once the ability to do this was achieved there was little variation with age. Although there was no case of perfect performance (no crosses omitted) at 6 years, from the age of 7 years 33 per cent were in this category and this proportion remained the same in adults. It would appear therefore to be a phenomenon tied to psychophysiological maturation.

Lesèvre also studied the evolution of the form taken by directed exploration, the number and type of eye-movements, as well as the duration of the pauses which separated them.

Given the task involved, a minimum of forty-eight movements in all was sufficient to carry out the instructions – forty-two movements of progression and six involving a return to the beginning of the line. All the subjects exceeded this number, but the number of redundant movements decreased rapidly with age, particularly between 6 and 8 years. The evolution of the total number of movements made when the task was carried out was as follows:

Table 22 *Number of movements made during the task (mean of individual performances)*

| Age (in years) | 6 | 7 | 8 | 9 |
|---|---|---|---|---|
| Number of movements per subject | 100·2 | 91·6 | 79·8 | 73·5 |
| Age (in years) | 10 | 11 | 12 | Adult |
| Number of movements per subject | 68·0 | 63·6 | 59·3 | 53·1 |

(After Lesèvre, 1964)

Lesèvre distinguished several categories of movements:

(a) L movements, involving the return to the beginning of a line. Of large amplitude, these were rarely precise and stopped on one side or the other of the first cross, which meant that a supplementary movement of adjustment was necessary.

(b) C, correction movements, after the return to the beginning of a line, in order to adjust fixation on the cross.

(c) Movements of progression, P, from one cross to another; these were divided into P+, or correct progression, the amplitude of which was such that the movement stopped exactly on the cross to be fixated, and P−, the amplitude of which was insufficient (hypometric) or excessive (hypermetric). These P− movements tended to be hypermetric in young children, hypometric in older children and adults.

(d) Small movements of adjustment, A, divided into movements A+ which followed a hypometric progression P−, and A− which followed a P− hypermetric progression.

(e) Verification movements, V, which went in the opposite direction to the progression, either to a cross which had been forgotten or already seen (V+), or to a point between two crosses (V−).

(*f*) Finally, those aberrant movements, Ab, which seemed to have no particular purpose; they were distinguished from movements of adjustment in that the latter were followed by a very short pause, whilst Ab movements preceded a long pause.

Only L and P+ type movements were exact, the others corresponding to an error of adjustment in relation to the target, such as the movements of the P−, V− and Ab variety, or otherwise having the function of correcting these errors, such as those of type R, A and V+. The decrease in the number of R, P−, V, A and Ab movements was a consequence of an improvement in visuo-motor exploration. The aberrant movements of progression or fixation were the first to disappear, their number decreasing rapidly between 6 and 9 years (sixteen at 6 years, eight at 9 years) with almost none from the age of 12 years (0·8 at 12 years, 0 in adults).

Movements of adjustment, verification and correction persisted at all age-levels, but they became less and less frequent.

## IV THE REGISTERING OF INFORMATION: THE DURATION OF A VISUAL FIXATION

Although the term 'visual fixation' is currently employed in the literature, and the duration of fixation has been measured by numerous investigators in a variety of tasks, the objective definition of a fixation is far from easy.

Implicit in the research carried out on visuo-motor activity is the postulate that a visual fixation is defined temporally by the time which elapses between voluntary and successive displacements of the eyes and spatially by the localisation of the fixation during the time of the pause. However, the visual micronystagmus is permanent and persists during the voluntary fixation of a point. It is therefore necessary to distinguish clearly between a voluntary displacement following a deliberate change of the fixation point and an involuntary displacement due to micronystagmus. This could be done by taking as a criterion the relative amplitude of movements of two sorts, namely what is expressed by the terms micro- and macro-movements of the eyes. We know that during a one-second fixation the mean displacement of the eye in adults is of the order of 3 minutes of arc (Heckenmueller, 1965), and that the largest movements do not exceed 50 minutes of arc and are relatively rare. By only treating as a voluntary movement visual displacements of an amplitude greater than 1°, any confusion with a micro-movement in a normal situation of visual exploration is

eliminated. It is possible that by counting as a voluntary movement only those where the amplitude exceeds 1° or 2°, or even 4°,
as is currently the practice, one is neglecting a certain number of
real exploration movements. Indeed, as far as we know, no one
has yet attempted to measure the minimal amplitude of a voluntary
displacement of the eye, for the very good reason that techniques
of recording such movements are subject to limitations. The
measurement of the amplitude of a voluntary eye-movement presupposes the possibility of neutralising any movement of the subject's head. However, this neutralisation is only relative and its
achievement continues to present one of the most serious technical
problems in research into visuo-motor activity. A method which
makes it possible to limit displacements of the head to a maximum
of 1°, and thus to regard as an eye-movement anything which
involves a visual displacement of 1·5° and more, can be considered
as satisfactory.

(a) *The duration of visual fixation in adults.* When a subject engages in free exploration of a picture or a printed page, he proceeds
by a series of inspection pauses linked by eye-movements. The
time taken by a displacement depends on the amplitude of the
movement; this is very slight by comparison with the time taken by
the pauses, so that very often the duration of the pauses is calculated on the basis of the duration of the exploration and the total
number of fixations, without taking account of the time taken by
the displacements themselves.

In adults the mean duration of a visual fixation is 250 ms in
reading (Anderson, 1937; Woodworth and Schlosberg, 1954) and
350 ms in the exploration of drawings, photographs, etc. (table 23).
Essentially this difference seems to be due to the fact that reading
is a very standardised task in which an optimal strategy can be
maintained and applied in every instance, with only slight adapta-
tions in response to the size of the characters and the presence of
pictures incorporated in the text. In the exploration of pictures
there is no optimal strategy, since it is a function of the task –
differentiation, identification, familiarisation – as well as the
characteristics of the picture itself. When the stimulus-objects
concerned are all of the same type, this facilitates the progressive
implementation of a single strategy; thus the duration of a fixation
goes from 370 ms in untrained radar operators to 250 ms in
trained operators (C. White and Ford, 1960), reaching compara-
bility with pauses in reading. Training in speed reading markedly
reduces the time taken to explore a printed page, but the increase
in speed is obtained by a reduction in the number of fixations, not

Table 23  *Duration of visual fixation during pattern exploration by adults*

| Authors | Task involved | Mean duration of a fixation (in ms) |
|---|---|---|
| Buswell, 1935 | Looking at representational pictures | 320–360 |
| Enoch and Fry, 1957 | Interpreting aerial photographs | 370 |
| White and Ford, 1960 | Watching a radar screen | 370 |
| Zusne and Michels, 1964 | Looking at representational forms | 333 |
| Lesèvre, 1964 | Fixating crosses arranged in rows, not equidistant | 365 |
| Gould and Schaffer, 1965 | Discovering one numeral amongst others | 310 |
| Mackworth and Bruner, 1966 | Looking at a photograph | 349–365 |

In all these researches a change of fixation was assumed when visual displacement exceeded an angle of 1°.

in their average duration (Thomas, 1962; Poulton, 1962). The amount of information registered during a visual fixation can therefore be increased through training; the concepts of enveloping centration (Piaget, 1961) and the useful field of view (Mackworth, 1965) correspond to this phenomenon. The period of 250 ms appears to constitute a physiological limit for the registering of information, and not the inertia of the visuo-motor system, since shorter periods have been recorded for fixations on a homogeneous, and thus non-informative, surface.

The relationships between visuo-motor and cognitive activities have been dealt with elsewhere (Vurpillot, 1969c) and we shall not discuss them further here.

If, as we think, the duration of a fixation is a function of the time necessary for registering information, we can predict that the younger the child, the more time will be needed to code the same amount of information as the adult. The mean duration of a fixation should thus decrease with age, which is in fact what we find.

(*b*) *Results obtained with young children.* Adults are capable of exercising a degree of self-control which eliminates head-movements: the accuracy of the data obtained thus depends essentially on the precision of the recordings and the interpretation – in the last analysis, qualities of the apparatus and the experimenter. However, it is not the same with children who until the age of 6 or 7 years at least, refuse to be bound by rigid constraints on mobility. All measurements are thus affected by a much greater degree of uncertainty than is the case in studies involving adults. Each research worker selects a technique and a margin of error compatible with the age of the children studied and the problem which he is attempting to resolve. In children over the age of 3 years, the definition of a visual fixation approaches that found in investigations involving adults, but the degree of precision is a function of the age of the subject. When the technique is a very exact one, children of less than 8 years have difficulty in accepting it (Piaget and Vinh-Bang, 1961b; Mackworth and Bruner, 1966).

The criteria for a fixation differ according to the author concerned. Piaget and Vinh-Bang (1961a) count as a fixation the maintenance of gaze on an area defined by an angle of 3 minutes. For Zinchenko, Van Chizi-Tsin and Tarakanov (1962) the criterion of fixation is the maintenance of gaze on an area which subtends an angle of less than 2°. Lesèvre (1964) has a displacement of less than 1° as his criterion. Vurpillot (1968) only counts as a movement the passage from one window to another in drawings of houses, which corresponds to an angular displacement of about 7°. Table 24 brings together a variety of data on the duration of fixation in children from 3 to 11 years. The differences which are found between different authors are due in part to the variation in the requirements of their criteria.

From these results obtained in a variety of situations it appears that, in a given task, the duration of a fixation generally decreases with age up to 7 years, although there are exceptions to this in certain tasks (Piaget and Vinh-Bang, 1961b; Zinchenko, Van Chizi-Tsin and Tarakanov, 1962). Children appear to be more sensitive than adults to the specific properties of the experimental material and setting.

We have seen that, in adults, prolonged training on very specialised material – radiographs, radar-screens – can reduce the mean duration of a visual fixation. The decrease with age of the duration of pauses in reading shows that in children also, familiarisation with the task and the material makes it possible to speed up the registering of visual information. Even during a relatively short experiment, the effects of familiarisation with pictures is apparent with older children. We have observed that in 9-year-old children the duration of a fixation decreases from the first to the sixth pair of pictures being compared (Vurpillot, 1968).

Table 24   *Mean duration of a fixation (in ms) in children from 3 to 11 years*

| Age (in years) | 3 | 4 | 5 | 6 | 7 | 9 | 11 |
|---|---|---|---|---|---|---|---|
| Piaget, Vinh Bang, 1961b: | | | | | | | |
| Figure I | | | | 170 | 292 | 267 | 292 |
|  | | | | (2) | (3) | (3) | (3) |
| Figure L | | | | 358 | 261 | 255 | 243 |
|  | | | | (2) | (3) | (3) | (3) |
| Lesèvre, 1964: | | | | | | | |
| On the crosses | | | | 365 | 365 | 365 | 365 |
|  | | | | (6) | (12) | (6) | (10) |
| Outside the crosses | | | | 225 | 225 | 225 | 225 |
|  | | | | (6) | (12) | (6) | (10) |
| Zinchenko, Van Chizi-Tsin and Tarakanov, 1962: | | | | | | | |
| Familiarisation | 833 | 417 | 435 | 250 | | | |
|  | (4) | (4) | (4) | (4) | | | |
| Recognition | 286 | 323 | 303 | 370 | | | |
|  | (4) | (4) | (4) | (4) | | | |
| Vurpillot, 1968: | | | | | | | |
| Differentiation | | 710 | 534 | | 457 | 405 | |
|  | | (18) | (20) | | (20) | (20) | |
| Buswell, 1922: | | | | | | | |
| Reading | | | | 660 | 432 | 316 | 252 |

Number of subjects in brackets.

Thus, in adults, training makes it possible to reduce the time taken by the central nervous system to register the information abstracted from a proximal stimulus (C. White and Ford, 1960); it also makes possible an increase in the amount of information registered during a visual fixation (Thomas, 1962; Poulton, 1962).

This increase appears to be due above all to the greater utilisation of peripheral vision. A number of factors lead one to believe that, in the young child, peripheral vision could well have as its sole function the triggering of the orientation reflex. The useful field of view (Mackworth, 1965) of the infant would be limited to foveal or perifoveal vision; one of the requirements for progress would be, over a period of years, to take into account further and further outlying peripheral information. But this is a hypothesis which has not yet been verified by experimental investigation, its plausibility being based on only a small number of observations. We know how difficult it is to get a young child to see something unless he is made to fix his attention by pointing with his finger or by turning his head in the right direction. As long as an object is only in peripheral vision the child appears incapable of recognising it. Finally, we can assume that if the points of fixation of a child are, on average, much closer together than those of an adult (Mackworth and Bruner, 1966) it is because, in order to abstract the same information, he needs to rely mainly on foveal and perifoveal vision; his proximal stimuli must therefore, to a large extent, be obscured.

# Chapter 10

# The Role of Perceptual
Activity in the Genesis
of Representational Structures

Two theories – Piaget's and the theory of the *image* (Wekker, 1966; Leontiev and Gippenreiter, 1966, etc.) – give prominence to perceptual activity in the perception and recognition of forms. In both theories, perceptual activity establishes links between sensory stimulation emanating from discrete proximal stimuli. The integration of these into perceptual or representational structures transforms a temporal sequence of 'sensory tableaux' (Piaget, 1936) into a simultaneous spatial structure.

Although Piaget's theory and that of the Russian school differ in many respects we shall concern ourselves here only with what they have in common. Both postulate that the perceptual activity of the subject is indispensable to the genesis of representational cognitive structures, which they describe as the internal model (Luquet, 1927a), the image (Wekker, 1966; Zaporozhets, 1966, etc.), representational schemata, mental images (Piaget and Inhelder, 1966, etc.). On the quantity and quality of perceptual activity depends the richness and precision of the representational model, and, in turn, the quality of this model determines the subject's identification and reproduction of the physical object.

If, in the account that follows, particular reference is made to the Russian theoretical approach, it is because it is based on an impressive number of experimental investigations whilst very few of the numerous investigations of the Geneva school have been devoted to the measurement of perceptual activities and their relationship with performances of identification (Piaget and Stettler, 1954), differentiation (Piaget and Vinh-Bang, 1961a, b), or reproduction. However, in demonstrating the influence of perceptual activity on their subjects' performances, Russian research confirms the predictions of Piaget as much as those of Wekker (1966), Leontiev (Leontiev and Gippenreiter, 1966), or Zaporozhets (1966).

## I  THE THEORY OF THE IMAGE

The Russian psychologists concerned with perception, basing their work on the theories of Sechenov and Pavlov, postulate that all mental processes are reflex in origin and that perception also includes efferent motor components as well as sensory afferent components. Mental processes constitute a form of activity which can be distinguished from overt action in two respects: firstly it involves the construction of models, programmes of action, which make it possible for the subject to orient himself in the physical world; secondly it involves an activity which is hidden from the external observer. These programmes of action have been called mental images; the present account of the theory of the image is, in its essentials, taken from Wekker (1966).

## 1  *Wekker's Hypotheses*

Wekker bases his theory on the concept of the reflex, but he is also influenced by cybernetics. Information theory, in its initial form of communication theory, he found unsatisfactory because it neglected the structural characteristics of information, only taking account of its quantity. In contrast, the concept of information in the form of structured units, operating a control function, constitutes an indispensable element in the theory of the image.

The adaptation of a human being to his environment involves the establishment of a correspondence between two structures, namely the characteristics of the stimulus and the characteristics of the subject, so that the actual reactions of the latter conform to the particular characteristics of the physical source of information.

Several types of correspondence between these two structures are conceivable. The simplest is an isomorphism which establishes a correspondence without taking account of the relationships between the components of each structure. In these terms one could establish a correspondence between measurements of the sensitivities of the receptors to intensities of stimulation. A simple coding process would thus make it possible to transform the conditions of the stimulus into the conditions of the subject and by this means obtain a series of signals; a second stage would involve a decoding process which would bring about a response to the signals. The major defect of such a system is that a signal or a group of signals is the code for *all* the stimulus-structures with which it is isomorphic. However, if no account is taken of the relationships that exist between the various parts of the stimulus, the number of isomorphic structures could be considerable and, during the decoding process, the probability that a response would be appropriate to a given stimulus-structure is slight. An adequate knowledge of the world, the necessary condition for the manifestation of adaptive behaviour, means that at the efferent level the action should be in unique agreement with the source of information, that is, that the signal be specific to this source only and not to a range of sources isomorphic to a range of conditions. In order to achieve such a level of operation, the spatial-temporal relationships that exist between the constituents of the stimulus source must be represented in the signal code.

The image is then translated into a code which preserves the spatio-temporal structure pattern of the characteristic elements in the stimulus-object; such an image is a special case of signal coding.

A coding process of this kind presupposes that in the transformation which takes place between the source and the signal, there has been a conservation of one or several invariants. The number of these varies with the degree of specificity demanded of the signal and there is a hierarchical series of representations of the source as a function of the levels of communality between the source and the signal.

At the lowest level, only the temporal sequence between components is conserved; then, to the extent that the number of spatial-temporal relationships between components increases, a correspondence is obtained which is in turn, topological, projective, affine, one based on similarity, and, finally, metric. In this way there is a progression from a code which satisfies a simple isomorphism, to a metric invariance which expresses perfect congruence between the source and its image.

When operative stimuli reach the receptors or, to use Pavlovian terminology, the peripheral analysers, they are transformed into neural excitations, signals in a frequency code; this first correspondence preserves only a simple isomorphism. It is at the level of the central system, of the cortical analysers, that the various recoding operations are performed which transform these simple coded signals into signal-images the structure of which is congruent with that of the object and capable of retaining the effecttive constituent of the reflex.

According to Wekker the programme of action to be effected

can only be registered in the image. It would seem to be impossible for it to occur at the level of neural connections because the range of movements which can be executed by each effector is enormous and only a co-ordination of such movements could decrease the number of degrees of freedom of the system. This co-ordination presupposes a certain number of choices; it is evident that these are rarely made on a chance basis – on the contrary, they seem to conform to a system, to a programme of action.

Principally this involves the elimination of redundant degrees of freedom in the motor activity, so that the spatial-kinetic organisation of the action conforms to the physical structure of the object. The signal image, intermediary between the stimulus-source and the response, only becomes an adequate programme of action to the extent that it conserves the individual geometry of the invariant source of information. There is thus a double correlation, firstly between the physical structure of the object and the geometry of the signal-image, secondly between this geometry and the structure of the movements which it controls; by this means the action response is integrated and adapted and the perceived object is similar to the physical object.

However, it is necessary to add that the geometry of a particular physical-spatial situation does not determine a single and specific motor solution, but a family of solutions all leading to the same final action – like, for example, touching an object with a finger but approaching it from different directions, all of which are compatible with the spatial characteristics of the situation. The choice from amongst these various motor solutions can be made either at the elementary level of sensory control or, voluntarily, at the superior level of intellectual control.

The total duration of the process is relatively long since it corresponds to the transformation of an information signal into a control signal. Within this perspective, the various stages of the perceptual act are as follows.

When the stimulus pattern emanating from the physical object impinges on the peripheral receptors, an initial neural coding converts the constituents of the continuous series of initial physical and physiological conditions into nerve impulses, the discrete elements of the frequency code. At the level of the cortical analyser, a series of decoding and recoding processes converts the nerve impulses into sensory quanta, the elements of a continuous mental image which faithfully reproduces the continuous initial state. In a final transformation the programme, contained within the signal image, controls the nerve impulses to the effectors and releases the sequence of actions.

Our knowledge of the physical world through the intermediary of images is neither immediate nor automatic; during the genesis of these images a particular form of activity, that of orientation and exploration, is preponderant.

## 2 *The Role of Perceptual Exploration in the Construction of the Image*

The Pavlovian orienting reflex, the observable orienting response of the sensory receptors to the stimulus-source, is accompanied by changes which are not directly observable, but which can be recorded by various means; these changes are manifest at the level of the electroencephalogram, muscular tension, and the functioning of the autonomic nervous system. The reaction of orientation (Sokolov, 1958, 1966; Berlyne, 1960) constitutes therefore a complex of events which play a double role, since it increases the organism's capacity for extracting information from the environment by heightening the sensitivity of the receptors, and it prepares the organism for rapid action. For Zaporozhets (1960) this orientation reaction is the objective equivalent of a process of conscious attention and the point of departure for an active examination of the object which has caused it. But a clear distinction must be made between the simple orientation of receptors and active exploration of the object. Only the latter makes possible the construction of a model, an adequate image, because a simple orientation towards the object provides insufficient information.

An individual part of an image reproduces the properties of an individual part of the object source, but a mental image, insofar as it is a structured and invariant unitary whole, must reproduce the totality of the structural properties of the source. But the field of an analyser is restricted by the extent of the receptor area; in order to construct an image of the entire object it has to be inspected and explored by the analyser. This inspection organises the spatial structure of the image whilst preserving the continuity of the temporal series of the initial conditions; there is a transformation of a successive temporal series into a simultaneous spatial structure.

Inspection thus appears to be the sole means of preventing the extent of the image being limited to that of the receptor screen. One can see immediately that the nature and extent of the exploration is going to determine the characteristics of the image. If this exploration is limited, if it only takes into account a proportion of the properties of the object, only a few invariants will be conserved and the correspondence between the geometry of the image and that of the stimulus will not attain the metric level but only an inferior one – topological or projective, for example. Or perhaps only one area of the object is explored and the image, incomplete like the exploration, will only represent this part.

In the course of his development the child acquires, through his contact with the environment and the influence of his social background, a certain number of perceptual 'operative structures' (Zaporozhets and Zinchenko, 1966), in effect, programmes of action for examining an object and evaluating its properties. These operative structures act as mediators for the child's actions in the same way as tools for practical activity or words for intellectual activity. Perceptual actions involve more than the reflection of a current situation; they anticipate the modifications which are liable to result from the practical action undertaken.

The developmental evolution of perceptual activities in the child is summarised by Zaporozhets (1965) in the following manner. During the first three months there is an orientation response differentiated as a function of the novelty, of the interest of the stimulus, but no perceptual structure is involved in the control of the behavioural response which is uncomplicated. An oriented activity, exclusively practical, begins with the emergence of coordination between prehension and vision; the characteristics of this practical activity determine those of perceptual actions; anticipation, for example, relates to the displacement of the object. The child discriminates the properties which are immediately visible and bound up in his actions, the rest remaining undifferentiated. From the second year anticipation is no longer limited to relationships between the subject and object but is also applied to certain relationships between objects; perceptual images cease to be fragmentary and become organised, the contour achieves unity, topological relationships are perceived. Between the ages of 3 and 7 years the exploration of the object and its integration into a structured whole develops. Faced with a new situation the child of this age gets to know it in the first place by means of practical activity; at a second stage he devotes himself to an increasingly exhaustive exploration of the object by displacing his sensory receptors and constructs an image of the object. During this period the tactile-kinaesthetic system is the first to be mobilised. Indeed the tactile-kinaesthetic analyser engages in direct interaction with the physical properties of the object, which are characterised by their macroscopic nature and are inseparable from its spatial-temporal structure. This direct interaction provides an adequate physical basis for the construction of an image. It follows that the cognizance of the formal properties of an object by the tactile-kinaesthetic receptors would seem to be the easiest. The first mental images will thus be tactile-kinaesthetic in origin; any other image formed on the basis of stimuli received by the more intermediate analysers, vision for example, would be constructed secondarily through the tactile-kinaesthetic modality.

Finally, at a third stage, perceptual actions are less apparent because the exploration becomes internalised.

## II  TACTILE MODELS AND VISUAL MODELS

Ananiev (Ananiev, Wekker, Lomov and Yarmolenko, 1959) postulates that the model constructed as a result of the encounter between the physical object and the receptors of a sensory modality can be utilised in other modalities. Tactile perception being ontogenetically more primitive than visual perception, tactile models of objects would be the first to be constructed and visual models could only be derived from them. An important series of investigations[1] has related tactile and visual performances with the aim of demonstrating that visual models present the same characteristics as tactile models because the former derive from the latter. Fairly recently a number of American psychologists have begun to investigate the transfer between visual and tactile modalities, and their results can be compared with those of the Russian workers.

## 1  *Recording Tactile Exploratory Activity*

Ananiev, Wekker, Lomov and Yarmolenko (1959) made a cine-recording of the way in which a blindfolded adult explored an object with both hands with the subsequent aim of reproducing it by drawing or identifying it from amongst other objects. A very elaborate analysis was made of the activity of each hand, the extent of the exploration, the rate of displacement of the hand or the objects, the point at which this rate slowed down, and the location of pauses. It emerged that the direction of exploration followed the sagittal axis of the body and that pauses occurred preferentially at the angles of objects. Reference to the available data on visual exploration reveals a striking analogy; vision also explores objects in a generally vertical direction and stops longest on the points of inflexion of the contour (Zusne and Michels, 1964). The theory of the image predicts that the reproduction should constitute a

---

[1]It is unfortunate that, because of our ignorance of the Russian language, we have only been able to acquaint ourselves with this research by means of summaries, the translation of which at times leaves something to be desired, and critical reviews by American authors (Berlyne, 1963; H. Pick, 1963, 1964).

graphic translation of the image of the stimulus, constructed during its exploration by an interaction between the object and the receptors. The results of Ananiev and his associates are in agreement with these predictions. The drawings reproduced the principal characteristics of the exploration. The points of inflexion where the hand had paused were shown, and the drawing was, in general, more elongated than the model along the vertical axis (the privileged direction of exploratory movements). The order followed during the exploration was also found when it came to the reproduction of the drawings.

Ginevskaya (1948) observed the tactile examination of objects by blindfolded children aged 3 to 7 years. At 3 years of age, a child was content to play with the object by rolling it, pulling it, tapping it, and so on. At 4 and 5 years, familiarisation activity was added to the playing, but it remained very crude, the child simply squeezing the object very hard with his hand. From the age of 6 years real exploratory activity developed in which the child followed the contour of the object with his finger, tested its degree of resistance to pressure, examined its texture – in short, analysed its properties.

Zinchenko and Ruzskaya (1960a, b) repeated the same study with the aid of cine-recording; they observed some exploratory handling of objects from the age of 4 years and carried out a precise analysis of the stages. The 3-year-old child seized hold of the object rather than handled it, and if the experimenter placed the palm of the child's hand on the edge of the object he was content to tap it with his finger tips without moving his palm. Between 4 and 5 years a preliminary contact activity between the hand and the object appeared, but limited to the palm of one hand, the fingertips playing no part. Between 5 and 6 years, the child began to use both hands and to follow the contour of the object, but this exploration remained partial and unsystematic; it was often limited to one part which was more distinctive than the rest, such as a hole or a projection. Really systematic, thorough exploration was not observed until after the age of 6 years.

A comparison of these results with those which have been obtained by the recording of eye-movements (Zinchenko, Van Chizi-Tsin and Tarakanov, 1962), reveals a striking analogy between the methods of exploration observed, at the same age, in both visual and tactile areas.

## 2   *Data Relating to Intermodal Transfer in Children*

Contrary to Ananiev's hypotheses (Ananiev, Wekker, Lomov and Yarmolenko, 1959) research investigations into intermodal transfer all demonstrate that a tactile model is not easier to construct than a visual model – quite the reverse. The existence of a dependent relationship between a tactile model and a visual model is not verified.

The term 'intermodal transfer' has been applied to two types of experiments, the first relating to the classic transfer of an initial learning effected in one sensory modality to a second task effected in another; another series of experiments measures, in one sensory modality, the recognition of objects presented in another modality.

Rudel and Teuber's (1964) experiment is an example of investigations of the second type. For their material they used three-dimensional objects, divided into two series: an easy one which consisted of five regular forms – a cube, a sphere, a cylinder, a cone and a pyramid – and a difficult one comprising four irregular forms, somewhat similar, and a flattened pyramid. In the visual-visual condition, one of the objects was shown to the child for a period of five seconds then removed; the five objects of the series were then presented, one at a time, with the instruction to say whether or not it was the same as the model. The tactile-visual condition differed from the preceding one only in the fact that the model was not seen but was handled during a five-second period. This was reversed in the visual-tactile condition where the model was seen for five seconds and the variables handled one after the other. In the tactile-tactile condition the child never saw the objects. This technique of successive presentation posed considerable difficulties for the youngest children; none of the 3-year-olds were able to carry out the task, and at 4 years judgments were only obtained for the easy series. In the latter instance the best performances were observed in the visual-visual condition; the tactile-tactile condition emerged as by far the most difficult and the two situations involving intermodal transfer were of intermediate difficulty. Five-year-old children were capable of identifying forms in both the easy and the difficult series, with successive presentation. Their performances were, of course, better with the easy forms but the differences between conditions were in the same direction for both series – the tactile-tactile task was more difficult than the other three, which seemed to be almost equivalent.

In order to obtain data on younger children, the authors limited themselves to the visual-visual and tactile-visual conditions, the objects for selection then being presented simultaneously with the instruction to indicate which one was identical to the model that had been seen or handled before but was now hidden. In this situation it was possible to obtain responses to the easy series at 3 years of age and to the difficult series at 4 years; at both ages the visual-

visual condition produced a better performance than the tactile-visual condition.

An experiment by Denner and Cashdan (1967) compared the relative influence of three modes of presentation on the recognition of forms by 3- to 4-year-old children. The child either simply saw the object or he saw it *and* manipulated it. This manipulation might directly involve the object, in which case it provided tactile information which supplemented the visual information. It was also possible to have a non-informative manipulation. In this situation the object was placed in a transparent plastic ball, that is, it was visible but the tactile stimuli related to the ball and not the object. The visual only presentation resulted in a poorer recognition performance than the presentations involving manipulation, but the two forms of the latter were equivalent. The facilitation would thus seem to be due to the level of gross motor activity, as the information provided by the handling of the object itself was not used.

A group of Russian psychologists has studied intra- and inter-modal transfer in children from 3 to 7 years, using as their material simple, asymmetrical forms carved on a piece of wood and derived from designs of Gaydos (1956); as with Rudel and Teuber (1964), the presentation and recognition of the model from amongst three choice-variables could be either tactile or visual, giving four experimental situations. Few details of the experimental designs are available and, unfortunately, it appears (H. Pick, 1964) that neither the order of presentation nor the effects of practice were controlled. However, the results do provide some interesting information, even as they stand.

From the results of a number of experiments (Zinchenko, 1960; Zinchenko and Ruzskaya, 1960a, b) it appears that before the age of 4 years recognition is better when presentation and recognition are made within the same sensory modality, but the number of correct responses is low (50 per cent error-rate). At the same age-levels tactile recognition after visual presentation seems to be impossible and, in the case of visual recognition after tactile presentation, responses appear to be distributed on a chance basis (70 per cent error-rate). From the age of 4 years intermodal transfer is in evidence and there is then no longer any systematic superiority of performances in intramodal situations over those obtained in intermodal situations. It is clear that the visual-visual condition is much the easiest; when tactile perception was involved, recognitions were often incorrect. The authors attributed the particular difficulty of those situations which involved the tactile-kinaesthetic modality to the fact that they depended to a greater extent on memory.

In order to verify this hypothesis, Lavrentyeva and Ruzskaya (1960) repeated the same experiment but substituted, in the recognition task, the simultaneous presentation of three choice-variables, instead of the successive presentation used in the first experiment. To their surprise performance was even worse, especially in the condition of tactile presentation followed by visual recognition.

### III  THE INFLUENCE OF TRÀINING ON EXPLORATION

By relating the data obtained from recording the exploratory activity of children during the examination and subsequent recognition of unfamiliar objects to the performances achieved during recognition, the above-mentioned investigators saw the errors as arising from inadequate exploration. In consequence they felt that by training the child to explore the stimulus-objects it would be possible to improve his recognition performance. The role attributed by Zaporozhets (1961) to voluntary movements in the development of cognitive performances led them to postulate that practical manipulatory activity could well be as effective as exploratory activity in familiarisation with objects. Consequently a group of experiments was devoted to comparing the effects of three types of training: the practical use of objects, their tactile exploration, and their visual exploration.

Tarakanov and Zinchenko (1960) divided their subjects into two groups. The children in the first group examined a stimulus by visual and tactile means and then had to recognise it in a group of three objects; for one sub-group this was done by means of touch, for the other it was done visually. The children in the second group played at placing the stimulus-object in the appropriate hole in a form-board and then carried out the same recognition tasks as those in the first group. This second group were clearly superior to the first, whether recognition was measured in terms of tactile or visual perception. Practical activity with a functional goal thus appeared to bring about a better perceptual knowledge of the object than a simple examination of it, a result which confirms the findings in many other experiments.

Still using the forms derived from Gaydos, Zinchenko and Ruzskaya (1960a) compared the relative value of four systematic methods of training. For one group familiarisation occurred by means of practical activity: the child learnt to insert the forms in a form-board. For the others training involved the activity of exploration: the child learnt to follow the contour of each form (training by touching) or to follow the contour visually (training by looking) or by means of visual and tactile exploration. In the visual training condition the experimenter traced the contour of the form with a stylus whilst the child followed the displacement with his eyes.

In the test task the children had to recognise from amongst some unfamiliar figures the one on which they had been trained. The comparison of performances as a function of the pretraining involved showed that in the youngest children practical activity was by far the most effective, training by tactile exploration the least so, and that, from 5½ years, visual exploration gave as good results as practical activity.

Table 25   *Percentages of errors made in a recognition task following four types of training*

|   | Training | *Age (in years)* | | | |
|---|---|---|---|---|---|
|   |   | *3– 4* | *4–5* | *5–6* | *6–7* |
| 1 | Visual | 50·0 | 28·5 | 0 | 2·5 |
| 2 | Tactile | 47·7 | 42·3 | 25·0 | 23·1 |
| 3 | Visual and tactile | 30·8 | 21·0 | 11·5 | 1·9 |
| 4 | Practical activity | 15·4 | 10·5 | 0 | 0 |

After Zinchenko and Ruzskaya (1960a), reproduced in Zaporozhets and Zinchenko (1966, p. 407).

Venger (1962) studied the activity of 2- to 3-year-old children with a form-board. They were given wooden pieces, geometric in form, which had to be placed in the corresponding holes which had been cut in the board.

All the children began by using a trial-and-error approach; the 2-year-olds did not get past this stage even after many repetitions, but at 3 years it was possible to see a development in the course of the activity. After a more or less protracted period of simple, trial-and-error, practical activity, the child began to make comparisons between the piece and the hole in the form-board; Venger observed that the child's gaze went from one to the other as if he were comparing the two objects before making a decision. Venger's observations, like those of other investigators cited by Zaporozhets and Zinchenko (1966), show that before the age of 3 years the child only compares objects by means of the action of one on the other, whilst from that age he becomes capable of predicting the result of this interaction on the basis of a comparison between successive perceptions.

The effects of practical activity with objects are also manifest in tasks involving the analysis and synthesis of complex structures.

Following active training with the component figures, children of 3 to 4 years were able to locate them in complex forms (embedded figures problems), which was impossible for children of the same age who had not had the same training (Sokhina, cited in Zaporozhets and Zinchenko, 1966). With a more difficult task in which the child had to choose, from amongst a group of objects, those which he would need to reconstruct a complex object, practical training was not equally effective at all ages. This training consisted of handling paper reproductions of the parts of various objects and placing them on the complex object; the child was thus able to verify whether the part selected was appropriate or not and in which position it could be placed. The 3-year-old children had great difficulty in following this form of training, and it did not improve their performance. In children from 4 to 5 years a positive transfer was obtained but it was limited to the complex object and to the components which had been handled, whilst between the ages of 5 and 7 years transfer generalised to other materials. In this experiment, therefore, practical activity brought about an improvement in the perceptual analysis of forms, notably the articulation between whole and parts.

Finally, Ruzskaya (1958) has shown that a pretraining involving perceptual activity also influences the acquisition of geometric concepts such as triangle and rectangle. A systematic pretraining, which associated the manipulation of cut-out forms, systematic exploration of the contour with a finger – at the same time counting the angles – and visual exploration, was followed by a number of categorical identification tasks involving triangular and rectangular forms presented visually. According to Ruzskaya, the child has acquired, progressively, an algorithm of exploratory activity which subsequently enabled him to identify the group of triangles as opposed to the rectangles, whatever their orientation and even when the contour was discontinuous (dotted).

## IV GRAPHIC REPRODUCTION AND EXPLORATORY ACTIVITY

The distribution of a child's perceptual activity amongst the stimulus-objects present during a discrimination learning task (White and Plum, 1964; Wright and Smothergill, 1967; Scott and Christy, 1968) or between a model and its copy in a task involving reproduction by drawing (Pêcheux and Stambak, 1969) evolves with age and with performance. The two last-mentioned authors related the quality of the copy to the way in which the child divided his time between the model drawing and the copy; they interpreted the observed evolution in terms of the extent of the repertoire of representative schemas the child possessed and his rapidity in constructing a new schema.

Pêcheux and Stambak (1969) measured the time during which the child looked at the model and at the reproduction he made, and also the number of movements from the model to the copy. The authors observed that the duration of the exploration of the model decreased with age between 5 and 10 years, and that the time spent looking at the reproduction decreased initially between 5 and 7 years but increased after that. In consequence, the total time taken to execute the task changed with age, the 5-year-old children devoting 40 per cent of the time to exploration of the model, the 10-year-olds giving it no more than 20 per cent. The number of movements from the model to the reproduction followed the same evolution as the time taken in making the copy: it decreased between 5 and 7 years and subsequently increased. These varying evolutions with age could be interpreted in the following way: the time necessary for gathering the information contained in the model decreases with age. Between 5 and 7 years the children were satisfied to reproduce what they had abstracted in an exploration of this model; becoming more and more skilful at drawing as they grew older, they took less and less time to execute their drawing. After the age of 7 years they became more exacting in what they required of their reproduction and so found it necessary to check by to-and-fro movements between their drawing and the model. Thus they also took the time which was necessary in order to reproduce all the relationships – metric as well as topological – of the drawing concerned. This was made up of a series of simple forms – circles, squares – linked up by lines into a complex structure. The quality of the copy developed with age and depended both on the internal models, or representative schemas, of simple forms which the child possessed before the beginning of the task, and on his capacities for constructing the more complex and unfamiliar model which corresponded to the drawing presented. Up to the age of 7 years, the child seemed content to use previously acquired models and to reproduce familiar structures – circles, squares, lines – without attempting to integrate them into a global structure. The parts of the complex model were therefore correctly reproduced from the age of about 6 years, but not their spatial relationships.

These results are in agreement with those of the Russian school of psychologists. A drawn reproduction gives an account of the properties of the representational model which the child has constructed during his perception of the form to be reproduced. When this – as a whole or at the level of certain of its parts – is familiar, the child has available, from the beginning, models previously acquired. He is thus content to identify the forms and reproduce them by referring simply to the representation he has made of them. The exactness of the reproduction depends on that of the representation. When the form to be reproduced is complex and unfamiliar, the child must construct his representational model during the task. The richness and precision of this model depends therefore on the perceptual activity of the child: the greater this is, the more the number of comparisons between the drawing and its reproduction will be increased, and the more the latter will be true to the model. In the investigation by Pêcheux and Stambak, it appears that the complex drawing is perceived as completely novel by the very young child, the reproduction then corresponding to a very limited and inexact internal model. Children a little older, those from 6 to 7 years, recognise in the structure the presence of familiar forms – squares or circles – for which they possess models; they content themselves with reproducing what they have identified without taking account of the spatial relationships between these structures and without feeling the need to check the result of their activity. Only the older children make a conscious attempt to construct an adequate model of the entire drawing, analysing both the parts and their relationships, hence the increased number of comparisons made between the stimulus and its reproduction.

## V  DISCUSSION AND INTERPRETATION OF THE DATA REPORTED

Zaporozhets and Zinchenko (1966) see in the results of these various investigations arguments in favour of the theory of the image (Wekker, 1966; Leontiev and Gippenreiter, 1966, etc.). An individual's ability to subsequently recognise or identify an object depends upon the model he has constructed of it; thus, when he is confronted with an unfamiliar object or event, which he expects to meet again, the individual sets about constructing a model of it since the degree of precision of a subsequent identification of the object is going to depend on the quality of this model. It seems that before the age of 3 years the child does not possess representational models separate from direct action on the object; these can only be held in reserve and used for the purpose of identifying what is already known in incorporating the stimulation to which the object gives rise within a set of actions – the aim of these being the establishment of functional relationships between objects. One can see in this parallels with Piaget's sensori-motor schema

(Piaget, 1936) and Bruner's concept of *enactive representation* (Bruner, 1964, 1966a, b, 1968).

From the age of 3 years strategies of comparison begin to detach themselves from immediate and practical activity; objects can be compared in a more mediational fashion, by comparing what is perceived with what is remembered. Representational models in the form of images then come to play an intermediate role between successive perceptions; for the Russian authors the perceptual activity of exploration is the means of constructing such models. Limited in their exploratory activity, 3-year-old children possess very inadequate models; 4- and 5-year-olds construct incomplete models, limited to a number of features of the objects; only the 6-year-olds, who carry out comprehensive explorations of the most informative part – the contour of objects – construct exact models. In a recognition task, identification rests on a comparison between the information currently obtained and the model formed previously. The youngest children operate randomly because their sketchy model gives them no real guide as to what information to look for; in consequence their performance is poor. Older children, of 4 or 5 years, look for the few specific features which they have included in their model, but this remains incomplete; errors are made which could be due to the fact that the model does not include an important area for differentiating between the forms to be recognised, or because, during recognition, the areas inspected are ill chosen. In short, in both instances error is the consequence of inadequate exploration, which can occur either at the level of the formation of the model or at the level of the information-search at the time of identification.

Not being concerned to construct an exact model, very young children spend little time familiarising themselves with an object but, because they only have rudimentary, incomplete models, they need a relatively long time, at the moment of recognition, in order to discover in the object with which they are presented that feature which can be related to a model; despite this their recognition is very often incorrect, since its degree of accuracy depends on that of the model. Older children, of 6 years, take the time they need in order to construct a model, which enables them, during recognition, to search for information where it is to be found and so to avoid examining uninformative areas; they are thus slower in familiarisation and quicker and more accurate in their identifications (Zinchenko, Van Chizi-Tsin and Tarakanov, 1962).

After considering all their results, Zinchenko and Ruzskaya (1960b) reached the conclusion that Ananiev's hypothesis (Ananiev, Wekker, Lomov and Yarmolenko, 1959), that manual exploration precedes the visual and acts as some sort of guide and model for it, is invalid. In this respect the results of A. Pick (1956; A. Pick, H. Pick and Thomas, 1966) and of Rudel and Teuber (1964) confirm those of Zinchenko and his associates. Transfer operations which involve the intervention of tactile perception are always more difficult than visual-visual transfer; as to intramodal tactile-tactile transfer, this is only possible relatively late in development and always produces performances inferior to the others. It therefore appears that visual models are established sooner and more easily than tactile models. This relative superiority of vision is certainly due in large part to the fact that the visual receptor system permits the simultaneous experience of multiple data, whilst the tactile receptor system only provides limited data in succession. The integration of the latter thus requires an intense and systematic perceptual activity; it is not surprising therefore that tactile models are even more inadequate than visual ones in the youngest children. The intervention of a model in the process of identification seems to be limited initially to the sensory modality in which it was acquired, and intermodal transfer appears only when there has been an integration of the subject's tactile and visual models. Finally, everything which brings about perceptual exploratory activity or an analysis of the properties of an object, having the effect of focusing attention on its characteristics, induces the construction of a model. But as a general rule the experimental results do not enable us to decide whether this model is a category (Bruner, Goodnow and Austin, 1956), an invariant based on distinctive features (E. J. Gibson, 1963), an image (Wekker, 1966; Zaporozhets and Zinchenko, 1966), or a figurative structure of the schematic type (Piaget, 1961).

## CONCLUSION OF CHAPTERS 9 AND 10

It would seem possible to make a rapid outline sketch of the development of perceptual activity in the child from 3 to 7 years by referring to Chapters 9 and 10 of the present volume, and to other sources for data concerning the baby (Vurpillot, 1966, 1972).

The baby manifests visuo-motor activity from birth; the utilisation of vision is a behaviour of the same kind as sucking. Initially this activity is satisfying in itself: 'Objects are first assimilated to the activity of looking itself; their sole interest is that they are capable of being looked at' (Piaget, 1963, p. 66). It does not follow from this that the visual fixations are distributed randomly, but, to begin with, their localisation seems to be determined solely by the physical properties of the stimulus.

During the first two months of his existence, the baby essentially manifests orientation reactions in response to stimulation. The orienting reflex is preferentially triggered by certain properties of the stimulus (Salapatek and Kessen, 1966), which results in differing durations of fixation according to the targets concerned.

However, there does not seem to be any deliberate choice in looking at one point rather than another, and the gaze tends to remain on or return to the same area (Ames and Silfen, 1965). Although predominant, the stimulus does not entirely control the infant's behaviour, however. When the same pattern of visual stimuli is presented repeatedly, it is looked at less and less often and for shorter and shorter periods of time. The phenomenon of habituation, distinct from sensory fatigue, shows that the baby can at least choose to look or not to look, that a new object is interesting because it is unfamiliar and that once it has become familiar it ceases to merit inspection. Habituation is established more quickly as the child becomes older (Kagan and Lewis, 1965; Fantz, 1966, 1967; Lewis, Bartels, Fadel and Campbell, 1966), a fact which seems to be linked to the progressive extension of the mnemonic field. During the course of the first two months the amount of time spent awake and, consequently, the amount of visual attention, increase markedly (B. White and Held, 1966); accommodation and binocular convergence are established and perfected, whilst fixation and visual pursuit become more rapid and precise.

From the age of two months the increased ability to differentiate visually and the progressive extension of the mnemonic field lead to an increase in the ability to identify and differentiate both successive and simultaneous stimuli. Instead of being stimulus-bound, as hitherto, the baby begins to choose to look in one place rather than another – what can properly be called visuo-motor activity.

This is increasingly refined up to about the age of 7 years; displacement-movements of the eye occur more and more rapidly (Lesèvre, 1964); anticipation of the amplitude of a movement as a function of the location of a target and the ability to stop the movement at the required point means the elimination of superfluous correction movements and the attainment of perfect precision in fixation, the signs of good sensori-motor co-ordination of the visual system (Lesèvre, 1964).

All of these attainments seem to be due largely to progressive maturation of the central nervous system in the form of the multiplication of neural connections, the acceleration of neural transmission, and so on. However, the strategies of exploration, evidenced in the choice of points fixated and the sequence of these fixations, appear to be determined by the child's decision criteria. If the role of perceptual exploration is to collect information from the physical world, the selection of this information can only depend on the use the individual proposes to make of it.

In the youngest children, those of 3 and 4 years, perceptual exploration – whether tactile or visual – is characterised by its limited nature. Presented with a new object, the child begins by incorporating it in a scheme of action, which is for him the best way of getting to know it. The visual or tactile exploration is extremely poorly organised and limited, the child making few exploratory movements and these being of restricted amplitude (Zinchenko, Van Chizi-Tsin and Tarakanov, 1962).

In the course of this exploration, the pauses are long ones. Since these pauses are used for registering the information obtained from the object through the medium of sensory stimulation, one can deduce that this processing takes a significantly longer time in older children. It also appears that, from amongst the information available in the proximal stimulus, only the most distinct – in other words, what is within foveal vision in the visual modality – is taken into consideration. In short, the very young child abstracts little information and processes it slowly; this information relates to a restricted area of the object and only those points which are close together are seen as being related.

The choice of the area to be explored seems to be determined initially by the physical properties of the stimulus, a function of their power of attracting inspection. However, from the age of 3 or 4 years the upper part of the visual field appears to possess a greater attraction than the lower part, and exploration is not entirely random; very soon the left-to-right and top-to-bottom directions appear as privileged ones.

Between 3 and 7 years perceptual activity is developing from all points of view. The area explored is extended, the amplitude of movements increases so that more and more information is obtained and relationships are established between parts more and more remote from each other – all of which is in agreement with the theories of Piaget. At the same time, the duration of a fixation decreases whilst the useful field of vision expands, which means that the amount of information processed per unit-time is accordingly increased. Finally, the selection of the information to be abstracted and the relationships to be established follows the evolution of the decision-criteria (Vurpillot, 1968, 1969; Vurpillot and Moal, 1970).

When the time comes for learning to read, the preferred strategy of left-to-right and top-to-bottom exploration is reinforced;

although rigid at first, it becomes more flexible after the age of 7 years.

The relationships between performance on identification tasks and the form and extent of perceptual exploration provide strong arguments in favour of the role of this exploration in the construction of a cognitive model of objects, representational in nature. In the very young child, a restricted exploration brings about the formation of very limited models and is accompanied by poor performance on recognition tasks.

In summary, the child's level of cognitive development determines the choice from amongst the potential information contained in the environment and hence the form of his perceptual exploration. Correspondingly, the poverty or extensiveness of this exploration has its effects on cognitive activity since it is by such means that it is provided with the substance of its activity.

# Chapter 11

# Identity Criteria of
# Equivalence and Difference

In the preceding chapters we have examined various possible explanations of poor performance on identification and differentiation tasks by children of preschool age. All of these interpretations account for a proportion of the results obtained on perceptual tasks. Thus, by diverting attention from small details, a globalist perspective goes with satisfactory identification performances but results in unsatisfactory performances of differentiation (cf. Chapter 5). The rigidity of the primary perceptual structures and the absence of articulation between a whole and its parts limit the possibilities for identification, since the same unit cannot be treated simultaneously as a whole and as part of a greater whole. Identification is thus a function only of the primary perceptual structures whose form is determined by the laws of Gestalt (cf. Chapters 1 and 5). The inability to abstract the properties of objects and to treat them as dimensions of differentiation or categorisation impedes and limits the acquisition of discrimination learning (cf. Chapters 6, 7 and 8). Inadequate perceptual activity influences performance in a number of ways. Its limited spatial extension means that the child identifies and differentiates objects on the basis of only a sample of the information contained in the environment (cf. Chapter 9). When perceptual activity is reduced, the establishment of relationships between stimuli tends to be limited to the content of a proximal stimulus (the 'field effect' of the Gestaltists or, in Piagetian terms, 'centration'). From this point of view the rigidity of primary structures is due largely to the absence of exploration in young children. The analysis of a whole into its parts, like the articulation between them, requires changes in the way they are seen, and hence exploration. In conclusion, it is our opinion that the representational structures of objects are destined to serve as models to which subsequent experiences are related, and that the construction of these models depends upon establishing active relationships between the various proximal stimuli emanating from the same physical object. The less the child has engaged in the activities of exploration and schematisation, the more restricted his repertoire of models, and the more crude and incomplete these will be; this is bound to affect the quality of his performance on identification tasks (cf. Chapter 9).

Each of the interpretations that have just been outlined is based on a large number of experimental findings; and far from contradicting each other they are, in fact, complementary. However, even when combined, they still do not provide a sufficient basis for the prediction of the behaviour of children of preschool age on perceptual tasks. As we have had cause to observe in passing, on a number of occasions, these interpretations would seem to postulate implicitly that the child formulates his judgments whilst employing the decision criteria of an adult. Yet, in differentiation tasks at least, the analysis of performance seems to show that the child's decision criteria evolve with age; and that around 6 years of age they become similar to those of the adult. Before this, whilst being quite capable of perceiving in what respects objects differ, or what they have in common, the child groups them in terms of partial equivalences and not according to logical relationships; he possesses neither real identity relationships nor real classes of equivalence.

The present chapter sets out to study the child's acquisition of the identity relationship and to examine to what extent his progression from judgments based on partial equivalences – the requirements of which increase with age – to the point where he employs a system of logical relationships of identity, equivalence and difference, makes it possible to explain certain aspects of performance on differentiation tasks which cannot be accounted for by the preceding interpretations.

## I THE RELATIONSHIP BETWEEN DIFFERENTIATION AND IDENTIFICATION

Starting with a small number of innate behavioural structures, the child gradually constructs classes of events which he is able to recognise when they recur. He becomes capable of operating on perceptual structures, of making comparisons between these structures – and hence of differentiating them – and of relating them to cognitive models for purposes of identification.

Identification and differentiation develop in a conjoint, complementary fashion, but the relationships between these two operations are not always clearly apparent. In part this seems to be due to the ambiguity of the terms employed. Thus, to identify an 'object' signifies recognition that the 'individual' in question is one that has been seen before, Mr X for example; but it is also a matter of deciding in which class of objects (e.g. men) it could be placed. The term 'identify' applies, therefore, both to a single object class and to a class of equivalence of multiple objects. In other words, 'identity' is used as much in respect of an individual who remains the same person, in spite of real or apparent changes, as it is with regard to two or more objects, distinct and separate but exactly similar. Yet the interaction between differentiation and identification differs according to the meaning that is given to 'identity' and 'identification'. If it is a matter of identifying a particular individual (individual identity), the important thing is to discover the essential constituents, those which remain invariant from one situation to another; the differences which do not reach this 'key' level can be treated as non-relevant variations and so ignored. If, on the other hand, identity relates to several objects, then it implies that no difference should be discovered between them; in this instance differentiation plays a determining role.

The study of the age-related development of the capacities of identification and differentiation in children, by means of performances obtained on perceptual tasks, requires an analysis of experimental settings and a clarification of the terminology employed.

## 1 Physical Identity and Perceived Identity

At the level of the physical world, two objects can only be identical or different. Physical identity is defined in terms of complete congruence: the two objects have the same values on all possible descriptive dimensions. When physical identity is not defined in absolute terms, that is to say in terms of the intrinsic characteristics of the object, but with a view to establishing a correspondence between physical identity and perceived identity, the role of context must be taken into consideration and in particular the relationship between the object and the observer. Consequently, it is necessary to establish whether physical identity, in whatever situational parameter, relates only to the intrafigural relations of each of the two objects or whether an identity of relationships with a frame of reference has to be added. In other words, are two rectangles of the same length and breadth, but one horizontal and the other vertical, considered as physically identical or different?

Although it is a simple matter to define unambiguously the criteria of identity and physical dissimilarity of two or more objects, the discovery, from a subject's responses, of whether he has established relationships of equivalence or identity and, in the latter case, the criteria on which it is based, is an extremely subtle procedure.

When two physically identical objects are presented to a subject, the information which enables him to compare them consists mainly of a series of proximal stimuli. The physical identity of these two objects can practically never be deduced from an identity between two proximal stimuli, an identity which would imply that the two objects were presented successively in the same spatial position, the subject maintaining exactly the same fixation point. In this privileged instance the only difficulty would be the comparison between the information presented in an actual proximal stimulus and the information which remained from the memory of the previous proximal stimulus.

One could imagine a case, even more special, where a subject kept his gaze fixed on a point situated between the two objects, at an equal distance from each of them. Apart from the fact that the projection of one would fall on one hemiretina, and that of the other on the other hemiretina, the corresponding parts of the proximal stimulus would be as similar as possible and no demands would be made on memory.

These artificial situations are only cited in order to demonstrate the extent to which physical identity cannot be perceived by means of an identity of sensory excitation. In the great majority of cases in everyday life, the identity of two objects can only be perceived by the intermediary of different proximal stimuli.

Short-term memory is almost always involved, whether it is a matter of comparing information gathered successively from two objects which have to be judged, or of integrating information obtained during visual fixations on different parts of the same object. The intervention of exploratory activity and the integration of sensory data, even in the relatively simple case where it is a a matter of saying whether two objects situated side by side are identical or different, makes very clear the continuity that exists between differentiation and identification. The perceived identity always derives from the conservation of an invariance despite the existence of certain differences; the invariant differs only in terms of the type of identity which is sought.

## 2   *The Meaning Of The Term 'Identity' in Some Perceptual Tasks*

(*a*)   *Perceptual invariants.* Perceptual constancies provide an example of when the identity of a particular object is maintained across modifications of its context: changes in the spatial relationships between the object and the subject, changes in illumination, and so on. The identity of an object and its intrinsic properties (size, form, colour, reflectivity) is conserved despite modifications in the proximal stimuli corresponding to different levels of illumination or different positions of the object. There is, as Poincaré (1902) observes, a distinction between changes of condition which attack the integrity of the object and changes of position which respect it. After a very long controversy, there is now agreement in recognising that it is a matter of perceptual invariance and not of a judgment based on previous knowledge. However, all psychologists concerned with perception know how ambiguous the measurement of perceptual constancy is, since the object that is moved nearer or further away, or turned in the fingers, or moved from the shade into the light, appears the same and yet different.

The conservation of a set of intrafigural relationships involves the invariance of what the psychologists concerned with form call a Gestalt, and which Bingham (1914) designated by the term *form* as opposed to *shape*. The *form* of a figure, or an object, would be defined solely in terms of internal relationships. The identity of a *form* would thus be maintained during rotations and translations within a plane, through changes in the absolute size, and even through rotation in space around one side of the figure (Fellows, 1968). From this point of view, a 'T' and a 'T' upside down, a triangle with the horizontal base at the top or the bottom, retain their identity of *form*, in the same way as a picture – of whatever kind – which has been doubled in size, or a melody which has been transposed one octave.

For Bingham (1914) *shape* would be defined in terms of the relationships between a figure, or an object, and its context, that is by a system of relations within a frame of reference. Thus all equilateral triangles would have the same *form*, whatever their size or orientation within a plane, but only those which had the same size and the same position would also have the same *shape*. There appears to be some disagreement between different authors concerning mirror images obtained by rotation through space and not within a plane. For one group only rotations within a plane conserve *form*, mirror images constituting a modification of the original form (Sutherland, 1961). For another group (Fellows, 1968) *form* is conserved in mirror images. Gellerman (1933) goes even further than Bingham, since he considers that an organism only discriminates a *form*, in Bingham's sense of the term, when it is subject to certain conditions. If we take the triangle as an example, these conditions would be as follows:

—The subject can learn to differentiate a triangle from other geometric forms.

—He conserves the distinction across rotation of the triangle.

—The discrimination is independent of the absolute or relative size of the forms with which he is presented.

—The subject generalises the learning to all triangles.

—He responds to line-drawings of triangles in the same way as to solid triangles.

—The discrimination is independent of the background on which the triangle is presented.

When all these conditions are respected, the form which has been learned is recognisable independently of its context and of modifications to all points other than those which define it; it can be described in terms of a set of relationships: a closed figure with three angles (or three sides). At this point it is no longer a matter of perceptual, but of conceptual invariance.

(b)   *Individual identity.* The response of identity (Bruner, Goodnow and Austin, 1956) is applied to a person or an object who or which, although subject to minor modifications, is nevertheless recognised as remaining the same. This elementary conservation is designated as individual or qualitative identity by Piaget (Piaget and Voyat, 1968), who in this way contrasts the conservation of an individual unit with that of a class (categorial identity) or with that of a quantifiable quality such as weight or volume. Recognising the same person, in spite of differences in clothing, hair-style, expression, and ageing, is an identity response. The acceptance of a certain amount of wear and tear is as applicable to objects as it is to people, only the margin of tolerance varies from one subject to another, and from one object to another.

In the permanence of an object, conserved during its temporary disappearance, Piaget sees the first manifestation of a conservation of individual identity. The object is only considered as permanent from the time when the child actively searches for it after its disappearance, and permanence is not really acquired until the child takes into account the displacements undergone by the object during its period out of sight. The object is then 'conceived as remaining the same whatever the unseen displacements . . .' (Piaget, 1937, 2nd edn, 1950, p. 75). Such an object is by its very nature representational; in consequence it is not surprising that its construction comes relatively late, being manifest towards the end of the first year (Piaget, 1936, 1937; Gouin-Décarie, 1962). It is, however, possible to demonstrate perceptual permanence much earlier than this (Bower, 1967b). Hence Piaget speaks of a permanence tied to action and relating to sensory tableaux, visual or tactile, encapsulated and unarticulated, with an invariant structure which alone can constitute the object.

Piaget and his associates have devoted a series of investigations to the concept of identity in the child (Piaget, Sinclair and Vinh-Bang, 1968), which demonstrate an evolution through three stages. In the first stage the form of the identity depends on his own body and his own actions: the object involved in this activity conserves its identity to the extent that it is assimilated into this activity. The beginnings of decentration appear during the second stage, when the child begins to distinguish modifications of the object in the course of his activity; a dissociation comes about between those properties which are modified and those which are conserved; the object acquires an individual identity, differentiated from and independent of action. Operational identity appears later, at the point in time when the child begins to grasp the principles of quantitative conservation and when his judgments become integrated into reversible group structures.

Since the identity of an object corresponds to the conservation of an invariance despite perceptual modifications, it is tempting to see in perceptual constancies a special case of individual identity. For Bruner (Bruner, Goodnow and Austin, 1956) every identity response is the result of learning, and is just exceptionally precocious in the case of the constancies.

At first sight, Bruner's position would seem to be the right one, but we must bear in mind that, in the case of the perceptual constancies, physical identity – defined in terms of the possibility of congruence between two objects or the absence of any intrinsic modification – is conserved, which is not the case when a person dyes his hair or when a plate is chipped. The invariance which is maintained is not the same in both cases: with perceptual constancies it is a matter of conserving a set of relationships which involve both the object and its context, whilst with individual identity conservation relates more to a certain number of essential properties, any modification to the other, less essential properties being tolerated.

(c) *Categorial identity.* The class of equivalence brings together in the same category discriminable objects to which the subject gives the same response. Even when they are perceived as different, several objects are considered as equivalent because they have certain properties in common. From the logical viewpoint a class of equivalence is defined in terms of both extent and comprehensiveness; however, categorisations and categorial identifications are manifest in the child long before he is capable of logical classification. Consequently some writers, reserving the term of class of equivalence and concept for those categorisations which obey the laws of logic, introduce other terms to take account of the regrouping of objects as a function of the same response, verbal or otherwise. Piaget speaks of preclasses, preconcepts (Piaget and Inhelder, 1959), of representational schemas (Piaget, 1961); Lépine (1966) distinguishes between responses of equivalence which would result from the use of a logical system of classification, and responses of proximity which would express a simple ordering of objects according to certain of their properties – two objects would thus be judged the same because they were close together in terms of their properties. We allow ourselves to use the terms 'category' or 'class of partial equivalence' in a very wide sense implying the grouping of objects which are physically different, perceptually discriminable, whatever the rule by which the child makes his regrouping.

(*d*)   *Judgments of identity or difference.* In the so-called tasks of perceptual differentiation, a response of perceived identity is correct only to the extent that it corresponds to the physical identity of the objects compared. However, there is a limit to the equation between a physical object and a perceived object, due to the characteristics of sensory receptor systems. In order to be perceived, a physical modification must exceed a certain liminal value; the determination of these values provides a stimulus for the study of sensory capacities and particularly their development with age, as well as the influence of certain variables of attitude, personality, and so on. Developmental research on perceptual differentiation has been preoccupied with determining the conditions for the acquisition of responses to stimuli (discrimination learning), the criteria of identity of difference and the strategies of comparison. Consequently, the physical differences introduced by the experimenter have been chosen at much above the sensory threshold of discrimination; in the case of very young babies, the value taken for this threshold of perceptual activity is usually the one for which the most precise information is available (Fantz and Ordy, 1959; Fantz, Ordy and Udelf, 1962; Gorman, Cogan and Gellis, 1957, 1959).

When the objects to be compared are presented simultaneously, the task is described as one of differentiation. When they are presented in succession, the task is described as one of recognition and the subject has to compare one or a number of objects present with an object seen previously but now absent. In the case of recognition the role of short-term memory is greater than in the case of simple perceptual differentiation, but it is only a matter of degree.

In two instances only – the perceptual constancies and perceptual differentiation – is it both possible and necessary for the perceived identity between two objects, a standard and a variable, to correspond to a physical identity; in both cases this perceived identity rests on the maintenance of a perceptual invariance across a series of proximal stimuli. In the case of specific or categorial identification, membership of the same category does not stem from a physical identity but from the presence of a limited number of properties, relative or absolute, common to all the objects of a class or to all the conditions of a particular object.

## 3 *The Logical Relationship of Identity*

Lépine (1965, 1966) adopts a formal, logical approach in defining the relationship of identity as a limited case of the relationship of equivalence. When objects possess one or more properties and can be substituted for each other in situations where these properties are involved, they can be said to present a relationship of equivalence. The relationship of identity corresponds to the extreme case where the objects can be substituted for each other in every situation where they could be involved. Relationships of identity or equivalence are therefore only distinguished by the exhaustiveness or otherwise of the possibilities of substitution.

These two relationships can be defined positively or negatively. Objects are described as identical when they have all their characteristics and properties in common, and equivalent when they have in common some part of their characteristics and properties (positive definition). They are also described as identical when they cannot be discriminated, and equivalent when they cannot be discriminated from the point of view of the properties which define the class of equivalence (negative definition). The relationship of identity rests on the establishment of a reciprocal correspondence of *all* the properties of the objects being compared, whilst a relationship of equivalence can arise from the establishment of a partial correspondence.

The only type of studies which would seem to make possible the investigation of the operation of the relationships of identity and difference are those concerned with perceptual differentiation. In such studies a judgment of identity requires a succession of operations, the first of which is a thorough analysis of the properties of the objects being compared, and the second the establishment of reciprocal comparisons of all the objects in respect of all their properties; if, following the establishment of all these correspondences, no difference is detected, the objects can be declared identical. Conventionally, a difference always excluded from the list of properties is the position of the object in relation to the subject. Since they cannot both be in the same place at the same time, they always differ from this point of view. It is accepted that the only differences of spatial localisation which will be taken into consideration are those relating to a frame of reference specified by the experimenter.

Giving the same response to physically identical objects can result from the use of a relationship of identity like that of a relationship of equivalence. Consequently only those judgments relating to objects which are physically different make it possible to distinguish between the two types of relationship. If these objects are judged as different it can be concluded that the subject makes use of the relationship of identity. If, on the other hand, he judges them as the same this could be due to the fact that he cannot discriminate them or because he ignores the differences in order to concentrate on the common properties, and so responds in terms of equivalence.

In order to carry out a task of comparison, the subject must be able to operate the relationships of identity, equivalence and difference and thus possess decision criteria appropriate to each of them; presented with a problem, he must be able to determine which type of judgment it must involve, which relationship must be employed, and so select an appropriate strategy.

## II   THE VERBAL RESPONSE 'THE SAME'

When a child responds 'the same' to two objects which are similar but not physically identical, we might consider whether this is due to a lack of specific verbal terms such as identical, similar, or different. It is difficult to answer this question, since there has been little research on this point. In an investigation of the concepts of identity and difference in children from 4 to 7 years of age, Oléron (1962) presented pairs of identical or different drawings which the child had to classify as a function of this relational property. The task was presented in a non-verbal manner to deaf and hearing children. Two models, one of which showed two men and the other a man and a woman, were each set out above a platform. The child was given pairs of other objects which could differ in terms of form, or colour, or size, or categorial membership, or weight, or speed. When the child placed identical stimulus-objects beneath the model with identical drawings, and different stimulus-objects beneath the model with different drawings, it was, the author suggests, because he responded as a function of the relationships of identity and difference. Correct choices were rewarded with a sweet, and one series of stimulus-objects replaced by another after a minimum of five correct responses or ten trials. Following the task the hearing children had to answer a certain number of questions, the purpose of which was to test whether the child, even when he had responded correctly, was capable of verbalising the rule governing his choices. However, Oléron found that none of the thirty-eight children questioned used the word 'identical' spontaneously and only one the word 'different'; the terms used were 'same' and 'not the same', and occasionally 'equal'. But even though the distribution of responses made by the 4-year-old children in this experiment was what one would expect on the basis of chance, the 5-, 6- and 7-year-olds quickly discovered the rule governing the response and conformed to it.

It does not seem, therefore, that success or failure in perceptual discrimination tasks can be attributed to the absence of specific verbal responses. The word 'same' accompanied by appropriate qualifiers would seem to be sufficient to determine clearly defined response categories: 'same' is the general term signifying that the task involves a comparison, 'exactly the same' corresponds to 'identical', 'almost the same' to 'similar', and 'not the same' to 'different'. When the experimenter used terms of this kind, he was satisfied to take those used by the child, and the categories determined in this fashion were employed to the extent that they belonged to the child's repertoire.

In the age-ranges studied by Oléron, that is, above the age of 4 years, the failure that involved giving a 'same' response to physically different stimulus-objects cannot be explained in terms of a straightforward verbal inadequacy. Without using the terms 'different' and 'identical' the older children employed the relationship of identity, whilst with the same vocabulary the younger children did not.

Nevertheless, examination of individual performances obtained in differentiation tasks reveals that the majority of 3-year-old children and a significant number of 4-year-olds did not understand verbal comparison instructions involving the judgment 'same' or 'not the same'. In all of the experiments of this type several children gave the same response to all the stimulus-objects presented, this response usually being 'same' but sometimes also 'not the same'. It would seem probable that some of the youngest children were still at the preverbal stage (Luria, 1957; T. Kendler and H. Kendler, 1969) but there is no way of deciding with certainty whether, when a child of 3 to 4 years describes all the pairs as 'the same', it is because according to his criteria he judges them the same, or whether it is because for him the word 'same' still lacks meaning.

### III   RELATIVE SENSITIVITY TO DIFFERENCES AND SIMILARITIES

The earliest child psychologists interested in perceptual development were concerned to discover whether young children were more attentive to the similarities than to the differences of objects, opting for one prediction as against the other according to their theoretical position *vis-à-vis* associationism. As we have already seen (Chapter 5), the proponents of associationism, believing that details were perceived prior to the structure of the whole, predicted that differences would be perceived much more easily, whilst supporters of syncretism, who held that the global aspect of an object was perceived before its details, predicted a greater awareness of similarities.

The earlier results seemed to support the former group: when children younger than 6 years were asked to say in what way two toys, such as a cart and a motor-car (Jonckheere, 1921), a cottage and a house (Segers, 1926a), a bee and a fly or a rose, or a rabbit, etc. (Claparède, 1918), were the same or different, the number of differences reported greatly exceeded the number of similarities. In Terman's (1916) test, the problem which involves indicating the differences between two objects – paper and card, for example – is at the 7-year level, whilst the one in which the child is asked to say what two objects have in common is at the 8-year level. These sorts of results indicate that to abstract a common characteristic of several objects requires a higher level of intellectual activity than indicating directly perceptible differences; they certainly do not allow us to draw the conclusion that the child responds as a function of differences rather than similarities in the objects he is comparing. On the contrary, investigations on perceptual differentiation show that if the child has to make a paired comparison between two objects, whether physically identical or physically different, his judgments of identical pairs are almost always correct, whilst in the case of differing pairs the number of correct responses increases markedly with age between 4 and 7 years. It follows from this that, with equal numbers of identical and different pairs, the number of 'same' responses is much greater than the number of 'not the same' or 'different' responses.

At 4 years 'same' responses account for rather more than two-thirds of the total, whilst at 6½ years there are as many 'not the same' responses as 'same' responses (table 26).

Table 26    *Percentages of 'same' responses in five percep-tual differentiation tasks*

|  | Age (in years and months) | | |
|---|---|---|---|
| Studies | 4y. | 5y. | 6y. 6m. |
| Vurpillot and Zoberman, 1965 | 60·2 | 62·3 | 55·9 |
| Vurpillot, 1968 | 64·4 | 69·2 | 57·5 |
| Vurpillot, 1969a: | | | |
| Exp. I | 73·3 | 58·9 | 50·5 |
| Exp. II | 71·8 | 61·7 | 58· 3 |
| Vurpillot and Moal, 1970 | 82·0 | 69·8 | 59·8 |

The percentages were calculated on the basis of the number of 'same' responses as against the total number of responses made to physically identi-cal and physically different pairs. Since, in all the experiments, the number of physically identical pictures was equal to the number of physically different pairs, the number of 'same' responses could be expected to equal the number of 'not the same' responses – that is, 50 per cent.

The results in table 27, taken from four of the present writer's experiments carried out on different populations with more or less different materials, show that from the age of 3½ years children judge identical pictures as 'the same' in 90 per cent of cases, whilst the number of 'not the same' responses given to differing pairs fluctuates around 50 per cent at 4 years, reaches approximately 75 per cent at 5 years, and does not exceed 80 per cent until 6½ years.

The fact that the youngest children judged the physically identical pairs correctly does not mean that one can say they responded as a function of an identity relationship, since they also judged physically different pairs as being the same.

## IV    EXPERIMENTAL DATA ON THE ACQUISITION OF THE IDENTITY RELATIONSHIP

### 1    *Paired Comparison Tasks*

Although many research workers have investigated those factors which influence the ability to differentiate two objects, very few have attempted to evaluate from what age it is possible, with appro-priate training, to get children to respond not to the identity of two specific objects, but to the identity relationship itself. Dis-crimination learning makes it possible for animals and children

Table 27   *Distribution of correct responses as a function of the type of pair (identical or different) and age in five perceptual differentiation experiments*

| Experiments | Age (in years and months) | | |
| --- | --- | --- | --- |
| | 4y. | 5y. | 6y. 6m. |
| Results obtained with physically identical pairs | | | |
| Vurpillot and Zoberman, 1965 | 90·0 | 100·0 | 94·0 |
| Vurpillot, 1968 | 74·1 | 95·0 | 93·3 |
| Vurpillot, 1969a: | | | |
| Exp. I | 96·7 | 95·6 | 97·8 |
| Exp. II | 88·3 | 93·3 | 98·1 |
| Vurpillot and Moal, 1970 | 96·0 | 97·3 | 97·0 |
| Results obtained with physically different pairs | | | |
| Vurpillot and Zoberman, 1965 | 69·0 | 75·0 | 81·0 |
| Vurpillot, 1968 | 42·6 | 56·7 | 78·3 |
| Vurpillot, 1969a: | | | |
| Exp. II | 49·9 | 77·8 | 96·7 |
| Exp. I | 46·7 | 70·0 | 81·6 |
| Vurpillot and Moal, 1970 | 32·0 | 57·7 | 77·3 |

The results are expressed as percentages of correct responses in each category. In all these studies equal numbers of identical and differing pairs were used.

to associate a specific response to a form, but transfer tasks show that this response is not attached to a single stimulus, but rather to a group of stimuli more or less similar to the one which has been learnt.

Possession of the identity relationship is manifested when the child attaches a 'same' response not just to a particular pair of objects, but to all the pairs which have the property of being physically identical and to none of the pairs which do not have this property. To discover whether a child possesses the identity relationship or not, the experimenter varies the objects presented and rewards systematically, and exclusively, 'the same' responses to identical stimulus-pairs and 'not the same' responses to differing stimulus-pairs; when the child responds correctly on a certain number of consecutive trials he is considered to have acquired the relationship. Oléron (1962) concluded from his experiment that the identity relationship appears at 5 years of age and that it hardly mattered what type of stimulus was employed; Babska (1965) is of the opinion that it is acquired around the age of 3½ years for simple tasks. This author employed a simple paired-comparison technique with children from 18 months to 5 years. She began by showing the child a box with a sweet or a small toy inside it and a picture on the lid, then she removed it and presented four boxes, one of which was identical to the model, the other three having different pictures on the lid. On each successive trial the model box as well as its counterpart in the series was changed and the experimenter no longer opened the model box in order to show the sweet. Thus the discovery of the sweet could not be due to the establishment of a specific link between a particular picture and obtaining a reward. Babska distinguished three stages in the evolution of the performance of the children concerned. In the first stage correct choices did not differ from a chance distribution; in 80 per cent of the series the child opened the box situated in a preferential position, and this occurred in more than 50 per cent of the trials with each series. At the second stage, success depended on a number of experimental variations; the lids could differ in terms of form or colour, could have representational or geometric drawings on them, could either have or not have verbal labels that went with them, and so on – all factors which influenced the number of successes. At the third stage the identity relationship was finally achieved.

In short, at stage one there would never be an identity relationship, whilst at stage three it would operate in all situations. At stage two it might be found in one situation and not in another.

Table 28 shows that the percentage of correct choices exceeded 60 per cent as early as the age of 3 years, and reached 93 per cent at 5 years.

Table 28 *Evolution of the number of correct choices as a function of age*

| Ages (in years and months) | 1y. 6m. | 2y. 3m. | 3y. | 3y.6m. | 4y. | 5y. |
|---|---|---|---|---|---|---|
| Percentage of correct choices | 27·5 | 37·5 | 62·2 | 68·0 | 80·2 | 93·3 |

(After Babska, 1965)

Oléron's results, and even less those of Babska, do not seem to justify the conclusion that responses of identity were involved rather than responses of equivalence. In Babska's experiment a picture of a chicken is grouped and compared with pictures of a horse, a cat, and a woman's head; a circle is compared with a square, a triangle, and a star; a red circle with blue, green and yellow ones. The involvement of an identity relationship is not absolutely necessary for success, categorisation being sufficient. In the series of pictures of living organisms, selecting the chicken could be a response to the class of birds as against quadrupeds, as well as a sign of the establishment of a correspondence between all the properties of the various drawings. In Oléron's experiment the responses could also be made in terms of categorical identity, as well as in terms of exact identity. In summary, this sort of experiment does not seem to allow definite conclusions to be drawn; only a test in which it was possible to distinguish responses made according to an identity relationship from those made according to a relationship of similarity or equivalence would provide unambiguous information. Oléron's and Babska's experiments show that between $3\frac{1}{2}$ and 5 years children can be induced to respond in terms of categorical identity. As to being able to operate an identity relationship in the way that we have defined it above, using the terms of Lépine (1965), this would not seem to be acquired until about the age of 6 to 7 years, when 'same' responses are given exclusively to physically identical stimulus-objects in a setting where the differences introduced by the experimenter do not lend themselves to the formation of sub-categories, and the group of objects being compared form a definite category.

## 2  Comparison Tasks with the Responses 'Same' and 'Not the Same'

In two different ways we have attempted to discover on what basis children between the ages of 4 and 7 years take the decision to judge two objects as the same or not the same; the first involved the investigation of the laws of correspondence between the information actually extracted from the objects and the judgment that was made, the second involved asking the children to justify their responses.

(a)  *The relationship between the information extracted and the judgment of identity or difference.* The recording of visuo-motor exploratory activity during the comparison of two pictures of houses (Vurpillot, 1968) has made it possible, within the limits of recording accuracy, to determine which windows had actually been looked at by the child when he gave his response. The analysis of the recordings showed that before the age of 6 years children were satisfied with a partial exploration. In the study of the criteria of judgment we did not take into account whether the child had looked at all or only part of the stimulus-objects before responding, nor the precision or lack of precision of this response. Each child had to judge six pairs of drawings of houses; three of the pairs of houses were physically identical, the other three differed in the contents of one, three or five homologous windows. Recall that two windows are described as homologous when they occupy the same position in both houses.

For each response of every child we noted on the recording which windows had been looked at and whether this sample contained only non-identical windows, or only pairs of homologous identical windows, or both pairs of identical and pairs of non-identical windows (fig. 51, p. 238/9). Then we looked to see whether the responses of the same child showed evidence of a systematic link between the content of the sample extracted from a pair and the fact that the judgment given was 'same' or 'not the same'. It was possible to demonstrate two types of correspondence between the information extracted and the judgment made and, on this basis, the children were divided into three groups A, B and C.

*Group A* – Two houses were judged the same if, in the sample extracted, each window in one house corresponded to a window in the other house with identical contents. Two houses were judged 'not the same' when two homologous windows had different contents, whether or not the sample contained other windows with identical contents.

*Group B* – Two houses were judged the same if, in the sample extracted, at least one window in one house corresponded to a window with identical contents in the other house, whether or not the sample contained other homologous windows with differing contents. Two house were only judged 'not the same' if the sample did not contain two windows with identical contents.

*Group C* – No systematic relationship was apparent between the content of the samples and the child's responses. Some children gave the same response, either 'same' or 'not the same', to the six stimulus-objects, whichever they were looking at; the others did in fact use the two responses but apparently at random.

In allocating the children to the three groups, we have included in groups A and B those subjects whose behaviour was consistent with the criteria at least five times out of six.

If the decision criteria of the subjects in group A and the subjects in group B are compared, it appears that for the subjects in group A identity is defined by the absence of a difference in content between the windows in both houses, compared two at a time, and non-identity by the presence of a difference in content between two homologous windows. However, for the group B subjects the identity of two houses results from a partial identity, constituted by the presence of a window with identical contents in both houses, whilst non-identity corresponds to the absence of partial identity.

Table 29   *Distribution of subjects amongst groups A, B and C as a function of age*

| | Age (in years and months) | | | |
|---|---|---|---|---|
| Group | 3y. 11m. | 5y.0m. | 6y. 6m. | 8y. 9m. |
| | % | % | % | % |
| A | (3) 16·67 | (10) 50 | (17) 85 | (18) 90 |
| B | (6) 33·33 | (10) 50 | (2) 10 | (0) |
| C | (9) 50 | (0) | (1) 5 | (2) 10 |

The figures in brackets relate to the number of subjects classed as A, B or C at a given age-level; the percentages were calculated from the ratio of this number to the total number of subjects at that age-level, that is, eighteen at 3y.11m. and twenty at the other ages.

An inspection of table 29 shows that group C behaviour is hardly seen at all except in the very youngest children, that group B behaviour becomes the exception after the age of 6 years, and that group A behaviour increases regularly with age. A relationship is evident between the child's decision criteria and the form of his visuo-motor exploration. Two of the parameters of this exploration have been abstracted: the number of windows fixated and the number of homologous comparisons (cf. pp. 240–243). At all ages group A subjects made their judgment after having inspected more windows, and thus having gathered more information and made more homologous comparisons than subjects from groups B and C (table 30). The older the child the clearer this relationship was; however, the very small number of subjects in groups B and C who were above the age of 6 years means that these observations cannot be given more than an indicative value.

(*b*)   *Verbal justifications of 'same' and 'not the same' judgments.* In Vurpillot and Moal's (1970) experiment the children were asked to justify their responses as they went along. The experiment has already been described (p. 114), and so it is sufficient to recall that twelve pairs of drawings of houses were presented in succession, that six of these pairs were physically identical, that in three other pairs differences were introduced by modifying the contents of homologous windows (differences of substitution), and the three remaining pairs by simple permutation between two windows (differences by permutation). When a pair was presented, the child

Table 30 *Comparison of the performances of groups A, B and C*

| Age (in years and months) | Grp. | N | Percentage of correct responses Identical pairs | Different pairs | Average number of windows fixated by pair and by subject Identical pairs | Different pairs | Average number of homologous comparisons by pair and by subject Identical pairs | Different pairs |
|---|---|---|---|---|---|---|---|---|
| | A | 3 | 100 | 55·5 | 7·55 | 7·44 | 1·44 | 1·11 |
| 3.11 | B | 6 | 88·9 | 38·9 | 6·11 | 6·33 | 0·61 | 0·83 |
| | C | 9 | 55·6 | 40·7 | 6·48 | 6·67 | 0·48 | 0·37 |
| | A | 10 | 93·3 | 73·3 | 7·53 | 6·60 | 2·17 | 1·20 |
| 5.0 | B | 10 | 96·7 | 40·0 | 6·70 | 6·60 | 1·80 | 1·17 |
| | C | 0 | | | | | | |
| | A | 17 | 96·1 | 86·3 | 11·00 | 8·61 | 4·57 | 2·94 |
| 6.6 | B | 2 | 100 | 33·3 | 7·33 | 5·67 | 2·00 | 1·17 |
| | C | 1 | 33·3 | 33·3 | 7·00 | 6·00 | 1·67 | 1·00 |
| | A | 18 | 100 | 100 | 11·44 | 7·81 | 5·67 | 4·00 |
| 8.9 | B | 0 | | | | | | |
| | C | 2 | 33·3 | 83·3 | 9·50 | 7·83 | 2·67 | 1·50 |

N=Number of subjects in each sub-group.

said whether the two houses were exactly the same or not and then the experimenter asked him why. Neither the exactness of the judgment given nor the soundness of the justification of it was questioned, and the experimenter passed on to the next pair.

Tables 31 and 32 show the breakdown of all the justifications made by the 150 children questioned, taking account of the nature of the response ('same' or 'not the same'), the nature of the stimulus-pairs (identical, differing by substitution, differing by permutation), the extent of the exploration (complete or incomplete), and the reasons given.

The exploration was described as complete when the child justified his response in terms of the establishment of a correspondence between all the windows of one house and those of the other house by a series of paired comparisons. It was described as incomplete when the child only justified himself in terms of one or two paired comparisons.

These paired comparisons could involve homologous windows, in other words those windows which occupied the same position in relation to the frame of reference constituted by the house to which they belonged. They could also involve non-homologous

Table 31   *Justification of 'same' responses*

| Age (in years and months) | 4y. | 5y. | 6y. 6m. |
|---|---|---|---|
| Number of 'same' responses made to identical pairs | 281 | 285 | 289 |
| *Complete exploration:* Justification in terms of the identity of all the homologous windows compared | | | |
| *Incomplete exploration:* Justification in terms of the identity of 2 homologous windows | 56 | 234 | 289 |
| | 225 | 51 | |
| Number of 'same' responses made to pairs differing by permutation | 137 | 115 | 65 |
| *Complete Exploration:* Justification in terms of the identity of all the windows without taking account of their position | 33 | 100 | 65 |
| *Incomplete exploration:* | 104 | 15 | |
| Justification in terms of: | | | |
| —the identity of the contents of 2 homologous windows | 54 | 6 | |
| —the identity of the contents of 2 non-homologous windows (that is, permutated windows) | 27 | 3 | |
| —the identity of the contents of 2 homologous windows and 2 non-homologous windows | 23 | 6 | |
| Numbers of 'same' responses made to pairs differing by substitution | 65 | 12 | 1 |
| *Incomplete exploration:* Justification in terms of the identity of 2 homologous windows | 42 | 8 | |
| 'Ambiguous' justification: the child said that there were some differences but concluded that the houses were the same | 23 | 4 | 1 |
| Total number of 'same' responses | 483 | 412 | 355 |

Table 32 *Justification of 'not the same' responses*

| Age (in years and months) | 4y. | 5y. | 6y. 6m. |
|---|---|---|---|
| Number of 'not the same' responses made to identical pairs | 8 | 6 | 9 |
| Justification in terms of differences in content in 2 non-homologous windows | | 5 | 6 |
| Nonsensical justification, after having established homologous correspondences | 8 | 1 | 3 |
| Number of 'not the same' responses to pairs differing by permutation | 9 | 34 | 83 |
| Justification: | | | |
| —in terms of a difference in the content of 2 homologous windows | 7 | 7 | |
| —in terms of a difference in the content of 2 non-homologous windows | | 3 | 3 |
| —in terms of a difference in the position of 2 windows with identical contents (permutated windows) | | 24 | 80 |
| —nonsensical (as for the identical pairs) | 3 | | |
| Number of 'not the same' responses to pairs differing by substitution | 82 | 138 | 149 |
| Justification: | | | |
| —in terms of a difference in the content of 2 homologous windows | 79 | 135 | 146 |
| —in terms of a difference in the content of 2 non-homologous windows | | 3 | 3 |
| —nonsensical | 3 | | |
| Total number of 'not the same' responses | 99 | 178 | 241 |
| No justification | 18 | 10 | 4 |

There was a total of 600 responses at each age-level, 300 to the identical pairs, 150 to the pairs differing by substitution, and 150 to the pairs differing by permutation. The number of failures to give a justification was very small.

windows, which thus occupied different positions relative to the frame of reference of the house.

The reasons given by a child for a 'same' or 'not the same' response could relate to the contents and to the position of the windows between which a correspondence was established.

The following facts emerge from an analysis of tables 31 and 32:

—Failures to justify responses were negligible at all age-levels and generally involved one pair, the first to be presented; only one 4-year-old child refused to give any justifications.

—The 'not the same' responses were almost always justified in terms of the contents in two homologous windows being different. Justifications of a 'not the same' response in terms of a comparison of two non-homologous windows were rare, being the prerogative of two subjects, aged 5 years and 6½ years respectively, who systematically compared symmetrical windows. Justification of a 'not the same' judgment in terms of the permutated pairs – two windows with the same contents but in different positions – did not appear until 5 years and was far from being the rule at 6½ years.

—Some of the 'not the same' responses have been classified as 'nonsensical', since they were based on a comparison between windows with identical contents. These instances were very rare.

—'Same' responses were always justified in terms of identity of the contents of windows in a paired comparison. With the 4-year-old children, the justification only related to one or sometimes two pairs of windows, that is, it was based on an incomplete exploration of the two houses and hence an incomplete establishment of correspondence between them. On the other hand, at 6½ years the 'same' judgment was always justified on the basis of a correspondence of all the windows in one house with all those in the other. With the physically identical pairs, the paired comparisons were always made between homologous windows, but, with the pairs differing by permutation, the comparisons relating to permutated windows only took into account their contents and not their position – consequently, in this particular case, they were made between non-homologous windows.

From the analysis of tables 31, 32 and 33 it can therefore be concluded that 4-year-old children judge the identity of two pictures on the basis of an incomplete exploration and without taking account of the position of the windows. Two houses are judged 'the same' when the contents of at least one window in one house are found in one of the windows of the other house, whether or not

Table 33 *Evolution with age of justifications of a 'same'*
*response based on the establishment of an ex-*
*haustive correspondence of the windows in the*
*houses being compared*
*(Complete exploration)*

| Age (in years and months) | 4y. | 5y. | 6y. 6m. |
|---|---|---|---|
| Total number of 'same' responses | 483 | 412 | 355 |
| Justification based on complete exploration | 18·4% | 81·1% | 99·7% |

it happens to be in the homologous position. Consequently, the pairs differing in terms of permutation are judged 'the same' except in those few cases where the child responds 'not the same' on the basis of a difference in content between two homologous windows. In these instances it is probably the limited extent of his exploration that has prevented him from discovering the window with identical contents, in a different position, in the second house.

By 5 years the criteria change; in the majority of cases the child responds 'the same' after having established a correspondence between all the windows of one house and all those of the other. At the same time the identical positioning of windows with identical contents begins, in a certain number of cases, to be a requirement for deciding on the identity of the houses.

Finally, by 6½ years, 'the same' judgments always result from exhaustive paired comparisons between the windows, and in more than half the cases a difference in position of two windows with identical contents leads to a judgment of difference.

The analysis of individual results makes it possible to show that in the course of the developmental evolution the requirement of an exhaustive correspondence precedes that of identity of position and even that of content (cf. table 34).

All the subjects were classified simultaneously on two dimensions: the extent of their exploration in 'same' judgments on all pairs, and their justification of a 'not the same' response relating to pairs differing by permutation.

On the exploration dimension, children were divided into three classes according to whether their justifications of 'same' responses were always based on a complete exploration (1st column), sometimes on a complete exploration and sometimes on an incomplete one (2nd column) and, finally, never on a complete exploration (3rd column).

On the justification dimension the children were also divided into three classes: those who always justified a 'not the same'

Table 34    *Classification of subjects as a function of the extent of their exploration when making 'same' judgments, and of the justifications of 'not the same' judgments made in respect of pairs differing by permutation*

|  | Exploration | | | |
|---|---|---|---|---|
| | *Always complete* | *Sometimes complete* | *Never complete* | |
| *Always in terms of contents* | 5 | 12 | 31 | 48 |
| Justifi-cations *Sometimes contents and sometimes position* | | | | 0 4y. |
| *Always in terms of position* | | | | 0 |
| | 5 | 12 | 31 | 48 |

(a)

|  | | | | |
|---|---|---|---|---|
| *Always in terms of contents* | 25 | 7 | 5 | 37 |
| Justifi-cations *Sometimes contents and sometimes position* | 10 | | | 10 5y. |
| *Always in terms of position* | 2 | | | 2 |
| | 37 | 7 | 5 | 49 |

(b)

|  | | | | |
|---|---|---|---|---|
| *Always in terms of contents* | 13 | | | 13 |
| Justifi-cations *Sometimes contents and sometimes position* | 23 | | | 23 6y. 6m. |
| *Always in terms of position* | 12 | | | 12 |
| | 48 | 0 | 0 | 48 |

(c)

For details of the construction of the double-entry tables see the text (pp. 299 and 301).

response made to a pair differing by permutation in terms of a non-identity of contents between windows (1st row), or else by a non-identity of the position of windows with identical contents (3rd row), or even sometimes by a non-identity of contents and sometimes a non-identity of position of two windows with identical contents (2nd row).

Almost all the children could be classified along these lines; only five out of 150 were eliminated from this distribution either because they had refused to give any justification (one child) or because they had systematically compared non-homologous windows (one child), or because their justifications had been classed as 'nonsensical' (three children).

The double-entry tables 34a, b, c give, at each age-level, the distribution of children according to the two dimensions given.

An examination of these tables shows that at each age-level, on either one or both dimensions, the children are distributed across the three given levels of performance, and that from one age to another the relative significance of these levels changes. It can be seen that four cells in these tables are empty at all ages, a fact which can be interpreted in the following fashion. There was no instance where a child whose exploration was not always complete stated that two houses were different because windows with identical contents were situated in different positions. It seems clear, therefore, that in the justification of a 'same' response, the need for the establishment of an exhaustive correspondence between the parts of the two structures being compared precedes, developmentally, the requirement of an identity of relationships between parts as well as that of an identity of their contents.

(c) *Discussion.* At first sight the results obtained in the two experiments which have been discussed (Vurpillot, 1968; Vurpillot and Moal, 1970) are not entirely consistent. On the one hand the complete exploration of the stimulus appears at an earlier age in the second experiment: on the other hand type B behaviour practically never appeared in the justifications of 'not the same' judgments. Several explanations can be put forward to account for these discrepancies, all of which amount to variations on the theme that the experimental setting is very different. This is true but it is not completely satisfactory.

In the experiment dealing with eye-movements the stimulus-objects were much larger but situated almost the same distance apart as those in the other experiment; it is, therefore, quite certain that in order to explore the houses in the 1968 experiment completely, the child had to manifest greater visuo-motor activity than

in the 1970 experiment. To that must be added the special requirement of the voluntary immobilisation of the head by keeping it
on a head-rest, which could have had an inhibiting effect; it is
after all a distinct possibility that the younger the child, the more
the movements of the head tend to accompany, indeed even to
take the place of, movements of the eyes. In summary, the later
appearance of a complete exploration in the 1968 experiment than
in the 1970 experiment could be explained in terms of the difference
between the experimental settings.

In the 1968 experiment the child was only using his eyes, but the
data on visuo-motor exploration (Lesèvre, 1964) show that before
the age of 6 years the child has great difficulty in fixating exactly
on precise points in a given order; however, if he can, at the same
time, point with his finger to the objects he is looking at, this acts
as a support accompanying the displacement of the eyes and greatly
facilitates the visuo-motor exploration. As we have already seen
(Chapter 9) deliberate paired comparisons do not appear until 5 years
and are not displayed by a majority until after the age of 6 years
(Vurpillot, 1968). It is therefore possible that the setting of the
1970 experiment not only favoured complete exploration but also
the correspondence of the pairs. Furthermore, it must be added
that in the 1968 experiment a number of children significantly
younger than those in the 1970 experiment were included in the
4-year-old group.

In both experiments the criteria of 'same' and 'not the same'
judgments were inferred from objective data, the nature of which
differed from one experiment to the other. In the 1968 experiment,
the criteria of judgment were inferred from the establishment of a
correspondence of all the information gathered by the child with
the judgment actually given. In one respect this technique provided very definite data: the information contained in those parts
situated outside the areas which were explored could not be involved in the child's responses.[1] If the physical difference or
differences presented in the stimulus had not been looked at, a
'same' response could be attributed to the fact that no difference
was perceived. When the sample extracted by the inspection of the
stimulus contained both identical and differing windows, a more
cautious interpretation of the response became necessary. Our
classification of subjects as A and B was based on the assumption
that the child had taken into account all the information extracted.
However, there is no way we can be sure that the child has used all

[1]As long as it is postulated that only those parts which had been seen in
foveal vision provided useful information and that peripheral vision was not
involved.

this information, and whether or not he is content to take into account only those windows he saw to begin with, or the ones he saw last. A number of analyses which led in this direction proved fruitless without, however, making it possible to draw any sort of conclusion.

The clarity of the verbal responses obtained in the 1970 experiment might lead one to think that none of the children used the criteria defined in the 1968 experiment under the B classification. But in both cases the experimenter only obtained incomplete information. The child who has answered 'not the same' justifies his response in terms of a non-identity of contents between two homologous windows and his 'same' response by an identity of content between one or more windows. He seems, therefore, to be employing criteria A. But how is one to know, when he replies 'the same' to a pair of houses differing by substitution, whether it is because – owing to a limited exploration – he has not seen any difference, or whether, having seen it, he considers (like the group B children in the 1968 experiment) that the presence of the difference does not mean that the houses are not the same? A further experiment, in which the houses only had four windows and where the experimenter ensured, by means of appropriate instructions that the child had looked at them all before giving his response, avoided only some of the ambiguities in the earlier studies (Berthoud and Vurpillot, 1970).

In this study, children in the age-range 3y. 4m. to 5y. 2m. were shown ten pairs of houses in which the number of differing windows varied from 0 (identical houses) to 4. All the differences were in terms of the content of windows which occupied homologous positions (substitution differences).

On the basis of the judgments made of physically different pairs, it was possible to classify the children in three groups. Some of them had answered 'the same' to both identical pairs and 'not the same' to all the differing pairs and consequently had made no mistakes (group I). Others had answered 'the same' to all the pairs (group II), even those which contained no identical pairs of windows – it would seem that these children did not find the instructions meaningful, unless it was that the identity of the configuration (a house with four windows) was sufficient for them. Finally, some children judged some of the physically different pairs as the same and others not the same (group III).

All of the 3-year-old children and four (out of eighteen) of the 4-year-old children came into group II, five of the 4-year-olds and twelve of the 5-year-olds came into group I, and nine of the 4-year-olds and six of the 5-year-olds into group III. The analysis of the individual results of the fifteen subjects in group III showed that none of them had answered 'not the same' to the pairs with 4 differences and 'same' to the pairs with 1, 2 and 3 differences, which would correspond to the pattern of the responses of group B subjects (Vurpillot, 1968). The doubt expressed on p. 303 as to the validity of the classification of A and B subjects is thus reinforced. In addition it is clearly evident that the number of correct 'not the same' responses increases in relation to the number of differences present (table 35).

Table 35   *Percentages of correct 'not the same' responses as a function of the number of differences between two houses*

| Number of differences | 1 | 2 | 3 | 4 |
|---|---|---|---|---|
| Percentage of correct responses | 36·7 | 53·3 | 78·3 | 93·3 |

The results were calculated on the basis of the responses of the fifteen children classed as group III (nine were 4 years old ± 2 months, six were 5 years old ± 2 months).

By making the child point with his finger to all the windows in turn during each comparison, the experimenter ensured that the child had registered all the useful information before giving his response; insufficient visual exploration could not therefore be held responsible for the incorrect responses and their variation with the number of differences. It could not be concluded categorically, however, that the children in group III based their judgments on the density of the differences, replying 'not the same' when the differing windows were relatively numerous and 'the same' when they were relatively rare. Indeed, as in the experiment involving the recording of eye-movements, it did not follow that because the

Table 36   *Percentage of correct 'not the same' responses as a function of the total number of windows and of the number of differences*

| Number of differences | 1 | 1 | 1 | 1* | 2 | 2 | 2* | 3* | 4* |
|---|---|---|---|---|---|---|---|---|---|
| Number of windows | 1 | 2 | 3 | 4 | 2 | 3 | 4 | 4 | 4 |
| Percentage of correct responses | 83·3 | 63·3 | 43·3 | 36·7 | 70·0 | 63·3 | 53·3 | 73·3 | 93·3 |

This table regroups the results of fifteen children from Berthoud and Vurpillot's (1970) experiment and fifteen children from the subsequent experiment. The columns marked with an asterisk relate to the results from Berthoud and Vurpillot's experiment.

child had looked at all the windows he necessarily took into account all that he had seen in order to formulate his judgment.

Consequently, a second experiment had the purpose of mini-mising reliance on memory. Pictures of houses were constructed, having a total of one, two or three windows; the number of differ-ences also varied. Thirty-six children aged 4 years ±6 weeks were asked to make 'same' or 'not the same' judgments of thirteen pairs of houses: three of these pairs were identical and ten different. As in the preceding experiment, we classified the children in three groups: those who made no mistakes and thus used adult decision criteria (eleven children), those who responded 'the same' and consequently did not give correct responses to the differing pairs (ten children), and those who made some correct responses and some incorrect ones (fifteen children). In the latter group the num-ber of correct responses to differing pairs increased, as it did in Berthoud and Vurpillot's (1970) experiment, in relation to the number of differences. But the total number of windows was also relevant; when all the windows were different, the number of cor-rect responses was less for the houses with two windows than for those with just one window.

In this last experiment the windows were few enough in number for the total number of parts which needed to be taken into con-sideration to be within the limits of the field of immediate appre-hension. In this instance it seems possible to draw some conclusions about the way in which the child uses the information he has extracted in formulating his judgments. The response category which we have designated as B and which is defined in the follow-ing way: 'same' responses to objects which have a part in common and 'not the same' responses to objects which do not have a part in common, would seem to be an artefact of analysis. Possibly our criterion (five consistent responses out of six) was inadequate and did not allow for a distinction to be made between type B judgments and judgments based on the density of the differences. At the point we have now reached, it would seem that between the period where the child judges all stimulus objects of the same category (such as our houses) as 'the same', and the period where he employs adult criteria in order to classify objects as 'the same' and 'not the same', there is a stage where he separates those which are alike from those which are not alike as a function of a quantitative evaluation of the degree of similarity and dissimilarity.

**V  CONCLUSION**

The analysis of the results obtained from the experimental studies of differentiation make it clear how difficult it is to draw any certain conclusions as to the criteria by which children of preschool age decide that two objects are the same or not. However, even if some uncertainties remain and some of the conclusions must still be regarded as tentative, a general line of development begins to emerge.

First of all, it is certain that the logically defined identity relationship is a relatively late acquisition and that before 6 years of age 'same' responses are based on partial equivalences. Two objects are declared to be the same because both of them have the same value on one dimension – for example red, or round – or else because they possess an identical part, such as a vase of flowers, or a cat, in a window, or again because they have the same meaning – that is, they can be related to an action (an object which can be banged or eaten) or to a representative schema (house, sailing-boat).

Whilst it is certainly the case that two objects are described as 'the same' because they are grouped into a category, this category is more a grouping in terms of proximity and similarity (Lépine, 1966) or an associative complex, Bruner and Olver, 1963) than an actual class of equivalence. Presented with a group of objects, the child selects certain attributes (part, property, name) but does not subordinate the whole of the group to a single attribute or a set of attributes. For example, stimulus A might be described as the same as B because both are round and the same as stimulus C because both of them have a vase of flowers. The use of such criteria demonstrates that children of preschool age possess neither the logical relationship of equivalence nor the logical relationship of identity, the same response ('the same') being applied to physically identical objects and to physically different objects, in which case it is based on the existence of a partial similarity between pairs of objects.

A judgment relating to the object as a whole is based on a consideration of only a part of its properties. It follows that, if a child feels himself able to judge objects as the same on the basis of only a sample of the available information, it is quite useless for him to explore them in full. The limited extent of visual exploration in comparison tasks would thus seem to be a consequence of the failure to use the identity relationship. Even though the visuo-motor activity of young children is slower, less accurate, and less organised than that of their elders, this slight sensori-motor inferiority cannot account for the limited area explored in the comparison experiments. The recordings demonstrate that even the youngest subjects are capable of movements of large amplitude and that, when their interest is aroused, they make as many visual displacements as the older ones. It is the same in those instances when, for example, the stimulus is a picture taken from a children's book, and where the number, the location and the sequence of the points of fixation are the same at all ages (Zaporozhets and Zinchenko, 1966). The main difference between the young children and the older ones rests on the fact that, with children above the age of 6 years, the extent of the area explored depends on the requirements of the task (recognition, categorisation, judgments of identity or difference) and the characteristics of the material (physical identity or non-identity), whilst with the youngest children the localisation of visual fixations is related to the value of attraction of the different points of the stimulus, and the number of fixations to the interest the stimulus arouses in the child. The development with age depends therefore not so much on exploratory activity itself as on the role which the child gives it in the resolution of a problem. In the last analysis it depends on the child's decision criteria.

It is far from being the case that all the properties of stimulus-objects are of equal importance in determining equivalence between them. As early as 3 years, and probably even before that, children perceive variations introduced by the experimenter into his material. They are sensitive to differences of form, colour, texture, size, etc.; they are also perfectly capable of detecting spatial displacements by reference to their retinal co-ordinates or to a simple frame of reference such as a human face or the outline of a house. But amongst all the differences which they perceive, some are considered as compatible with an equivalence and others incompatible. In a 'same' judgment the number of differences which are tolerated decreases with age, whilst the necessary conditions increase according to a progression which is found in all tasks and for all children. Differences of form seem to be the first to be considered incompatible with a 'same' judgment (Vurpillot, 1969b). In the case where the objects being compared are configurations of discrete parts, the identity of the form of the configurations is a later requirement than the identity of form of the parts themselves (Pineau, 1969). As a general rule, the relational properties – such as size or the spatial setting – are the last to be taken into consideration in the elaboration of a 'same' or 'not the same' judgment.

Between 5 and 6 years the child acquires adult criteria which determine what amount of information must be gathered before a judgment is formulated. Thus a 'same' response is given after all the parts of one object have been matched with all the parts of the other object, whilst a 'not the same' response is justified by a single comparison if this should reveal a difference. However, to begin with, the reciprocal correspondences which are established take into account only the intrinsic properties of the parts, and the spatial relationships between them are neglected.

In the experiments involving permutations (Moal, 1969; Lécuyer, 1969; Vurpillot and Moal, 1970) the form of the configurations remained invariant and the only difference between two pictures related to the spatial location of the parts. From the age of 5½ years the great majority of children proceeded to establish a reciprocal correspondence of all the windows of the houses or of all the objects in the configurations and concluded that they were the same when each part of one picture corresponded to a part of the other picture which was identical in respect of all its intrinsic characteristics. Thus the 'same' response is reserved for those structures which are exactly isomorphic, except for the spatial relationships between the parts (Vurpillot and Moal, 1970). A comparison between the experiments involving permutations (Lécuyer, 1969; Moal, 1969) and those dealing with displacements (Pineau, 1969) shows that there is an interactive effect; when the displacement of a part modifies the form of the configuration it brings about the response 'not the same' at an earlier age than when this form is respected.

Table 37   *Comparison between displacements and per-mutations*

| Age (in years and months) | 4y. | 4y. 6m. | 5y. | 5y. 6m. | 6y. 6m. |
|---|---|---|---|---|---|
| Displacements | | 2·1 | | 53·6 | |
| Permutations | 3·1 | | 26·7 | | 81·9 |

The results are expressed as percentages of the 'not the same' responses made to physically different pictures. The figures can only be taken as indicative since they are the result of a regrouping of the internal and external displacements (Pineau, 1969) and of the horizontal and non-horizontal permutations (Moal, 1969). However, the percentages of correct responses are very different according to whether a displacement is external or internal, a permutation horizontal or non-horizontal.

The concept of things being 'the same' can be demonstrated as early as 3 years of age in simple paired comparison tasks with the correct responses positively reinforced (Babska, 1965), but consistent 'same' or 'not the same' judgments in a comparison task with verbal instructions are hardly in evidence until the age of 4 years. Before that the child either does not make a response, or if he selects one of the responses which are open to him, this choice appears to bear no relation to the characteristics of the stimulus.

The first 'same' judgments express a communality of representational meaning between two objects; there does not appear to be any extraction of a common part or attribute. Two pictures or two objects are judged the same because their perceived form represents the same thing. For example, all pictures identified as 'houses' are described as the same, whilst a picture identified as 'a house' and another one identified as 'a duck' are described as 'not the same'. It must be acknowledged that, at the present moment, there are no studies which might tell us what it is in the perceived object that makes it possible for the 2- to 3-year-old child to identify the house or the duck.

At a second level, the child proceeds to a sort of intensive quantification of the similarity of objects being compared; thus he judges two objects 'the same' when they seem to him to be more similar than they are different, and 'not the same' if they seem to him, on the whole, to be different. This evaluation of the relative similarity and dissimilarity of objects compared is gross and involves neither a complete exploration nor a careful analysis of the characteristics of the objects.

At a third level, the child, like the adult, comes to define things as 'the same' by the absence of relevant differences and 'not the same' by the presence of at least one relevant difference. But this level is characterised by a sampling strategy; perceptual exploration is limited to one area of the object and, from amongst the differences to which the sensory receptors are sensitive, only certain of them, the number of which increases with age, are considered as relevant.

At a fourth level, at about the age of $5\frac{1}{2}$, perceptual exploration is exhaustive; the child no longer allows himself to judge two objects as the same without having established a reciprocal correspondence of all their parts. But the objects are still treated as additive sets of parts and not as articulated structures; provided that each part of one of these sets has an identical homologue in the other, it is of little importance that these parts do not maintain the same spatial relationships within the two sets. Finally, at a fifth level, the identity of spatial relationships also becomes a requirement; the criterion of the 'same' response is physical identity.

It must be added, further, that the justifications of their responses given by children in the permutations experiment (Vurpillot and Moal, 1970) lead one to think that the 'same' responses are independent of the 'not the same' responses – whilst in the adult they are organised into a single structure. Thus the fact that 'same' judgments depend, even in many of the 6½-year-old children, only on the contents of the windows might lead one to think that the children are indifferent to their position; consequently it seems surprising that the justifications of 'not the same' responses are based so rarely on the establishment of a correspondence between non-homologous windows. There is an apparent contradiction in this which disappears if one allows the independence of judgments of identity and difference and the existence of a hierarchy of the properties of the parts compared. Observation of the children's behaviour in the tasks studied shows that, when the child compares two houses, he goes initially from a window in one house to the one occupying the homologous position in the other house; if he finds there a window with identical contents he can stop at that point and conclude that they are the same or, if he has reached the level where a complete exploration is required before reaching a conclusion of identity, he can go on to establish correspondence between the other homologous windows. When he encounters, in the homologous position, a window with differing contents, he can decide right away that that is sufficient to answer 'not the same', or else ignore the factor of position and look for a window with the same contents in another position. If he does find one, he concludes that the two houses are identical. If he does not find one, he concludes that they are different.

The identity of content is the dominant criterion, and if it is satisfied it determines the 'same' response; it is only when this is no longer the case that position plays a role and is mentioned in the justification. It would seem that this dominance of content might be linked to, and to some extent explained by, the selection of a strictly positive definition of identity. We have seen that, from the logical point of view, the relationship of identity can be defined as much in positive terms by the existence in one object of all the properties present in another object, as in negative terms by the absence of differences between these two objects. However, it seems that the young child does not use the negative definition; it appears in none of the justifications that we obtained. Even those children who carried out a complete exploration and took into account the identity of position as well as content always justified their response by a series of identities between windows, never by the absence of a difference.

What might seem to us equally paradoxical is that the existence of a difference, recognised as such, does not prevent the young child from reaching a conclusion of identity. Windows with different contents, situated in homologous positions, do indeed constitute a difference for him, but if he is able to find, for each window in one house, a window with the same contents in the other house, he feels himself justified in concluding, all the same, that they are identical. Judgments of difference and judgments of identity remain to some degree independent until after the age of 7 years.

Thus, it can be hypothesised that during an initial period the decision process remains in a state of flux when there exists, conjointly, identity between certain properties or parts and differences between others. It is only when a hierarchy is determined, which renders even an incomplete identity dominant, that coherent and systematic judgments can be established. A stage of uncertainty is succeeded by a stage of categorisation in which the discovery of similarities determines the decision. The identity relationship is only truly acquired when a positive definition of 'same' in terms of the communality of the properties and parts is added to a negative definition in terms of an absence of differences.

*The figures and tables in Part Three have been reproduced with the kind permission of the following authors and publishers:*

Fig. 44  Zinchenko, V. P., Van Chizi-Tsin, V. and Tarakanov, V. V. *Psychological Research in the U.S.S.R.*, 1966, pp. 396, 397, 399.

Figs 45, 46, 51 and 53  Vurpillot, E. *Journal of Experimental Child Psychology*, 1968, **6**, pp. 634, 643–644, 649–650.

Table 19  Vurpillot, E. *Journal of Experimental Psychology*, 1968, **6**, p. 644.

Table 20  Elkind, D. and Weiss, J. 'Studies in perceptual development: III. Perceptual exploration', *Child Development*, The Society for Research in Child Development, Inc., 1967, **38**, 533–561, p. 558.

Table 25  Zinchenko, V. P. and Ruzskaya, A. G. *Psychological Research in the U.S.S.R.*, 1966, p. 407.

# General Conclusions

1   When the same task is presented to children of differing ages, the most usual finding is that the older the child the better the performance. Those responses classed as correct by the experimenter increase in number and, at the same time, progress takes place in that the decision criteria become more stable.

However, some performances are as good in 4-year-old children as they are in 7-year-olds; this is the case, for example, with judgments of identity relating to identical objects or pictures (Vurpillot and Zoberman, 1964; Vurpillot, 1968, 1969a; Vurpillot and Moal, 1970). But it would be extremely unwise to infer from an identity of performance an identity of decision criteria and strategies; correct solutions could rest on false reasoning.

When the psychologist compares results on a given task obtained from groups of children of differing ages, the improvement in performance appears to be progressive, the slope of the developmental curve being more or less steep depending on the task concerned. This appearance of continuous progress afforded by the study of performance means (obtained from widely varying performances) is deceptive. If the individual results are compared – in those cases where the experimental design makes it possible – it is usually feasible for the children, at each age-level, to be divided into several response categories, the balance of these changing with age. Thus, in Gottschaldt-type embedded figures tasks, the results from the different age-groups show a progressive increase between 4 and $6\frac{1}{2}$ years in the number of successes in problems involving the discovery of secondary structures (Chapter 1). The individual results show that at each age-level these successes are attributable to a few subjects (the number of these increasing with age) who were successful on all or almost all of the problems in the category, whilst the others were successful on none of them. In a perceptual differentiation task (Vurpillot and Moal, 1970) the number of consistent subjects, that is, those who used consistent criteria of judgment and applied them systematically, was extremely high since ultimately it reached almost 90 per cent. Out of thirty-two children at each age-level, two at 4 years, fifteen at 5 years and thirty-one at $6\frac{1}{2}$ years justified their responses in terms of a complete correspondence of the parts of the pictures being compared. The 'same' response was given on the basis of an identity of both form *and* position of the parts of the two pictures by none of the 4-year-old children, by only two of the 5-year-olds, and by twenty-one at $6\frac{1}{2}$ years.

In a comparison of the performances of children of different ages in learning transfer tasks involving reversal or non-reversal shift, the results of the groups showed that non-reversal shift learning was acquired more rapidly in children under the age of 5 years (T. Kendler, H. Kendler and Wells, 1960), reversal shift learning more rapidly in older children and adults (H. Kendler and d'Amato, 1955), with an equal rate of learning for reversal and non-reversal shifts in children between the ages of 5 and 7 years (T. Kendler and H. Kendler, 1959). This equality, observed at the group level, simply expresses the existence of a number of subjects who learned a reversal shift more quickly than a non-reversal shift, and an equal number for whom the difference is in the opposite direction.

Indeed, as a general rule it seems that a change in performance expresses either the adoption of a new decision criterion or a new method of execution, that the period of uncertainty during which the child hesitates between two methods or two criteria is very brief, and that the new cognitive instruments are very quickly applied to all the problems presented. Although it is certain that every change has a fairly long period of preparation, and advance signs of this can be detected by careful observation, the modification to be seen at the level of the child's response proceeds more by mutation than by evolution. One of the more spectacular examples of this is when, under the very eyes of the experimenter, the child passes from the non-conservation to the conservation of quantity (Piaget and Inhelder, 1941).

During the various stages of childhood the number and importance of the changes observed is particularly impressive. Thus, in the baby the co-ordination of prehension and vision, the establishment of the occipital alpha rhythm, and the differentiation between the spontaneous electro-physiological activity of different areas of the cortex (Dreyfus-Brisac and Blanc, 1956, 1957) all appear at about 3 months of age.

During the second year of life, walking, which allows greater autonomy and increases the range of possibilities for getting to grips with the environment, together with the means of communication afforded by language, change the system of relations between the child and his surroundings. But the fundamental change is the one that involves the appearance of the semiotic function, that is, the ability to represent an object or an event by a signifier – word, mental image, imitative play or movement, etc. – detached from the signified.

Finally, between the ages of 6 and 8 years begins the period of the concrete operations of thought: the conservation of quantity, seriation, classification, etc. The appearance of operational structures brings about modifications in the resolution of perceptual tasks as much as in more specifically intellectual tasks. It is not by chance that, during this period from 6 to 8 years, we find the development of the articulation between the whole and the parts in tasks of identification (Elkind, Koegler and Go, 1964), that in terms of perceptual organisation the primary structures can be taken apart and secondary structures constructed (Vurpillot and Flores, 1964), and that, in differentiation tasks, adult criteria of identity are established (Vurpillot, 1968; Vurpillot and Moal, 1970).

2   The behaviour of the child is never random; if it appears to be so, it is because it does not always conform to the same rules as those governing adult behaviour, and the major concern of developmental research is the discovery of the particular behavioural structures of children and their interdependent relationship in the course of development.

As indicated in the introduction, the study of perceptual development undertaken in this book is based exclusively on the analysis and interpretation of the observable activities of children in standardised situations.

Amongst these activities, some appear to be entirely dependent upon external stimuli, in the sense that their form is often specific to one stimulus and that the subject can neither trigger them nor inhibit them. A proportion of those behaviours which can be called involuntary are the neurologically-based reflexes, Pavlovian and second-order conditioning (S. Miller and Konorski, 1928). In the present work they have been seen only as a means of measuring the sensory capacities of very young children.

The voluntary or involuntary status of other activities is somewhat ambiguous. On the one hand, certain simple actions, such as sucking or the fixation of gaze in the baby, can either be triggered by an external stimulus – and consequently without any decision on the part of the subject – or they can be deliberate. On the other hand, sequences of actions, each unit of which was initially independent, can be linked together and then become automatic, so that, in the end, only the initial mobilisation is voluntary – as is the case with walking and with sensori-motor habits in general, and, in the last analysis, with instrumental conditioning.

Finally, action can be the outcome of a decision in which the physical state of the subject is involved, his previous experience, the representation of the desired goal and the means of attaining it, as well as the presence of this or that external stimulation. Thus the subject decides to undertake an action or a series of actions, determines a goal and also the means by which to achieve it.

Some learning theorists, Watson (1919) for example, have proposed the economical hypothesis that all behaviours can be reduced to chains of conditioned reflexes, in which case the subject's decision would be an illusory phenomenon. Without going as far as this, S-R learning theorists do uphold the existence of semi-automatised behaviours in which every action is considered as a response to a stimulus. In order to account for the complexity of human behaviour one need only conceive of sufficiently complex chains and sufficiently subtle categories of stimuli and responses. Cognitive theorists do not accept this reduction, a mechanistic conceptualisation which is demeaning for man; they recognise the existence of sensori-motor sequences in which one action serves as a stimulus to the following one, but give their entire attention to those activities in which anticipation and representation are more important than the link between a unit of stimulation and the unit of response associated with it.

From the first we have made it clear that our preferences are for the cognitive approach. Consequently it is from this point of view that we have attempted to interpret the results obtained in the perceptual tasks which have been reviewed in the preceding chapters.

When the psychologist designs an experiment he determines the setting and the instructions, and he selects the independent and dependent variables as a function of a particular 'model'. When the child tackles this task, he also works on it as a function of a model which he selects from his available repertoire. To the extent that his responses are ratified, in other words when some of them bring about an agreeable event – a sweet, a light that comes on, the experimenter's approval – whilst others bring about a disagreeable event, such as the experimenter's disapproval or the absence of an agreeable outcome, the child seeks to satisfy the requirements of the experiment. In other words, he tries to find out what the experimenter's model is (S. White, 1964) and in order to do that he tries out, in succession, the models in his personal repertoire. In this respect he is simply like the rats of Lashley (1929) and Krechevsky (1932) which formed hypotheses and put them to the test. It is important to emphasise the fact that these hypotheses are not relative to the setting itself, which can always be interpreted in a number of ways, but to the manner in which the experimenter regards the setting, which is not necessarily the most obvious or the most satisfactory one for the subject. The selection of the variables depends, above all, on the model of the setting which the individual has constructed; there is no *a priori* reason which obliges the subject to make the same selection as the experimenter.

When the subject succeeds, that is to say, when he responds in the manner predicted by the experimenter, the latter is always tempted to conclude that the subject has done so in accordance with the model which the experimenter himself constructed of the setting. But this is only true to the extent that there is only one way of succeeding on the task. However, one of the main difficulties is the development of tests devoid of ambiguity and with a single solution; in order to do that the psychologist relies on the results from previous tests and on his own intuitions, a procedure which, in animal or child psychology, has many pitfalls. Consequently the interpretations which are proposed are extremely tentative.

When certain consequences follow each of the child's responses, a change in performance in the direction desired by the experimenter indicates either that the child has discovered the experimenter's model and is acting in accordance with it, or that he has found another one compatible with the system of responses selected by the experimenter. When the responses bring about no consequences, or the consequences are undifferentiated, such as 'Very good, carry on', one could assume that the child might execute every task as a function of the same model (Levine, 1966).

The experimenter can never claim that he possesses an exhaustive set of the models which could explain a child's behaviour. What he can do, by varying the experimental settings and increasing theii number, is to eliminate from the models which could account foɪ a first set of data, those which prove to be incompatible with new· data. Thus 'same' responses given to physically identical stimuli could indicate the use of a logical identity relationship with a one-to-one correspondence of all the properties of the objects compared and an absence of difference, but it could also indicate the selection of a criterion of judgment which allows the conclusion as to identity to be drawn on the basis of a single property in common. If the comparison of physically identical objects does not make it possible to decide which of these models the child is acting in accordance with, the comparison of physically different objects does allow the elimination of the former (decision based on the logical relationship of identity) when the child declares as 'the same' stimuli whose differences greatly exceed his perceptual threshold.

An examination of the data at present available seems to us to support an interpretation of child behaviour in terms of the use of models, and, if one gives the term 'model' a wide enough meaning, it is possible to speak of babies making use of models, as well as older children. A number of authors, notably Piaget, Zaporozhets (1961), Miller, Galanter and Pribram (1960), attach particular importance to voluntary actions and propose a theory of behaviour in terms of plans and images. According to Miller, Galanter and Pribram (1960), a plan is a programme of action, analogous to that given to a computer – a set of instructions which prescribes a series of actions and the order in which they must be linked together; an image is the equivalent of the computer's memory store, containing the information gathered and recorded through the contacts between the subject and his environment. A learning experiment involves the transmission of the experimenter's programme of action to the subject. In the case of adults and older children, the strategy to be followed can be communicated verbally, its implementation being perfected by practice. With animals and very young children this verbal communication is not possible; the plan is learnt by trial and error and so, for these authors, always remains incomplete. Thus Miller, Galanter and Pribram (1960) make the acquisition of plans dependent on a certain level of verbal behaviour corresponding to what others (T. Kendler, 1963) have called verbal mediators.

Zaporozhets (1961) is also of the opinion that it is only from about the age of 4 years that the child's actions are planned. Planning implies the conjoint representation of the situation and of the actions to be accomplished, the two together constituting an image. This image therefore has two aspects: the static one seems to correspond to what Tolman (1948) called a cognitive map, and the other, kinetic, one relates to the programme of action. Although agreeing with Miller, Galanter and Pribram (1960) in placing the beginning of the use of plans and images at around 4 years, Zaporozhets (1961) differs from them in attributing the development of these plans to the child's exploratory activity and not to verbalisation.

Piaget employs somewhat different terms but it seems to us that his theory is capable of encompassing the essentials of the hypotheses of the authors just quoted, and we would hope not to misrepresent his position by setting out the way in which we envisage this question of plans and images.

To begin with, reaffirming that the behaviour of young children is not haphazard but systematic and organised, we believe that, from birth, the child possesses a number of programmes of action which are built into his neural structures.

The programmes of action can be divided into two categories: chains, within which each segmentary action is triggered by the one immediately preceding it and which itself serves as the stimulus to the one that follows; and structured wholes, within which the

318   *The Visual World of the Child*

sequences are not rigid and where each segment is determined more by the goal to be attained than by the immediately contiguous parts of the sequence. The programmes in this second category always involve a more or less detailed representation of the whole situation and set of actions. In order to avoid any confusion, the programmes of action in the first category will be called sensori-motor schemas[1] and those in the second category, strategies.

The reflex schemas of visual fixation, sucking and grasping are sequences of actions, just as the sensori-motor schemas which will derive from them (Piaget, 1936). The first action schemas – and the younger the baby the more inflexible these are – are built into the central nervous system and can be said to be predetermined. Contact with the environment enriches them and makes them more flexible. Numerous schemas are constructed, the linking of actions within them being acquired by the repetition of stimulus-action sequences; their progressive automatisation is evidence in support of the existence of neurophysiological structures, no longer predetermined as for the reflexes and the schemas, but acquired. The existence of sensori-motor habits, whose sequence of actions unfold without the apparent intervention of conscious will, is universally accepted, and can be accounted for without engaging in an interpretation in S-R, or other, terms.

It appears that, at least during the first year of life, the child only possesses programmes of this kind and that his repertoire of models only amounts to a series of sensori-motor schemas which he applies to each new situation (Piaget, 1936).

During this period, most actions are specific responses to stimuli, i.e. they are *stimulus-bound*. Visual fixations are localised in areas determined by certain physical properties (Kessen, 1967; Fantz, 1958, 1961, 1963 etc.). Visual pursuit can be maintained by the displacement of a target until the baby is almost exhausted, as if he were unable to detach himself from it (Wolff and White, 1965). The infant repeats interminably certain cycles of activity.

With the emergence of the semiotic function and the possibility of representation, a new category of models becomes available; these differ from simple sensori-motor chains in that the sequence of actions is integrated in a representation of the situation and the goal to be attained, and is accompanied by the ability to anticipate the results of an action. From this point onwards it is not only the sensori-motor schemas the child possesses which a new situation brings into play; response systems are tried out which are adapted to the situation, that take into account the results of actions, and which demonstrate the existence of hypotheses. S. White (1964)

[1]In the sense of a motor habit.

observes that, during a discrimination learning task, 2- to 3-year-old children employ a model where the independent variable is the position of the object, a fact noted by all child psychologists and which constitutes one of the greatest obstacles in experimentation. However, White analysed this behaviour and found that it was modified with age. The youngest children formed a hypothesis as to position – the left, for example – and held to this choice whatever the outcome of their response. As the child grew older he used simple alternation, then he took the outcome into account but in a different manner from the experimenter, that is, if his response was followed by a favourable outcome, he continued to select the same position, whilst if it had an unfavourable outcome, he changed it. Relationships of this type between the response and its consequences cannot bring about success in a discrimination learning task; they manifest the existence of a model which is unsatisfactory because it neglects one of the terms (the nature of the stimulus) in the relationship stimulus–response–consequences. It is, however, still true to say that there is a programme of action and a representation of the situation.

When the task concerned does not have a predictable outcome, or the outcome is unrelated to the responses, the child operates in terms of one of his own models and it can be assumed that he employs, from amongst these, the one which is most readily available. The degree of availability can be a function of the recency of acquisition; this is why the systematic left-to-right, top-to-bottom exploration of a visual field is most frequent between 6 and 7 years, at the time when the child is learning to read and has a strict strategy of exploration, being replaced after the age of 8 years by more complex and more varied forms of exploration (Elkind and Weiss, 1967). During this same period certain recently acquired models (or *learning sets*) take a rigid form and are applied scrupulously, even when the situation no longer justifies it, as in the case of observing responses in the trials which follow the attainment of the learning criterion (Wright and Daehler, 1966).

A model can also be employed in preference to another because it is economical, because it has been possible to apply it in a large number of situations. Finally, if with Levine (1966) we think that, in the absence of a negative outcome, the child retains his hypothesis (or model), one negative outcome is not sufficient for it to be rejected. It appears from learning studies that a certain proportion of positive outcomes is sufficient to satisfy the very young child, and that, unlike his elders, he does not always try to get things right.

Briefly, our interpretation of the data described in the preceding chapters rests on the following postulates. The child's responses are organised in terms of coherent systems called models. These imply the existence of a representation of the problem which is presented – thus, of the experimental setting – together with the desired result and the sequence of actions likely to lead to this result. In a perceptual differentiation task, involving the responses 'same' or 'not the same', the model comprises a representation of the situation which can be expressed as 'a comparison from the point of view of whether or not they are the same', as well as the information necessary to make this decision, and a programme of action or strategy which prescribes where the gaze must be directed and in what order. In a task which involves copying a drawing, the model comprises a representation of the situation 'make a drawing like the model', and so also includes a criterion of 'the same'; to this is added a programme of exploratory activities in order to construct a representation of the drawing, or simply to compare it with a representation already in the child's possession, and an action programme for drawing the reproduction.

When learning is involved, the desired result is an increase in the number of positive outcomes. If the first model the child tries out does not achieve this end, he tries another; if the situation involves no particular outcome, the goal is simply the setting in motion of a series of responses which the subject judges to be satisfactory.

3   We have taken the view that for a living organism to get to know his environment involves both the gathering of information, effected through the intermediary of organs of sensory reception, and the processing of this information at the level of the central nervous system. We have stressed the fact that the disproportion between the amount of information available and the capacity for processing it is such that a usable knowledge can only be acquired by means of a selection of the information and its organisation into structured units.

The capacity for selecting and organising information is built into the nervous system; certain types of organisation – such as the organisation of visual stimuli into primary perceptual structures – even seem to be predetermined in their form and independent of the number and nature of the encounters between an organism and his environment. It must nonetheless be added that when these encounters are artificially suppressed right from birth, in those situations involving early sensory deprivation, for example, the neurophysiological bases of these structures deteriorate and the subsequent restoration of visual stimulation does not bring about the restoration of these structures (Chow, Riesen and Newell, 1957; Wiesel and Hubel, 1963; Fantz, 1965b).

As the child grows, under natural conditions of stimulation, new, acquired structures are added to those which are predetermined and modify them slightly. Involved in the development of these acquired structures is the frequency with which one pattern of stimulation rather than another is encountered and the rules to which the subject conforms in selecting from amongst the information that which he judges to be relevant.

The number of studies devoted to children's capacities for processing information is extremely limited; however, a few general strands can be disentangled.

The amount of information which can be registered simultaneously and made ready for immediate use increases with age, and the extent of this can be measured by assessing short-term memory or by relating discrimination performance to a unit analysis of the complexity of the material. The number of figures repeated correctly in Binet and Simon's test (1908) goes from two at 3 years, to three at 4 years, five at 8 years, and seven at 15 years. When the solution to a problem depends upon the processing of a small amount of information (two to three units), performance is as good at 3 years as it is at 4 or 5 years, but if this quantity increases, even slightly, then the younger the child the greater the number of errors (Santa Barbara and Paré, 1965).

The time necessary for processing the information extracted from a proximal stimulus, a measure of which is provided by the duration of a visual fixation, decreases very markedly between 3 and 9 years (see table 24, p. 255).

Finally, the temporal and spatial extent of the information selected and brought together within a given structure, perceptual, representational or mnemonic, increases with age. To begin with, the organisation is limited to the content of a temporal and spatial field, which Piaget calls the field of centration (Piaget, 1955, 1961); it involves only the stimulation deriving from a particular proximal stimulus, a sensory tableau (Piaget, 1936). Then, gradually, there is a temporal and spatial extension of the collection of stimuli which can be assembled in a common organisation.

The youngest children hardly relate any but a very few elements which are close together, as is shown by the restricted extent of their visual displacements (Zinchenko, Van Chizi-Tsin and Tarakanov, 1962; Mackworth and Bruner, 1966) and the relatively circumscribed area of their useful field of fixation (Mackworth, 1965).

One of the forms of progress observed with age – or with practice on one kind of material in a specific situation, as in learning to read – involves the extension of what Mackworth calls the useful field of fixation. It is almost certain that all the information contained in a proximal stimulus which brings about an excitation of the sensory receptors, is transmitted to the central nervous system, apart from those losses entailed in the transmission due to the anatomical conjunctions between the conductive fibres. This information is divided into two categories, depending on the part of the retina involved, foveal or peripheral, and it seems that the selection between the information which is retained and the information which is rejected depends to some extent on a topographical factor. Foveal information will be selected in preference to peripheral, the latter simply being divided into the interesting and the uninteresting. When classed as interesting, it determines the localisation of a subsequent fixation and is thus transformed into foveal vision (Mackworth and Morandi, 1967). The question of knowing on what indices the classification of extrafoveal information operates remains open. Sustained practice, such as training in speed reading, makes it possible to process peripheral information directly and considerably increases the extent of the useful field, whilst the introduction of an excess of information to process within a very short space of time and within a single proximal stimulus restricts this field to foveal vision alone (*tunnel vision*, Mackworth, 1965). The increase in the useful field, measured by the surface area of the proximal stimulus within which the information is selected, corresponds, in Piaget's terminology, to the appearance of enveloping centrations.

Whilst we await the availability of more extensive data concerning children, it is reasonable to hypothesise the following picture of the evolution of development. The young child can process only a very limited amount of information at a time, and it takes him a relatively long time to do that. Moreover the information which can be combined and organised must be close together in space and time; it is therefore extremely probable that, in the area of vision, only foveal or immediately perifoveal information is involved. The consequences of these limitations are that the very young child is particularly sensitive to any increase in the information density, useful or not, and any reduction in the time of presentation. Furthermore, by using foveal vision almost exclusively he can only link up the contents of successive proximal stimuli by multiplying his points of fixation and bringing them close together. But he is equally limited by the restricted extent of his field of temporal apprehension. The result of this is that, in order to gather all the information he wants, he needs more time and more fixations than the adult, whilst two successive units of information will only have a chance of being integrated if their temporal distance apart is much less than would be needed by an adult. We are inclined to think that this set of constraints is at least partly responsible for the inadequate exploratory activity of the very young child, since a complete exploration is of little use if he lacks the means of relating the information gathered in the latter part of the exploration to that gathered at the beginning.

The child's limited capacity for processing information makes it vitally necessary for him to organise it into a small number of units and to use very simple rules to determine what is relevant and thus to be retained.

Various writers such as Werner (1940), Piaget (1936, 1937, etc.), and Spitz (1958) postulate that the child's development takes place in the direction of a progressive differentiation from a primitive state of relative globalism, or undifferentiation, at the same time as a hierarchical organisation, which Werner (1947) subsumes under the heading of the orthogenetic law. Although the available evidence is certainly in agreement with the hypothesis of a progression in terms of differentiation and organisation, it categorically belies the description of the infant as totally undifferentiated (Spitz, 1958). At birth the baby possesses a very limited repertoire of voluntary actions since he can scarcely do anything except suck, look, turn his head, grasp an object which touches the palm of his hand and display a global disorganised activity; but he is already capable of using these few behaviours in a manner which is differentiated according to the nature of the stimulation. Investigations of visual perception in babies (see Vurpillot, 1966, 1972) have shown in an incontrovertible fashion that the duration and number of visual fixations vary according to certain specific properties of the objects presented; the study of sucking behaviour reveals clear differences between sucking for nourishment and sucking for its own sake, when a teat as opposed to a rubber tube is involved (Lipsitt, 1967). Almost from birth the baby's behaviour is differentiated as a function of the nature of the stimulation. This differentiation, gross to begin with, becomes refined with age and is always accompanied by an organisation of the information selected. It seems probable that the development of the process of differentiation, like that of organisation, does not take place uniformly and simultaneously from all points of view, and is not a matter of a gradual transition from a complete lack of organisation to perfect organisation, with intermediate levels where all structures and all contents are of equal value.

To begin with there are islets of organisation which are gradually linked together and integrated into unitary structures; the influence of proximity is thus particularly great in the case of the youngest children and is manifested not only in perception but also in intellectual activities. The first categories the child constructs are very restricted groupings, in pairs, or in chains, in which object A, for example, is associated with B on the basis of a common property *m* and with C by property *n*, whilst B and C are associated by a third property *p* (Bruner and Olver, 1963; Olver and Hornsby, 1967).

The first structures are sensori-motor and perceptual. The organisation of the stimuli which takes place seems to be determined first of all by the physical properties of the stimulus alone, and one might be tempted to consider these primary perceptual structures as innate and a function of the properties of the central nervous system.

A distinction between homogeneous and heterogeneous stimuli is present from birth (Fantz, 1958a, 1963, etc.; Hershenson, 1964, etc.), manifested by a preference for patterned as against plain surfaces. But this differentiation seems to correspond more to the primitive segregation between figure and ground envisaged by Hebb (1949) than that of the Gestaltists, for whom it also included the perception of organised form. The limited amount of data (Bower, 1965a, 1967a, etc.) available at the present moment encourages one to think that if the various laws of organisation are not perhaps effective at birth, they take effect very early, during the first year of life, and make it possible, at the age-levels which interest us, to predict into what sort of units diverse stimuli are going to be regrouped and articulated.

The first units isolated by the child are certainly three-dimensional objects; in the case of the pictorial material which forms the basis of so many experiments, it would seem probable that the drawing is initially perceived as a single unit, indissociable, but differentiated from the sheet of paper. The limitations of our techniques of investigation make it impossible to demonstrate, before the age of 4 years, the segregation of a drawing into several individualised units. It cannot necessarily be concluded from this that it does not occur. All that can be said is that at 4 years, three-quarters of the children can isolate overlapping figures (Piaget and Stettler, 1954; Ghent, 1956a; Vurpillot and Florès, 1964).

These first perceptual structures, three-dimensional objects or figure drawings, which we have called primary units, are, above all, indissociable, in the sense that one of their parts or one of their properties cannot be abstracted from them – which does not mean that the whole is undifferentiated. If we take the example of the property of colour, a differential sensitivity to colour can be demonstrated during the first few days of life (Chase, 1937); matching of objects of the same shade can be carried out by children from two to three years of age (Cook, 1931). At this age-level a child has the words corresponding to several simple colours and may speak of her tartan dress or her blue jacket; however, if she is asked to indicate something blue, or to say what colour her dress is, there is complete failure. The property 'blue' or 'tartan' cannot be considered independently of the object which has this characteristic, i.e. the colour cannot be abstracted from the object and treated as a dimension of differentiation on which the objects can be located to serve as a basis for a systematic categorisation. The same is true for other physical properties of objects such as texture or size. This inability to analyse an object in terms of its properties is what differentiates very young children from older ones in their performance on learning transfer tasks. Young children, like older ones, are able to learn to associate specific responses to stimulus-objects, although it takes them a much larger number of trials. When a second discrimination learning can be acquired with the same relevant dimension of differentiation being conserved (reversal shift learning), it is facilitated for the older children but not for the younger ones who have not analysed the objects and have thus not discovered the dimensions of differentiation (H. Kendler and T. Kendler, 1962).

The ability to abstract a property and to compare several objects on this basis seems to appear around the age of 3 years. But it is not applied immediately to all the qualities in terms of which an object can be described. Certain dimensions of differentiation such as thickness (L. Tighe and T. Tighe, 1966) or brightness (T. Kendler and H. Kendler, 1959) are abstracted at an earlier age than others such as size (T. Kendler and H. Kendler, 1959) or the vertical or horizontal orientation of stripes (L. Tighe and T. Tighe, 1966).

The same phenomenon of indissociability exists between the parts of an object, and is manifested either at the level of identification or at the level of perceptual reorganisation. If one part of a drawing is perceived and identified as 'a banana', it is no longer available to take the part of a leg in a whole identified as a skier (Dworetzki, 1939). The part in question can only belong to a single perceptual or semantic unit. This is not to say that when the child interprets one part as a banana the remainder of the lines in the drawing cease to exist for him. It is more a matter of a rigidity phenomenon: when a line belongs to one figure, when an object is placed within one category, for the moment its fate is sealed; it belongs to this figure or this category and cannot enter into another. This rigidity is temporary: certain figures, certain categories are in general more probable than others; but these others can, at another time, become more readily available, and the drawing organises itself in another fashion. But then the new units which are formed suppress the existence of the preceding ones; if the drawing is seen as a skier, with legs, it is impossible for one of these to be a banana.

The possibility of a double identification of the same ambiguous (Dworetzki, 1939; Elkind, Koegler and Go, 1964) or reversible (Elkind and Scott, 1962; Elkind, 1964) drawing only appears around the age of 6 to 7 years.

It is in this same rigidity of perceptual structures that the inability of young children to resolve embedded figures problems (Gottschaldt, 1926) originates. Whatever the model that has to be found, before 6 years of age the child can only break down a complex figure into its primary units, the form of which can be predicted in terms of exact laws of organisation (Ghent, 1956a; Vurpillot, 1964a; Vurpillot and Florès, 1964 and Chapter 1 of the present volume).

Within this perspective the old controversy about syncretism no longer has any point and all the examples of the dominance of the parts (pointillism) or of the whole (globalism) cease to be contradictory. Every set of stimuli is organised into a limited number of perceptual structures or units determined by certain laws. With the exception of some special cases, relatively rare in the natural environment, the probability of appearance of a particular form or organisation is extremely high; the structures formed in this way are thus coercive and the whole is perceived in the same fashion by everyone. These structures are the only ones likely to be perceived by the youngest children; from this point of view their perception is very rigid. When the situation is sufficiently ambiguous for two different sets of perceptual structures to have an effectively equal probability of arising from the same set of stimuli, then there is an alternation between the two forms of organisation, although this alternation is slower in the child than in the adult (Elkind and Scott, 1962).

For the very young child the primary structures are indissociable, either into their detachable elements or parts, or into their properties, and from this point of view perception can be described as globalist; but the fact that they are unanalysable does not mean that they are confused – on the contrary they are strongly organised. Moreover, the globalist characteristic is independent of size of the structures. Global perception does not mean that the perceived structure encompasses all the lines of a drawing; the physical characteristics of the drawing determine that the most probable organisation will involve either a part, or the whole of the lines. A perception of a few details rather than the whole of the drawing is perfectly consistent with the globalist character of the structure, as Meili (1939) has made clear.

Finally, identification itself is oriented both by the perceptual organisation of the drawing and by the child's interests and repertoire of categories. Only those structures which are perceived are identified, hence the role of the organisation into primary units; but these structures seem to be treated by the very young children as simple cues and, as we shall see later on, the margin within which a child makes an inference from a part to a whole is very large; their identifications, unlike their perceptual structures, will therefore be extremely varied and sensitive to their interest of the moment.

The representational structures undergo an evolution which is in part analogous to that of perceptual structures; initially rigid and impoverished, they become richer and more adaptable with age. Drawn reproductions, despite the distortions of their motor origin, appear to be one of the best ways of gaining evidence of the form of a representational image structure, designated – according to the writers concerned – by the term internal model (Luquet, 1927a), representational image (Bruner, 1964, 1966a, etc.), representational schema (Piaget, 1961), mental image (Piaget and Inhelder, 1966), or image (Wekker, 1966; Leontiev and Gippenreiter, 1966; Zaporozhets, 1960; Zaporozhets and Zinchenko, 1966). Studies of the development of children's drawings have shown the degree of rigidity of the internal model to which the child conforms in his interpretation of external reality; each drawing of a man, reduced to the bare essentials, amounts to a sort of statement of what, for the child, constitutes a human being. Thus one can follow, stage by stage, the modifications – in the form of additions or specifications – of the representation of what the child sees. Of course, perception itself is certainly infinitely richer, and the amount of information lost in the passage from perception to representation is very great, but it is reasonable to assume that the child retains in his model what is, for him, the most important.

In the construction of a representational model as well as in increasing the flexibility of perceptual structures, perceptual exploration appears to be the essential factor for a number of research-workers in this area (Piaget, 1961; Zaporozhets and Zinchenko, 1966). The amount of information extracted depends on the extent of the exploration; consequently the more exhaustive this is, the greater the amount of information. On the other hand, one can find in the work of authors as different as Hebb (1949), Piaget (1961) and Zaporozhets (Zaporozhets and Zinchenko, 1966) the idea that the form of the structure constitutes an internalisation of the exploration of the object, and that the relationships brought about by the displacement of the receptors between the various parts are incorporated, so to speak, in the perceptual or representational structure.

Only Hebb (1949) fails to distinguish between primary and secondary perceptual structures, since for him they are all acquired by means of exploratory activity. Piaget, on the other hand, generally establishes a distinction between the two. A very large number of experimental results show that tactile as well as visual exploration increases markedly with age, at the same time as it becomes more and more systematic. Piaget and his students have given their attention to the perception of very simple, geometric figures and have proceeded to the investigation of size perception. The important series of publications stemming from their research has shown that the parts likely to be integrated into a single structure become more and more numerous and further and further apart. Relating, by means of perceptual activity, units of information formerly treated as separate wholes, organised as primary units, involves both the construction of new secondary units (as in the case of linking up the separate lines in an incomplete drawing) and the modification of the primary structures involved.

The main object of the researches of the Russian school has been to establish a correspondence between the form of the exploration, such as that which takes shape in the sequential recording of the points of visual fixation or the areas of tactile contact, and that of a drawn reproduction. Here also the bulk of the data obtained shows that the richness of the representational model increases with the extent of the exploration, in the same way that the exactness of this model depends on the systematisation of the exploration.

An accurate drawn reproduction, an exact recognition, is only achieved at around the age of 6 years, when, during the familiarisation of a form, the child proceeds to a systematic and orderly exploration of its contour.


4   Limited in his capacity for gathering, recording and processing information, the child, even more than the adult, finds himself obliged to make a selection from the totality presented by the environment. But, as he possesses limited powers of abstraction and a restricted number of cognitive categories, he relies on a few simple criteria. The relatively large and varied amount of data which we have available on the behaviour of children in the age-range 3 to 7 years on tasks of perceptual differentiation makes it possible to disentangle the main strands of the observed development and the characteristics of the stages.

The sensitivity of the visual receptors to the variations of the physical dimensions of stimulation (such as brightness, the texture or heterogeneity of the intensities of the various parts of the proximal stimulus, colour, the size and certain parameters of form) exists from birth and during the first few months of life it reaches a level close to that found in adults. Recent researches carried out on babies and very young children show that they are capable of perceiving the differences introduced by the experimenter into his material. On this point the data relating to fixation times on varying targets are quite conclusive.

However, the performances of young children on tasks of perceptual differentiation, paired comparison, or discrimination learning are poor. We have tried to show that before the age of 6 years the child does not possess logical relationships of identity, of equivalence and the ordering of classes, and that his judgments are always of the categorial type and based on partial equivalences.

Placed in a world of great complexity, bombarded by a variety of constantly changing stimuli, the child can only adapt and manifest purposive behaviour if he introduces a certain order by gathering into a few large classes the events which it is in his interest to recognise when they recur. Even though his receptors are, above all, sensitive to change, and thus to differences, his central nervous system seems to be constructed to organise the multiple excitations received by the receptors into a small number of structured units.

These units – perceptual and representational structures, intellectual categories, etc. – combine the various elements on the basis of common properties and constitute the invariants of a stable world.

The child comes into possession of perceptual invariants very early, since size constancy can be demonstrated before the age of 6 months, as well as categories. These latter are not logical classes of equivalence but constitute, for the child, an effective means of gathering together objects or events in terms of making a common response to them. In a differentiation task, whether it is a matter of learning or simple judgment, the objects to be compared all possess several common properties; some of them are physically identical in the sense that each value taken by one of them on a physical dimension of differentiation corresponds to the same value, on the same dimension, for the other. Two identical objects therefore have equal values for all their properties. Two different objects, on the other hand, are objects which present different values in respect of at least one of their properties. For a subject who employs the logical relationship of identity, the response 'identical' can only be given to physically identical objects; the presence of a single difference, whatever the property it applies to, invokes the response of non-identity.

It is, however, quite clear, that in children of preschool age the presence of a difference does not necessarily prevent two objects from being judged as identical. This is the first point that emerges from the study of the responses of children from 3 to 5 years of age; if two objects are judged as being 'exactly the same' it is because they have some properties in common and not at all because there is no difference between them. To a certain degree, judgments of difference and judgments of identity are independent, the two areas separate, and two objects can be simultaneously 'the same' and 'not the same'. This is the case, of course, when the task is one of categorisation, since, in ordering objects in terms of their colour, one knows very well that they have neither the same form nor the same size, for example, and thus are different. The great difference between the child above the age of 7 years and the preschool-age child is that the former chooses to conform either to a relationship of equivalence, or to a relationship of identity, and that in categorising he follows the rules of logical classification and class inclusion, whilst the latter always judges in terms of partial equivalence, and his categories do not obey logical rules.

The analysis of the performances and the justifications of their responses given by children showed that between the ages of 3 and 7 years they used levels of equivalence which were progressively more exacting.

At a first level, two objects are judged 'the same' because they have something in common, this being a detail or a part which could be considered as detachable, rather than a property that could be abstracted such as colour, for example. In comparing pictures of houses (Vurpillot, 1968, 1969a; Vurpillot and Moal, 1970) or familiar objects (Vurpillot, 1969a), the justification of a 'same' response by a 4-year-old child is always of this type: 'The two houses are the same because there is a vase of flowers (house on the left) and there is a vase of flowers here as well (house on the right)', or else 'You can easily see the two fisherman are the same – there's a fish there and one there as well'.

This level is characterised above all by a very incomplete exploration of the objects being compared. The child extracts only a sample of the available information, a sample limited spatially to one area of the stimulus, and he feels himself able to judge the whole on the basis of this fragment. But the limitation is not only spatial; within the area which is inspected, the presence of differences does not inevitably bring about the response 'not the same'. To take the example of the fisherman again, the fish, indicated by the child in support of his judgment of identity, is precisely what contains the difference introduced by the experimenter, since its orientation is not the same in both drawings.

At a second level, reached between the ages of 5 and 6 years, the child ceases to think that he can judge after having seen only a part, exploration becomes complete and correspondence is established between each part of one object and each part of the other. Two objects are judged 'the same' when, for each part of one object, there is a corresponding identical part in the other, but the spatial relationships between the parts within the whole are not taken into consideration. Thus, in the experiment involving permutations (Vurpillot and Moal, 1970), if it was possible to find, for each window in one house, a window with identical contents in the other house, it was of little significance that the positions occupied by the windows were not homologous, and the two houses were judged as being the same. There is certainly a one-to-one correspondence between parts, and the requirement of the physical identity of these parts, but the judgment still involves an equivalence since the spatial relationships between these objects can differ from one object to the other.

It is only at the third level, which is reached between the ages of 6 and 8 years, that the use of a real identity relationship appears, defined positively by the identity of all the values on all the properties and negatively by the absence of differences.

Some judgments of difference appear even in the youngest children, although these are few in situations where the task is the simple decision between 'same' and 'not the same' or where the response is followed by a particular outcome. These responses can therefore be due to the fact either that the sample extracted contained no identical parts in both objects, or that the sample did in fact contain identical homologous parts but the child, in establishing correspondence, did so with non-homologous parts; or even that the differences, perceived as such, were considered as preventing the objects from being the same.

As we have already observed, the child very soon begins to organise the physical world in terms of invariant objects. At an early age he becomes accustomed to neglecting a certain number of the differences which he perceives but which he needs to ignore for the invariance of the object to be respected. Thus his sensory receptors transmit, simultaneously, data concerning the difference in size and form of the retinal projections of objects, and the density and density gradient of the texture of their surfaces ((Gibson, 1950) as well as the degree of illumination. Nevertheless he perceives, as a function of all these indices, objects which remain invariant from the point of view of their intrinsic properties, but whose spatial relationships with the subject change. Very soon he makes the indispensable distinction between those transformations of the proximal stimulus compatible with a conservation of the physical object (Gibson's 'transformations of perspective', 1950) and those which are not and express a modification of the object itself. The material presented in perceptual tasks usually consists of representational drawings of actual objects, and the child therefore applies to these pictures the same distinction between conserving and non-conserving transformations as to the objects themselves. To begin with, only those modifications which interfere with the integrity of the object are considered to amount to non-identity – for example, the open/closed topological transformations and changes of form which are incompatible with the representational schema, the internal model of the object. From this point of view, the more numerous and elaborate the models, the more likely it is that a modification will be seen as non-conserving. On the other hand, changes of size, spatial displacements and all those transformations of what is called perspective do not affect the integrity of the object and are treated as conserving.

As the child grows older, the number of his representational schemas and categories increases, at the same time as his capacity for abstracting the properties of an object, which means taking into consideration more and more numerous and progressively finer differences so that these categories are not confused. Repeated encounters with the physical environment and the pressures of cultural norms, oblige him to make distinctions which, to begin with, did not compel recognition; consequently he needs to pay attention to some differences which he previously neglected, although capable of responding to them from the point of view of sensory sensitivity. Thus, in the process of learning to read, the orientation of a form or of one of its parts relative to a frame of reference must be taken into account.

5   Several explanations, none of which is sufficient on its own, have been proposed to account for the developmental evolution of children's performances.

The first is biological. If the performances of young children are inferior to those of older children, it is because their central nervous system is not mature.

The consequences of the immaturity of the neurones of the various parts of the nervous system and of the fibres involved in transmission are a limited sensitivity to excitation, a slowness in all processes and, at the level of simple transmission and the various chemical syntheses, a deficiency of connective relationships due to the inadequacy of the connector elements such as the dendrites.

All child psychologists recognise the influence of neural maturation. It is quite clear that a certain level of maturity must be attained before a particular task can be carried out; but this is only a necessary, not a sufficient, condition. Consequently, the younger the child, the more important the influence of neural maturation, this being particularly marked during the first year. No one would deny that the increase in perceptual acuity between 0 and 6 months results from changes taking place in the retinal neurones, that the increase in the speed of visuo-motor reaction time and visual pursuit is due to the maturation of the paths of transmission, and that the ability to co-ordinate prehension and vision marks the appearance of new connective fibres. At more subtle and less accessible levels, the decrease in the duration of a visual fixation indicates a decrease in the time necessary for processing a given amount of information and must itself be attributable to organic changes.

All this being granted, there can be no question of seeing in the immaturity of the nervous system the explanation of all the deficiencies of very young children. So far as the sensory receptors are concerned, maturation is reached well before the age at which we have seen our youngest subjects; acuity and accommodation are excellent, only the pupil of the eye has not reached its maximum size and presumably the restriction of the useful field of vision could be partially due to this fact. Let us also concede that the extension of the mnemonic field has a neurophysiological basis and that the spatial and temporal distances within which the relationships between distinct units of information can be established are limited by the speed of transmission and the proliferation of connections.

It is to S. White (1966, 1968, 1969) that we owe an interesting attempt to establish a relationship between the changes observed in the behaviour of children from 5 to 7 years and neural maturation. His thesis rests on a collection of evidence gathered in very diverse areas, but all having in common the demonstration of the concomitant appearance of neurophysiological changes and changes in behaviour.

Thus the evolution of IQ with age, and likewise the change in the sensitivity to pathological disorders both provide evidence of a decrease in the child's intellectual and neurological vulnerability. The stabilisation of the IQ (Bloom, 1964), the resistance to nervous disorders and illnesses (S. White, 1968), both observed from the age of 7 years, would depend on maturational development.

A second hypothesis stems from a comparison between the behaviour of children and the behaviour of very old people. A number of investigations have demonstrated marked similarities between the development of the child of preschool age and the involution of the elderly person. The behavioural analogy between the very young and the very old would be explained by an analogy in terms of neural structures. The emergence during the process of ageing of the cognitive systems of the young child would be in accord with the explanation of development in terms of ontogenetic corticalisation proposed by Hughlings Jackson. Around the age of 7 years, and due to neural maturation, cognitive mechanisms of a lower order would be subordinated to higher-order mechanisms; the latter would disappear in the elderly person, as a result of the effects of an inverse process of neurological regression, disinhibiting the lower-order cognitive system which would have continued to exist since childhood (S. White, 1966, 1969).

A third hypothesis derives from anatomical and pathological investigations carried out on children and adults. Cortical maturation seems to be reached by the age of 6 years in the parietal, occipital and temporal lobes (E. Milner, 1967), but that of the frontal areas goes on beyond this age. The important change observed in all behaviour between 5 and 7 years would thus coincide with the mature organisation of the temporal, occipital and parietal cortex. Taking a different approach, a number of analogies can be drawn between the responses of preschool-age children and those of adults who have suffered brain lesions, on various tasks such as Bender's (1938) test or the finger localisation test (Benton, 1959), to quote just two examples.

S. White concludes that if neural maturation cannot be considered as the only factor involved, it certainly accounts in part for the changes in behaviour which take place between 5 and 7 years.

The degree of neurophysiological maturation of an organism determines the limits between what it cannot possibly do and what it could do; it does not determine in a direct fashion what the child actually will do. Maturational progress displaces an impassible barrier, but it does not explain how, from within these limits, the child passes from one behaviour to another.

In marked contrast to the few for whom all progress in performance is to be found in some organic change (and who see the impossibility of demonstrating the cogency of this hypothesis as being due to the inadequacies of techniques of investigation) are the proponents of modern empiricism. Learning theorists undertake to explain changes in performance with age by the same mechanisms as the development of performance on a task under the influence of repetition within a limited period of time in a laboratory. In short, provided that the organism possesses the sufficient anatomo-physiological characteristics, one could teach anything to anybody; it would take a longer time in the child than in the adult, but the learning mechanism itself would not change. This position does not seem to us to be confirmed by the facts.

It is true that a sensori-motor habit presents the same characteristics of acquisition and evolution at all ages, and even in all animal species. Provided that the stimuli to which a response has to be made and the acts which have to be accomplished are within the limits of an individual's sensory and motor capacity, the sensori-motor habit can be acquired. Within the term 'habit' we include Skinner's complicated programmes of skill acquisition, as well as simple discrimination learning.

However, if at the end of a discrimination learning task everyone reaches the same level of performance, there are, nonetheless, considerable differences in the way in which this acquisition is going to affect the subsequent behaviour of the subject. In the youngest children, a learning is specific to a particular situation and particular material; if new material, a new situation is presented, there is no transfer. The child, in this case, has acquired a rigid habit which he will forget more or less quickly, but his other behaviour will not be changed. Unless we suppose that our childhood is spent acquiring a large enough number of habits to make it possible to respond to every situation which could ever present itself to us, it is difficult to see how such mechanical acquisitions could account for intelligent and adapted behaviour in novel circumstances.

Older children, on the other hand, not only learn an initial discrimination quickly, but take into account what they have learnt when they come to resolve subsequent problems. Instead of establishing a rigid connection between a stimulus and a response, or a chain of stimuli and responses, they analyse the stimuli, seeking a law of correspondence between the ordered stimulus-values and the response-values and, from amongst the information available, select the one that relates to the relevant dimension of differentiation. In a subsequent task their behaviour is influenced by what they have just learnt; they also do better when the same dimension remains relevant than when the reverse is the case.

Some learning theorists have preferred to see, in this selection of a part of the information, the simple acquisition of an intermediate response, intercalated between the stimulus-object and the choice-response. They have believed that by this means the behaviour of older children could be accounted for in the same way as the behaviour of younger children – in terms of an S-R type theory. To call the focusing of attention on just one part of the available information, or the abstraction of a dimension of differentiation, a 'response', would seem rather artificial. Nothing in the data makes it possible to demonstrate that a response is really involved and, in particular, that the links between a mediational response and the final outcome are of the same order and react in the same way to the different variables as the observable choice-responses (Mackintosh, 1965).

With these qualifications, it is nonetheless certain that all behaviour is affected by practice. The nature of the environment and, hence, the child's encounters with the physical world, their frequency, the positive or negative nature of the consequences of actions – which relate to cultural norms and social pressures as well as physical laws – mean that certain forms of behaviour bring about more beneficial results than others. The number and nature of the categories formed depend, therefore, on the child's experience and the context within which it has been acquired. But the capacity for categorising exists outside any learning; the capacity for abstracting properties from objects and organising responses as a function of them cannot be inculcated in a child of 2-3 years, whatever the number of learning trials, yet it is present from the first trial in the 9-year-old. Learning has the effect of determining which dimension will be abstracted in a given situation, not that of making abstraction appear. In short, learning and development must not be confused.

We fully endorse Piaget's theoretical position; we think that the child's development takes place according to a certain order, that at each stage a certain form of structure predominates, to which all behaviour conforms, and that, in the passage from one stage to the next, all of these behaviours undergo a reorganisation as a function of the new structure which characterises this stage and which includes the preceding structures. Between 5 and 8 years, the child passes from the pre-operational period to the period of concrete operations, his intellectual structures henceforth obeying the logic of classes and relations. In every area the characteristics of this structure are found; from the point of view of perceptual organisation it is then that the articulation between the whole and its parts appears; each perceptual structure can be considered both as a unit and as part of a larger unit, identified therefore either as a whole or as part of another whole, in the same way that in the logic of classes an object can belong simultaneously to several inclusive classes. In the area of perceptual differentiation, at these same ages, the child no longer dissociates judgments of difference and identity or bases the latter on partial equivalences. Capable of using real classes of equivalence, he also defines identity logically in terms of the absence of difference as well as by the presence of common properties.

Whilst in the young child the influence of context on an object is imposed rigidly and externally – hence his sensitivity to what are called primary field effects – from the age of 6 years he places each part in relation to the others within a single system of relationships. He can then voluntarily decide to take account of only one part or one relationship and to consider the others as irrelevant without being unaware of their presence.

From this point all behaviours are characterised by a hierarchical articulation of all the parts within inclusive structures.

Speaking in terms of models, we would say that at each stage of his development the child has at his disposal a certain number of them, that the actual number and the content of these models depend on the nature of his environment and, in the main, on his acquired experience. But these models all belong to the same family, characterised by a communality of structure: the sensori-motor schemas of the baby, the models based on partial equivalence of the 4-year-old child, the class-inclusive models of the 7-year-old. Every task presented to a child is resolved by him as a function of the type of models he possesses; if a learning task is involved where the experimenter tries to get the child to adopt his own model, he can only succeed if it belongs to the child's family of models. The experimenter will be able to get 5-year-old children to discover the relevant dimensions of differentiation, but not 3-year-olds, as is shown by the effects of overlearning in learning tasks involving reversal or non-reversal shift.

Faced with a new task, the child begins by assimilating it to the models in his repertoire, then, if the result is not satisfactory, he tries to modify his model, to accommodate it to the new situation. But this accommodation is only possible if the modification it involves is not too great.

# Bibliography

Amato d', M. R. and Jagoda, H. 'Overlearning and position reversal', *J. Exp. Psychol.*, 1962, **64**, pp. 117–122.

Ames, E. W. and Silfen, C. K. 'Methodological issue in the study of age differences in infants' attention to stimuli varying in movement and complexity'. *Paper presented to the Society for Research in Child Development*, Minneapolis, U.S.A., 1965.

Ananiev, B. G., Wekker, L. M., Lomov, B. F. and Yarmolenko, A. V. *Osyazanie v protsessakh poznaniya i truda* (Touch in the processes of learning and action), Moscow: Publishing House of the Academy of Pedagogical Sciences, U.S.S.R., 1959.

Anderson, I. H. 'Studies in the eye movements of good and poor readers', *Psychol. Monogr.*, 1937, **48**, No. 215, pp. 1–35.

Andrieux, C. 'Contribution à l'étude des différences entre hommes et femmes dans la perception spatiale', *Année Psychol.*, 1955, **55**, pp. 41–60.

Antonovsky, H. F. and Ghent, L. 'Cross-cultural consistency of children's preferences for the orientation of figures', *Amer. J. Psychol.*, 1964, **77**, pp. 295–297.

Attneave, F. 'Some informational aspects of visual perception', *Psychol. Rev.*, 1954, **61**, pp. 183–193.

Aubert, H. 'Eine scheinbare beteunde Drehung von Objekten bei Neigung des Kopfes', *Virchows Arch.*, 1961, **20**, p. 381.

Babska, Z. 'The formation of the conception of identity of visual characteristics of objects seen successively', *Monogr. Soc. Res. Child Dev.*, 1965, **30**, pp. 112–124. In: P. E. Mussen (ed.) *European research in cognitive development*.

Bartley, S. H. *Principles of perception*, New York: Harper, 1958.

Bender, L. *A visual motor gestalt test and its clinical use*, New York: American Orthopsychiatric Association, 1938.

Benton, A. L. *Right-left discrimination and finger localization*, New York: Hoeber, 1959.

Berlyne, D. E. *Conflict, arousal, and curiosity*, New York, Toronto, London: McGraw Hill, 1960.

Berlyne, D. E. 'Soviet research on intellectual processes in children'. In: J. C. Wright and J. Kagan (eds) 'Basic cognitive processes in children', *Monogr. Soc. Res. Child Dev.*, 1963, **28**, Monogr. 86, pp. 165–183.

Berthoud, M. and Vurpillot, E. 'Influence du nombre de différences sur les réponses "pas pareil" chez l'enfant d'âge préscolaire', *Enfance*, 1970, **23**, pp. 23–30.

Beyrl, F. 'Ueber die Grössenauffassung bei Kindern', *Z. Psychol.*, 1926, **100**, pp. 344–371.

Bijou, S. W. and Baer, D. M. 'Some methodological contributions from a functional analysis of child development'. In: L. P. Lipsett and C. C. Spiker (eds), *Advances in child development and behavior*, Vol. 1, New York, London: Academic Press, 1963, pp. 197–231.

Binet, A. 'Perception d'enfants', *Rev. Philos.*, 1890, **30**, pp. 582–611.

Binet, A. and Simon, Th. 'Le developpement de l'intelligence chez les enfants', *Année Psychol.*, 1908, **14**, pp. 1–94.

Bingham, H. C. 'Size and form perception in *gallus domesticus*', *J. Anim. Behav.*, 1913, **3**, pp. 65–113.

Bingham, H. C. 'A definition of form', *J. Anim. Behav.*, 1914, **4**, pp. 136–141.

Birch, H. G. 'Dyslexia and the maturation of the visual function.' In: J. Money (ed.) *Reading disability*, Baltimore: John Hopkins Press, 1962.

Birch, H. G. 'Dyslexia and the maturation of the visual function'. In: *Monogr. Soc. Res. Child Dev.*, 1963, **28**, No. 83, No. 5.

Bloom, B. S. *Stability and change in human characteristics*, New York: Wiley and Sons, 1964.

Bobbitt, J. M. 'An experimental study of the phenomenon of closure as a threshold function', *J. Exp. Psychol.*, 1942, **30**, pp. 273–294.

Botha, E. 'Practice without reward and figure-ground perceptions of adults and children', *Percept. Mot. Skills*, 1963, **16**, pp. 271–273.

Botzum, W. A. 'A factorial study of the reasoning and closure factors', *Psychometrika*, 1951, **16**, pp. 361–386.

Bower, T. G. R. 'Discrimination of depth in pre-motor infants', *Psychon. Sci.* 1964, **1**, p. 368.

Bower, T. G. R. 'The determinants of perceptual unity in infancy', *Psychon. Sci.*, 1965a, **3**, pp. 323–324.

Bower, T. G. R. 'Stimulus variables determining space perception in infants', *Science*, 1965b, **149**, pp. 88–89.

Bower, T. G. R. 'Phenomenal identity and form perception in an infant', *Percept. Psychophys.*, 1967a, **2**, pp. 74–76.

Bower, T. G. R. 'The development of object-permanence: some studies of existence constancy', *Percept. Psychophys.*, 1967b, **2**, pp. 411–418.

Braine, L. Ghent. 'Age changes in the mode of perceiving geometric forms', *Psychon. Sci.*, 1965a, **2**, pp. 155–156.

Braine, L. Ghent. 'Disorientation of forms: an examination of Rock's theory', *Psychon. Sci.*, 1965b, **3**, pp. 541–542.

Brandner, M. 'Das bildnerische gestaltende Kind: II. Der Umgang des Kleinkindes mit Würfeln bis zu den fruhesten Formen des Bauens', *Neue Psychol. Stud.*, 1939, **8**, p. 216.

Brandt, H. F. *The psychology of seeing*, New York: The Philosophical Library, 1945.

Brault, H. 'Étude génétique de la constance des formes', *Psychol. Franç.*, 1962, **7**, pp. 270–282.

Brian, C. R. and Goodenough, F. L. 'The relative potency of color and form perception at different ages', *J. Exp. Psychol.*, 1929, **12**, pp. 197–213.

Broadbent, D. E. *Perception and communication*, London, New York, · Paris: Pergamon Press, 1958.

Bruner, J. S. 'Les processus de préparation à la perception', In: J. S. Bruner, F. Bresson, A. Morf and J. Piaget (eds) *Logique et perception*, Paris: Presses Universitaires de France, 1958 pp. 1–48.

Bruner, J. S. 'The course of cognitive growth', *Amer. Psychologist*, 1964, **19**, pp. 1–15.

Bruner, J. S. 'On cognitive growth. I.' In: J. S. Bruner, R. R. Olver and P. M. Greenfield (eds) *Studies in cognitive growth*, New York, London, Sydney: John Wiley and Sons, 1966a, pp. 1–29.

Bruner, J. S. *Toward a theory of instruction*, Cambridge, Mass.: Harvard University Press, 1966b.

Bruner J. S. *Processes of cognitive growth: Infancy*, Worcester, Mass.: Clark University Press, 1968.

Bruner, J. S., Goodnow, J. J. and Austin, G. A. *A study of thinking*, New York: John Wiley and Sons, 1956.

Bruner, J. S. and Olver R. R. 'Development of equivalence transformations in children'. In: J. C. Wright and J. Kagan (eds) 'Basic cognitive processes in children', *Monogr. Soc. Res. Child Dev.*, 1963, **28**, Monogr. 86, pp. 125–141.

Bruner, J. S., Postman, L. and Mosteller, F. 'A note on the measurement of reversals of perspective', *Psychometrika*, 1950, **15**, pp. 63–72.

Brunswick, E. *Perception and the representative design of psychological experiments*, Berkeley and Los Angeles: University of California Press, 1956.

Brunswik, E. and Kamiya, J. 'Ecological cue-validity of "proximity" and of other Gestalt factors', *Amer. J. Psychol.*, 1953, **66**, pp. 20–32.

Burzlaff, W. 'Methodologische Beiträge zum Problem der Farbenkonstanz', *Z. Psychol.*, 1931, **119**, pp. 177–235.

Buss, A. H. 'Rigidity as a function of reversal and nonreversal shifts in the learning of successive discriminations', *J. Exp. Psychol.*, 1953, **45**, pp. 75–81.

Busse, K. 'Die Austellung zur vergleichenden Entwicklungsgeschichte der primitiven Kunst bei den Naturvölkern, den Kindern und in Urzeit', *Kongr. f. Aest. u. allg. Kunstwiss.*, 1914.

Buswell, G. T. 'Fundamental reading habits: a study of their development', *Suppl. Educ. Monogr.*, 1922, Suppl. 21.

Buswell, G. T. *How people look at pictures: a study of the psychology and perception of art*, Chicago: University of Chicago Press, 1935.

Campione, J., Hyman, L. and Zeaman, D. 'Dimensional shifts and reversals in retardate discrimination learning', *J. Exp. Child Psychol.*, 1965, **2**, pp. 255–263.

Cantor, G. N. 'Effects of three types of pretraining on discrimination learning in preschool children', *J. Exp. Psychol.*, 1955, **49**, pp. 339–342.

Cantor, J. H. 'Transfer of stimulus pretraining to motor paired-associate and discrimination learning tasks'. In: L. P. Lipsitt and C. C. Spiker (eds) *Advances in child development and behavior*, Vol. 2. New York, London: Academic Press, 1965, pp. 19–58.

Capaldi, E. J. and Stevenson, H. W. 'Response reversal following different amounts of training', *J. Comp. Physiol. Psychol.*, 1957, **50**, pp. 195–198.

Chase, W. P. 'Color vision in infants', *J. Exp. Psychol.*, 1937, **20**, pp. 203–222.

Chow, K. L., Riesen, A. H. and Newell, F. W. 'Degeneration of retinal ganglion cells in infant chimpanzees reared in darkness', *J. Comp. Neurol.*, 1957, **107**, pp. 27–42.

Claparède, E. 'Exemple de perception syncrétique chez un enfant', *Arch. de Psychol.* (Geneva), 1907, **7**, pp. 195–198.

Claparède, E. *Psychologie de l'enfant et pédagogie expérimentale*, Geneva: Kundig, 1909.

Claparède, E. 'La conscience de la ressemblance et de la différence chez l'enfant', *Arch de Psychol.* (Geneva), 1918, **17**, p. 67.

Claparède, E. 'Sur la perception syncrétique', *L'Éducateur*, 1925, p. 42.

Claparède, E. 'A propos d'un cas de perception syncrétique', *Arch. de Psychol.* (Geneva), 1938, **26**, pp. 367–377.

Colby, M. C. and Robertson, J. B. 'Genetic studies in abstraction', *J. Comp. Psychol.*, 1942, **33**, pp. 385–401.

Compayré. Preface to: J. Sully, *Études sur l'enfance*, Paris: F. Alcan, 1898.

Cook, F. M. 'Ability of children in color discriminations', *Child Dev.*, 1931, **2**, pp. 303–320.

Corah, N. L. 'Color and form in children's perceptual behavior', *Percept. Mot. Skills*, 1964, **18**, pp. 313–316.

Corah, N. L. 'The influence of some stimulus characteristics on color and form perception in nursery-school children', *Child Dev.*, 1966a, **37**, pp. 205–211.

Corah, N. L. 'The effect of instruction and performance set on color-form perception in young children', *J. Genet. Psychol.*, 1966b, **108**, pp. 351–356.

Corah, N. L. and Gospodinoff, E. J. 'Color-form and whole-part perception in children', *Child Dev.*, 1966, **37**, 837–842.

Corah, N. L. and Gross, J. B. 'Hue, brightness, and saturation variables in color-form matching', *Child Dev.*, 1967, **38**, pp. 137–142.

Cramaussel, E. *Le premier eveil intellectuel de l'enfant*, Paris: Alcan, 1909.

Cramaussel, E. 'Ce que voient des yeux d'enfant', *J. Psychol. Norm. Pathol.*, 1924, **21**, pp. 161–169.

Cramaussel, E. 'Expériences au jardin d'enfants', *J. Psychol. Norm. Pathol.*, 1927, **24**, pp. 701–718.

Cruikshank, R. M. 'The development of visual size constancy in early infancy', *J. Genet. Psychol.*, 1941, **58**, pp. 327–351.

Davidson, H. P. 'A study of reversals in young children', *J. Genet. Psychol.*, 1934, **45**, pp. 452–465.

Davidson, H. P. 'A study of the confusing letters *b, d, p* and *q*', *J. Genet. Psychol.*, 1935, **47**, pp. 458–468.

Debot-Sevrin, M. R. *Étude du sens du regard*, Liège: Vaillant-Carmane, 1962.

Decroly, O. *La fonction de globalisation et l'enseignement*, Brussels, 1929.

Demoor, J. and Jonckheere, T. *La science de l'éducation*, Brussels, Paris: M. Lamertin, F. Alcan, 1920.

Denis-Prinzhorn, M. 'Perception des distances et constance des grandeurs (étude génétique)', *Arch. de Psychol.* (Geneva), 1960, **37**, pp. 181–309.

Denner, B. and Cashdan, J. 'Sensory processing and the recognition of forms in nursery-school children', *Brit. J. Psychol.*, 1967, **58**, pp. 101–104.

Descoeudres, A. 'Couleur, forme ou nombre?', *Arch. de Psychol.* (Geneva), 1914, **14**, pp. 305–341.

Dickerson, D. J. 'Performance of preschool children on three discrimination shifts', *Psychon. Sci.*, 1966, **4**, pp. 417–418.

Djang, S. S. 'The role of past experience in the visual apprehension of masked forms', *J. Exp. Psychol.*, 1937, **20**, pp. 29–59.

Dreyfus-Brisac, C. and Blanc, C. 'Electroencéphalogramme et maturation cérébrale', *L'Encéphale*, 1956, **45**, pp. 205–241.

Dreyfus-Brisac, C. and Blanc, C. 'Aspects E.E.G. de la maturation cérébrale pendant la première année de la vie', *E.E.G. Clin. Neurophysiol.*, 1957, Suppl. No. 6, pp. 432–440.

Dworetzki, G. 'Le test de Rorschach et l'évolution de la perception. Étude expérimentale', *Arch. de Psychol.* (Geneva), 1939, **27**, pp. 233–396.

Eimas, P. D. 'Comment: comparisons of reversal and nonreversal shifts', *Psychon. Sci.*, 1965, **3**, pp. 445–446.

Elkind, D. 'Ambiguous pictures for study of perceptual development and learning', *Child. Dev.*, 1964, **35**, pp. 1391–1396.

Elkind, D., Koegler, R. R. and Go, E. 'Effects of perceptual training at three age levels', *Science*, 1962, **137**, pp. 755–756.

Elkind, D., Koegler, R. R. and Go, E. 'Studies in perceptual development: II. Part-whole perception', *Child Dev.*, 1964, **35**, pp. 81–90.

Elkind, D., Koegler, R. R., Go, E. and Van Doorninck, W. 'Effects of perceptual training on unmatched samples of brain-injured and familial retarded children', *J. Abnorm. Psychol.*, 1965, **70**, pp. 107–110.

Elkind, D. and Scott, L. 'Studies in perceptual development: I. The decentering of perception', *Child Dev.*, 1962, **33**, pp. 619–630.

Elkind, D. and Weiss, J. 'Studies in perceptual development: III. Perceptual exploration', *Child Dev.*, 1967, **38**, pp. 553–561.

Enoch, J. M. and Fry, G. A. *Opthalmographic studies of search*. Unpublished manuscript, 1957, reported in Mackworth and Bruner, 1966.

Fantz, R. L. 'Pattern vision in young infants', *Psychol. Rec.*, 1958, **58**, pp. 43–47.

Fantz. R. L. 'The origin of form perception', *Scientific American*, 1961, **204**, pp. 66–72.

Fantz, R. L. 'Pattern vision in newborn infants', *Science*, 1963, **140**, pp. 296–297.

Fantz, R. L. 'Visual perception from birth as shown by pattern selectivity'. In: H. E. Whipple (ed.) 'New issues in child development', *Ann. N.Y. Acad. Sci.*, 1965a, **118**, pp. 793–814.

Fantz, R. L. 'Ontogeny of perception'. In: A. M. Schrier, H. F. Harlow and F. Stollnitz (eds) *Behavior of non-human primates*, Vol. II., New York, London: Academic Press, 1965b, pp. 365–403.

Fantz, R. L. 'Pattern discrimination and selective attention as determinants of perceptual development from birth'. In: A. H. Kidd and J. L. Rivoire (eds) *Perceptual development in children*, New York: International Universities Press, 1966, pp. 143–173.

Fantz, R. L. 'Visual perception and experience in early infancy: a look at the hidden side of behavior development'. In: H. W. Stevenson, E. H. Hess and H. L. Rheingold (eds), *Early behavior. Comparative and developmental approaches*, New York, London, Sydney: John Wiley and Sons, 1967, pp. 181–224.

Fantz, R. L. and Ordy, J. M. 'A visual acuity test for infants under six months of age', *Psychol. Rec.*, 1959, **9**, pp. 159–164.

Fantz, R. L., Ordy, J. M. and Udelf, M. S. 'Maturation of pattern vision in infants during the first six months', *J. Comp. Physiol. Psychol.*, 1962, **55**, pp. 907–917.

Fellows, B. J. *A theoretical and experimental analysis of visual discrimination performance*. Unpublished doctoral thesis, University of Bristol, 1965.

Fellows, B. J. *The discrimination process and development*, London: Pergamon Press, 1968.

Fraisse, P. 'De quelques comportements dits "spontanés"', *Enfance*, 1968, pp. 161–181.

Fraisse, P. and Vurpillot, E. 'Effet de l'orientation de l'attention sur l'étendue du champ d'appréhension', *Année Psychol.*, 1956, **56**, pp. 433–436.

Fraisse, P., Ehrlich, S. and Vurpillot, E. 'Études de la centration perceptive par la méthode tachistoscopique', *Arch. de Psychol.* (Geneva), 1956, **35**, pp. 193–214.

Francès, R. 'L'apprentissage de la ségrégation perceptive', *Psychol. Franç.*, 1963, **8**, pp. 16–27.

Furth, H. G. and Youniss, J. 'Effect of overtraining on three discrimination shifts in children', *J. Comp. Physiol. Psychol.*, 1964, **57**, pp. 290–293.

Gaines, R. 'Color-form preferences and color-form discriminative ability of deaf and hearing children', *Percept. Mot. Skills*, 1964, **18**, p. 70.

Galifret-Granjon, N. 'L'élaboration spatiale au cours du développement d'après Henri Wallon', *Education Nouvelle*, Special Edition, 1964, pp. 39–46.

Gassel, M. M. and Williams, D. 'Visual function in patients with homonymous hemianopsia: II. Oculo-motor mechanisms', *Brain*, 1963, **86**, pp. 1–36.

Gaydos, H. F. 'Intersensory transfer in the discrimination of form', *Amer. J. Psychol.*, 1956, **59**, pp. 107–110.

Gellermann, L. W. 'Form discrimination in chimpanzees and two-year-old children: I. Form (triangularity) *per se*', *J. Genet. Psychol.*, 1933, **42**, pp. 3–27.

Van Gennep, A. 'Dessins d'enfant et dessin préhistorique', *Arch. de Psychol.* (Geneva), 1911, **10**, pp. 327–337.

Gessell, A. and Amatruda, C. S. *Developmental diagnosis; normal and abnormal child development, clinical methods and pediatric applications*, New York: Paul B. Hoeber, 1947 (2nd edition).

Gesell, A., Thompson, H. and Amatruda, C. S. *Infant behavior. Its genesis and growth.* New York, London: McGraw Hill, 1934.

Ghent, L. 'Perception of overlapping and embedded figures by children of different ages', *Amer. J. Psychol.*, 1956a, **69**, pp. 575–587.

Ghent, L. 'The child's choice of "upsidedownness"; description of a new phenomenon', *Paper presented to the Eastern Psychological Association*, Atlantic City, 1956b.

Ghent, L. 'Recognition of pictures in various orientations by children of different ages', *Paper presented to the Eastern Psychological Association*, New York, 1957.

Ghent, L. 'Recognition by children of realistic figures presented in various orientations', *Canad. J. Psychol.*, 1960, **14**, pp. 249–256.

Ghent, L. 'Form and its orientation: a child's-eye view', *Amer. J. Psychol.*, 1961, **74**, pp. 177–190.

Ghent, L. 'Stimulus orientation as a factor in the recognition of geometric forms by school-age children', *Paper presented to the Eastern Psychological Association*, 1963.

Ghent, L. 'Effect of orientation on recognition of geometric forms by retarded children', *Child Dev.*, 1964, **35**, pp. 1127–1136.

Ghent, L. and Bernstein, I. 'Influence of the orientation of geometric forms on their recognition by children', *Percept. Mot. Skills*, 1961, **12**, pp. 95–101.

Ghent, L., Bernstein, L. and Goldweber, A. M. 'Preferences for orientation of form under varying conditions.' *Percept. Mot. Skills*, 1960, **11**, p. 46.

Gibson, E. J. 'Perceptual development', In: H. W. Stevenson, J. Kagan and C. Spiker (eds) *Child psychology*. The Sixty-second Yearbook of the National Society for the Study of Education. Chicago: The University of Chicago Press, 1963, pp. 144–195.

Gibson, E. J. 'Learning to read', *Science*, 1965, **148**, pp. 1066–1072.

Gibson, E. J. *Principles of perceptual learning and development*, New York: Appleton-Century-Crofts, 1969.

Gibson, E. J., Gibson, J. J., Pick, A. D. and Osser, H. 'A developmental study of the discrimination of letter-like forms', *J. Comp. Physiol. Psychol.*, 1962, **55**, pp. 897–906.

Gibson, E. J. and Yonas, A. 'A developmental study of visual search behavior', *Percept. Psychophys.*, 1966, **1**, pp. 169–171.

Gibson, J. J. *The perception of the visual world*, Boston: Houghton Mifflin Company, 1950.

Gibson, J. J. 'Perception as a function of stimulation'. In: S. Koch (ed.) *Psychology: a study of a science*, Vol. I, New York, Toronto, London: McGraw Hill Book Co. Inc., 1959, pp. 456–501.

Gibson, J. J. 'The concept of the stimulus in psychology', *Amer. Psychologist*, 1960, **15**, pp. 694–703.

Gibson, J. J. 'The useful dimensions of sensitivity', *Amer. Psychologist*, 1963, **18**, pp. 1–15.

Gibson, J. J. *The senses considered as perceptual systems*, Boston: Houghton Mifflin Company, 1966.

Gibson, J. J. and Gibson, E. J. 'Perceptual learning: differentiation or enrichment?', *Psychol. Rev.*, 1955, **62**, pp. 32–41.

Ginevskaya, T. O. 'Development of hand movements in touch', *Izvestia Akademii Pedagogicheskikh Nauk U.S.S.R.*, 1948, vypusk 14 (quoted in Zaporozhets and Zinchenko, 1966).

Gollin, E. S. 'Developmental studies of visual recognition of incomplete objects', *Percept. Mot. Skills*, 1960, **11**, pp. 289–298.

Gollin, E. S. 'Tactual form discrimination: developmental differences in the effects of training under conditions of spatial interference', *J. Psychol.*, 1961, **51**, pp. 131–140.

Gollin, E. S. 'Factors affecting the visual recognition of incomplete objects: a comparative investigation of children and adults', *Percept. Mot. Skills*, 1962, **15**, pp. 583–590.

Gollin, E. S. 'Perceptual learning of incomplete pictures', *Percept. Mot. Skills*, 1965, **21**, pp. 439–445.

Gollin, E. S. 'Serial learning and perceptual recognition in children: training, delay, and order effects', *Percept. Mot. Skills*, 1966, **23**, 751–158.

Gollin, E. S. 'Word labels and perceptual recognition', *Psychon. Sci.*, 1967, **7**, pp. 63–64.

Goodwin, W. R. and Lawrence, D. H. 'The functional independence of two discrimination habits associated with a constant stimulus situation', *J. Comp. Physiol. Psychol.*, 1955, **48**, pp. 437–443.

Gorman, J. J., Cogan, D. G. and Gellis, S. S. 'An apparatus for grading the visual acuity of infants on the basis of optokinetic nystagmus', *Pediatrics*, 1957, **19**, pp. 1088–1092.

Gorman, J. J., Cogan, D. G. and Gellis, S. S. 'A device for testing visual acuity in infants', *Sight Saving Rev.*, 1959, **29**, pp. 80–84.

Gotteschaldt, K. 'Ueber den Einfluss der Erfahrung auf die Wahrnehmung von Figuren: I. Ueber den Einfluss gehäufter Einprägung von Figuren auf ihre Sichtbarkeit in umfassenden Konfigurationen', *Psychol. Forsch.*, 1926, **8**, pp. 261–317. English translation in: W. D. Ellis (ed.) *A source book of gestalt psychology*, London: Routledge and Kegan Paul, 1950, pp. 109–122.

Gottshalk, J., Bryden, M. P. and Rabinovitch, S. 'Spatial organisation of children's responses to a pictorial display', *Child Dev.*, 1964, **35**, pp. 811–815.

Gouin-Décarie, Th. *Intelligence et affectivité chez le jeune enfant*, Paris, Neuchâtel: Delachaux & Niestlé, 1962.

Gould, J. D. and Schaffer, A. 'Eye-movement patterns during visual information processing', *Psychon. Sci.*, 1965, **3**, pp. 317–318.

Graham, C. H. 'Area, color and brightness difference in a reversible configuration', *J. Gen. Psychol.*, 1929, **2**, pp. 470–483.

Guignot, E., Macé, H., Savigny, M. and Vurpillot, E. 'Influence de la consigne sur une mesure de constance de forme', *Bull. de Psychol.*, 1963, **16**, pp. 619–629.

Guilford, J. P. and Hunt, J. M. 'Some further experimental tests of McDougall's theory of introversion-extraversion', *J. Abn. Soc. Psychol.*, 1931, **26**, pp. 324–332.

Guillaume, P. *La psychologie de la forme*, Paris: Flammarion, 1937.

Hanawalt, N. G. 'The effect of practice upon the perception of simple designs masked by more complex designs', *J. Exp. Psychol.*, 1942, **31**, pp. 134–148.

Harrow, M. and Friedman, G. B. 'Comparing reversal and non-reversal shifts in concept formation with partial reinforcement controlled', *J. Exp. Psychol.*, 1958, **55**, pp. 592–598.

Harway, N. I. 'The judgment of distance in children and adults', *J. Exp. Psychol.*, 1963, **65**, pp. 385–390.

Hebb, D. O. *The organization of behavior*, New York: John Wiley and Sons, 1949.

Hecaen, H. and Ajuriaguerra, J. de *Les gauchers. Prévalence manuelle et dominance cérébrale*, Paris: Presses Universitaires de France, 1963.

Heckenmueller, E. G. 'Stabilization of the retinal image: a review of method, effects, and theory', *Psychol. Bull.*, 1965, **63**, pp. 157–169.

Heilbronner, K. 'Zur klinisch-psychologischen Untersuchungstechnik', *Mschr. Psychiat. Neurol.*, 1905, **17**, pp. 115–132.

Helson, H. 'The psychology of Gestalt', *Amer. J. Psychol.*, 1926, **37**, pp. 25–62.

Hermelin, B. and O'Connor, N. 'Recognition of shapes by normal and subnormal children', *Brit. J. Psychol.*, 1961, **52**, pp. 281–284.

Hermelin, B. and O'Connor, N. 'Effects of sensory input and sensory dominance on severely disturbed, autistic children and on subnormal controls', *Brit. J. Psychol.*, 1964, **55**, pp. 201–206.

Hershenson, M. 'Visual discrimination in the human newborn', *J. Comp. Physiol. Psychol.*, 1964, **58**, pp. 270–276.

Hertz, M. 'Wahrnehmungspsychologische Untersuchungen am Eichelhäher', *Z. Vergl. Physiol.*, 1928, **7**, pp. 144–194.

Hill, M. B. 'A study of the process of word discrimination in individuals beginning to read', *J. Educ. Res.*, 1936, **29**, pp. 487–500.

Hochberg, J. E. 'Figure-ground reversal as a function of visual satiation', *J. Exp. Psychol.*, 1950, **40**, pp. 682–686.

Honkavaara, S. 'A critical reevaluation of the color and form reaction, and disproving of the hypotheses connected with it', *J. Psychol.*, 1958, **45**, pp. 25–36.

Hooker, D. 'Early fetal activity in mammals', *Yale. J. Biol. Med.*, 1936, **8**, pp. 579–602.

Hooker, D. 'Early human fetal behavior, with a preliminary note on double simultaneous fetal stimulation', *Res. Publ. Ass. Nerv. Ment. Dis.*, 1954, **33**, pp. 98–113.

Horn, G. 'Physiological and psychological aspects of selective attention'. In: D. S. Lehrman, R. A. Hinde and E. Shaw (eds) *Advances in the study of behavior*, Vol. I. New York, London: Academic Press, 1965, pp. 155–215.

House, B. J. and Zeaman, D. 'A comparison of discrimination learning in normal and mentally defective children', *Child Dev.*, 1958, **29**, pp. 411–416.

House, B. J. and Zeaman, D. 'Visual discrimination, learning and intelligence in defectives of low mental age', *Amer. J. Ment. Defic.*, 1960, **65**, pp. 51–58.

Hubel, D. H. and Wiesel, T. N. 'Receptive fields of single neurones in the cat's striate cortex', *J. Physiol.*, 1959, **148**, pp. 574–591.

Hubel, D. H. and Wiesel, T. N. 'Receptive fields, binocular interaction and functional architecture in the cat's visual cortex', *J. Physiol.*, 1962, **160**, pp. 106–154.

Hubel, D. H. and Wiesel. T. N. 'Receptive fields of cells in striate cortex of very young, visually inexperienced kittens', *J. Neurophysiol.*, 1963, **26**, pp. 994–1002.

Hubel, D. H. and Wiesel, T. N. 'Receptive fields and functional architecture in two nonstriate visual areas (18 and 19) of the cat', *J. Neurophysiol.*, 1965, **28**, pp. 229–289.

Hubel, D. H. and Wiesel, T. N. 'Receptive fields and functional architecture of monkey striate cortex', *J. Physiol.*, 1968, pp. 195, 215–243.

Hull, C. L. 'Knowledge and purpose as habit mechanisms', *Psychol. Rev.*, 1930, **37**, pp. 511–525.

Hull, C. L. 'The problem of stimulus equivalence in behavior theory', *Psychol. Rev.*, 1939, **46**, pp. 9–30.

Hull, C. L. *Principles of behavior*, New York: Appleton Century Crofts, 1943.

Huttenlocher, J. 'Children's ability to order and orient objects', *Child Dev.*, 1967a, **38**, pp. 1196–1176.

Huttenlocher, J. 'Discrimination of figure orientation: effects of relative position', *J. Comp. Physiol. Psychol.*, 1967b, **63**, pp. 359–361.

Jakobson, R. and Halle, M. *Fundamentals of language,* The Hague: Mouton & Co., 1956.

James, W. *The principles of psychology*, New York: Henry Holt, 1890.

Janet, P. *L'automatisme psychologique. Essai de psychologie expérimentale sur les formes inférieures de l'activité humaine*, Paris: Félix Alcan, 1889.

Jenkin, N. and Feallock, S. M. 'Developmental and intellectual processes in size-distance judgment', *Amer. J. Psychol.*, 1960, **73**, pp. 268–273.

Johannsen, D. E. 'Black-white relation of figure and ground in nursery school children's figure perception', *Percept. Mot. Skills*, 1960, **10**, pp. 23–26.

Johnson, M. S. 'Factors related to disability in reading', *J. Exp. Educ.*, 1957, **26**, pp. 1–26.

Jonckheere, T. 'Notes sur la psychologie des enfants arriérés', *Arch. de Psychol.* (Geneva), 1903, **2**, pp. 253–268.

Jonckheere, T. 'Mémoire visuelle remarquable chez un enfant', *Arch. de Psychol.* (Geneva) 1908, pp. 84–85.

Jonckheere, T. *La pédagogie expérimentale au jardin d'enfants*, Brussels: Maurice Lamertin, 1921 (5th ed, 1949).

Kagan, J. and Lemkin, J. 'Form, color, and size in children's conceptual behavior', *Child Dev.*, 1961, **32**, pp. 25–28.

Kagan, J. and Lewis, M. 'Studies of attention in the human infant', *Merrill-Palmer Quart.*, 1965, **11**, pp. 95–127.

Katz, D. 'Studien zur Kinderpsychologie', *Wiss. Beitr. Pädag. u. Psychol.*, 1913, p. 4.

Katz, P. A. 'Effects of labels on children's perception and discrimination learning', *J. Exp. Psychol.*, 1963, **66**, pp. 423–428.

Kelleher, R. T. 'Discrimination learning as a function of reversal and non-reversal shifts', *J. Exp. Psychol.*, 1956, **51**, pp. 379–384.

Kendler, H. H. and d'Amato, M. F. 'A comparison of reversal shifts and non-reversal shifts in human concept formation behavior', *J. Exp. Psychol.*, 1955, **49**, pp. 165–174.

Kendler, H. H. and Kendler, T. S. 'Effect of verbalization on reversal shifts in children', *Science*, 1961, **134**, pp. 1619–1620.

Kendler, H. H. and Kendler, T. S. 'Vertical and horizontal processes in problem solving', *Psychol. Rev.*, 1962, **69**, pp. 1–16.

Kendler, H. H. and Kendler, T. S. 'Selective attention versus mediation: some comments on Mackintosh's analysis of two-stage models of discrimination learning', *Psychol. Bull.*, 1966, **66**, pp. 282–288.

Kendler, H. H. and Kendler, T. S. 'Mediation and conceptual behavior'. In: K. W. Spence and J. T. Spence (eds) *The psychology of learning and motivation*, Vol. 2, New York: Academic Press, 1968, pp. 197–244.

Kendler, H. H. and Kendler, T. S. 'Discrimination learning in children: some significant issues', *Paper presented to the 19th International Congress of Psychology*, London, 1969.

Kendler, T. S. 'Development of mediating responses in children'. In: J. C. Wright and J. Kagan (eds) 'Basic cognitive processes in children', *Monogr. Soc. Res. Child Dev.*, 1963, **28**, Monogr. 86, pp. 33–48.

Kendler, T. S. 'Verbalization and optional reversal shifts among kindergarten children', *J. Verb. Learn. Verb. Behav.*, 1964, **3**, pp. 428–436.

Kendler, T. S., Basden, B. and Bruckner, J. 'Dimensional dominance and continuity theory', *J. Exp. Psychol.*, 1970, **83**, pp. 309–318.

Kendler, T. S. and Kendler, H. H. 'Reversal and non-reversal shifts in kindergarten children', *J. Exp. Psychol.*, 1959, **58**, pp. 56–60.

Kendler, T. S., Kendler, H. H. and Learnard, B. 'Mediated responses to size and brightness as a function of age', *Amer. J. Psychol.*, 1962, **75**, pp. 571–586.

Kendler, T. S., Kendler, H. H. and Silfen, C. K. 'Optional shift behavior of albino rats', *Psychon. Sci.*, 1964, **1**, pp. 5–6.

Kendler, T. S., Kendler, H. H. and Wells, D. 'Reversal and non-reversal shifts in nursery school children', *J. Comp. Physiol. Psychol.*, 1960, **53**, pp. 83–88.

Kessen, W. 'Sucking and looking: two organized congenital patterns of behavior in the human newborn'. In: H. W. Stevenson, E. H. Hess and H. L. Rheingold (eds) *Early behavior. Comparative and developmental approaches*, New York: John Wiley and Sons, 1967, pp. 147–179.

Kessen, W., Salapatek, P. and Haith, M. M. 'The ocular orientation of newborn human infants to visual contours'. *Paper presented to the Psychonomic Society*, Chicago, 1965.

Klimpfinger, S. 'Die Entwicklung der Gestaltkonstanz vom Kind zum Erwachsenen', *Arch. ges. Psychol.*, 1933, **88**, pp. 599–628.

Koffka, K. *Principles of gestalt psychology*, London: Routledge and Kegan Paul, 1935.

Köhler, W. *Dynamics in psychology*, New York: Liveright Publishing Corporation, 1940.

Köhler, W. and Fishback, J. 'The destruction of the Müller-Lyer illusion in repeated trials: I. An examination of two theories', *J. Exp. Psychol.*, 1950a, **40**, pp. 267–281.

Köhler, W. and Fishback, J. 'The destruction of the Müller-Lyer illusion in repeated trials: II. Satiation patterns and memory traces', *J. Exp. Psychol.*, 1950b, **40**, pp. 398–410.

Köhler, W. and Wallach, H. 'Figural after-effects. An investigation of visual processes', *Proc. Amer. Phil. Soc.*, 1944, **88**, pp. 269–357.

Komaki, J. 'The facilitative effect of overlearning in discrimination learning by white rats', *Psychologia*, 1961, **4**, pp. 28–35.

Krechevsky, I. ' "Hypotheses" in rats', *Psychol. Rev.*, 1932, **39**, pp. 516–532.

Kretshmar, J. 'Kinder Kunst und Urzeitkunst', *Z. Pädag. Psychol.*, 1910, **11**, p. 354.

Kuenne, M. R. 'Experimental investigation of the relation of language to transposition behaviour in young children', *J. Exp. Psychol.*, 1946, **36**, 471–490.

Kurtz, K. H. 'Discrimination of complex stimuli: the relationship of training and test stimuli in transfer of discrimination', *J. Exp. Psychol.*, 1955, **50**, pp. 283–292.

Lambercier, M. 'Recherches sur le développement des perceptions: VI. La constance des grandeurs en comparaisons sériales', *Arch. de Psychol.* (Geneva), 1946a, **31**, pp. 1–204.

Lambercier, M. 'Recherches sur le développement des perceptions: VII.

La configuration en profondeur dans la constance des grandeurs',
*Arch. de Psychol.* (Geneva), 1946b, **31**, pp. 287–323.

Lamprecht, K. 'De l'étude comparée des dessins d'enfants', *Rev. de
Synthèse Historique*, 1905, **11**, p. 54.

Lamprecht, K. 'Les dessins d'enfant comme source historique', *Acad.
Roy. de Belgique, Bull. de la Cl. des Lettres et de la Cl. des Beaux-
Arts*, 1906, pp. 457 et seq.

Lamprecht, K. 'Einführung in die Ausstellung von parallelen Entwick-
lungen in der bildenden Kunst', *Kongr. f. Aesth. u. allg. Kunstwiss.*,
Stuttgart, 1914, p. 75.

Lang, A. 'Perceptual behavior of 8- to 10-week-old human infants',
*Psychon. Sci.*, 1966, **4**, pp. 203–204.

Lashley, K. S. *Brain mechanisms and intelligence, A quantitative study
of injuries to the brain*, Chicago: University of Chicago Press, 1929.

Lashley, K. S. 'The mechanism of vision: XV. Preliminary studies of the
rat's capacity for detail vision', *J. Gen. Psychol.*, 1938, **18**, pp. 123–193.

Lashley, K. S. 'An examination of the "continuity theory" as applied to
discriminative learning', *J. Gen. Psychol.*, 1942, **26**, pp. 241–265.

Lavrent'Eva, T. V. and Ruzskaya, A. G. 'Sravnitel'nyi Analiz osyazaniya
i zreniya. Soobschenie: Odnovremennoe intersensornoe sopostavlenie
formy v doshkol' nom vozraste (Comparative analysis of touch and
vision: V. Simultaneous intersensory comparison of forms in preschool age children)', *Dokl. Acad. Ped. Nauk. U.S.S.R.*, 1960, 4(4),
pp. 73–76.

Lawrence, D. H. 'Acquired distinctiveness of cues: I. Transfer between
discriminations on the basis of familiarity with the stimulus', *J. Exp.
Psychol.*, 1949, **39**, pp. 770–784.

Lawrence, D. H. 'Acquired distinctiveness of cues: II. Selective association in a constant stimulus situation', *J. Exp. Psychol.*, 1950, **40**,
pp. 175–188.

Lawrence, D. H. 'The nature of a stimulus: some relationships between
learning and perception'. In: S. Koch (ed.) *Psychology: a study of a
science*, New York, San Francisco, Toronto, London: McGraw-Hill,
1963, vol. 5, pp. 179–212.

Lécuyer, R. 'Effet de singularisation, exploration oculo-motrice et
critère d'identité chez l'enfant', *Mémoire de psychologie expérimentale* (Master's thesis), Paris, Sorbonne, 1969.

Leeper, R. W. 'A study of a neglected portion of the field of learning:
the development of sensory organisation', *J. Genet. Psychol.*, 1935,
**46**, pp. 41–75.

Leibowitz, L. and Menghini, K. 'Shape perception for round and
elliptically shaped test-objects', *J. Exp. Psychol.*, 1966, **72**, pp. 244–249.

Leontiev, A. N. and Gippenreiter, Y. B. 'Concerning the activity of
man's visual system' (trans. from the Russian). In: *Psychological
research in the U.S.S.R.*, Moscow: Progress Publishers, 1966, pp. 361–
392.

Lépine, D. 'La réponse "pareil" chez l'enfant: identité ou équivalence?',
*Année Psychol.*, 1965, **65**, pp. 57–76.

Lépine, D. 'Critères de la réponse d'identité chez l'enfant', *Année Psychol.*, 1966, **66**, pp. 417–446.

Lesèvre, N. *Les mouvements oculaires d'exploration: étude electro-oculographique comparée d'enfants normaux et d'enfants dyslexiques.* Doctoral thesis in psychology (third stage), duplicated format, Paris, 1964.

Lesèvre, N. 'L'organisation du regard chez les enfants d'âge scolaire, lecteurs normaux et dyslexiques (étude électro-oculographique)', *Rev. Neuropsychiat. Infantile*, 1968, **16**, pp. 323–349.

Levine, M. 'Hypothesis behavior by humans during discrimination learning', *J. Exp. Psychol.*, 1966, **71**, pp. 331–338.

Lévy-Bruhl, L. *Les fonctions mentales dans les societés inférieures*, Paris: Alcan, 1910.

Lévy-Schoen, A. 'Détermination et latence de la réponse oculo-motrice à deux stimulus simultanés ou successifs selon leur excentricité relative', *Année Psychol.*, 1969, **69**, pp. 373–392.

Lewis, M., Bartels, B., Fadel, D. and Campbell, H. 'Infant attention: the effect of familiar and novel stimuli as a function of age', *Paper presented to the Eastern Psychological Association*, New York, 1966.

Lipsitt, L. P. 'Learning in the human infant'. In: H. L. Stevenson, E. H. Hess and H. L. Rheingold (eds), *Early behavior. Comparative and developmental approaches*, New York, London, Sydney: John Wiley and Sons, 1967, pp. 225–247.

Lovell, K. 'A follow-up study of some aspects of the work of Piaget and Inhelder on the child's conception of space', *Brit. J. Educ. Psychol.*, 1959, **29**, pp. 104–117.

Luquet, G. H. *Les dessins d'un enfant*, Paris: Félix Alcan, 1913.

Luquet, G. H. *Le dessin enfantin*, Neuchâtel, Paris: Delachaux & Niestlé, 1967 (1st edition, 1927a).

Luquet, G. H. 'Le réalisme intellectuel dans l'art primitif', *J. Psychol. Norm. Pathol.*, 1927b, **24**, pp. 765–797; 888–927.

Lurçat, L. 'Étude des facteurs kinesthétiques dans les premiers tracés enfantins', *Psychol. Franç.*, 1962, **7**, pp. 301–311.

Luria, A. R. 'The role of language in the formation of temporary connections'. In: B. Simon (ed.), *Psychology in the Soviet Union*, Stanford, California: Stanford University Press, 1957, pp. 115–129.

MacCaslin, E. F., Wodinsky, J. and Bitterman, M. E. 'Stimulus-generalization as a function of prior training', *Amer. J. Psychol.*, 1952, **65**, pp. 1–15.

Mackintosh, N. J. 'The effects of overtraining on a reversal and a non-reversal shift', *J. Comp. Physiol. Psychol.*, 1962, **55**, pp. 555–559.

Mackintosh, N. J. 'The effect of irrelevant cues on reversal learning in the rat', *Brit. J. Psychol.*, 1963a, **54**, pp. 127–134.

Mackintosh, N. J. 'Extinction of a discrimination habit as a function of overtraining', *J. Comp. Physiol. Psychol.*, 1963b, **56**, pp. 842–847.

Mackintosh, N. J. 'Overtraining and transfer within and between dimensions in the rat', *Quart. J. Exp. Psychol.*, 1964, **16**, pp. 250–256.

Mackintosh, N. J. 'Incidental cue learning in rats', *Quart. J. Exp. Psychol.*, 1965a, **17**, pp. 292–300.

Mackintosh, N. J. 'Selective attention in animal discrimination learning', *Psychol. Bull.*, 1965b, **64**, pp. 124–150.

Mackintosh, N. J. 'The effect of attention on the slope of generalization gradients', *Brit. J. Psychol.*, 1965c, **56**, pp. 87–93.

Mackworth, N. H. 'Visual noise causes tunnel vision', *Psychon. Sci.*, 1965, **3**, pp. 67–68.

Mackworth, N. H. and Bruner, J. S. *Selecting visual information during recognition by adults and children.* Duplicated format, Harvard Center for Cognitive Studies, 1966.

Mackworth, N. H. and Morandi, A. J. 'The gaze selects informative details within pictures', *Percept. Psychophys.*, 1967, **2**, pp. 547–552.

Mandes, E. J. and Ghent, L. 'The effect of stimulus orientations on the recognition of geometric forms in adults', *Paper presented to the American Psychological Association*, Philadelphia, 1963.

Marsh, G. 'Effect of overtraining on reversal and nonreversal shifts in nursery school children', *Child Dev.*, 1964, **35**, pp. 1367–1372.

Meili, R. 'Les perceptions des enfants et la psychologie de la Gestalt', *Arch. de Psychol.* (Geneva), 1931, **23**, pp. 25–44.

Meneghini, K. A. and Leibowitz, H. W. 'Effect of stimulus distance and age on shape constancy', *J. Exp. Psychol.*, 1967, **74**, pp. 241–248.

Michotte, A. *La perception de la causalité*, Louvain: Publications Universitaires, 1946.

Miller, G. A. 'The magical number seven, plus or minus two: some limits on our capacity for processing information', *Psychol. Rev.*, 1956, **63**, pp. 81–97.

Miller, G. A., Galanter, E. and Pribram, K. H. *Plans and the structure of behavior*, New York: Holt, Rinehart and Winston, 1960.

Miller, N. E. 'Theory and experiment relating psychoanalytic displacement to stimulus-response generalization', *J. Abnorm. Soc. Psychol.*, 1948, **43**, pp. 155–178.

Miller, N. E. and Dollard, J. C. *Social learning and imitation*, New Haven: Yale University Press, 1941.

Miller, S. and Konorski, J. 'Sur une forme particulière des réflexes conditionnels', *C. R. Soc. Biol.*, 1928, **99**, pp. 1155–1157.

Milner, E. *Human neural and behavioral development*, Springfield, Ill.: Charles C. Thomas, 1967.

Moal, A. 'Évolution génétique des critères d'identité dans une tâche de différenciation perceptive', *Mémoire de psychologie experimentale* (Master's thesis), Paris, Sorbonne, 1969.

Monroe, M. 'Methods for diagnosis and treatment of cases of reading disability', *Genet. Psychol. Monog.*, 1928, **4**, pp. 333–456.

Mooney, C. M. 'A factorial study of closure', *Canad. J. Psychol.*, 1954, **8**, pp. 51–60.

Mooney, C. M. 'Age in the development of closure ability in children', *Canad. J. Psychol.*, 1957a, **11**, pp. 219–226.

Mooney, C. M. 'Closure as affected by viewing time and multiple visual fixations', *Canad. J. Psychol.*, 1957b, **11**, pp. 21–28.

Moses (Mme). 'Observation d'un timbre-poste de 5 centimes', *Bull. Soc. libre pour l'étude psychologique de l'enfance*, 1913, **31**, pp. 184–190.

Mouchly, R. Quoted by W. Köhler in: *Dynamics in psychology*, New York: Liveright Publishing Company, 1940.

Muller, G. E. 'Über das Aubertsche Phänomen', *Z. Psychol.*, 1916, **49**, pp. 109–244.

Mumbauer, C. C. and Odom, R. D. 'Variables affecting the performance of preschool children in intradimensional, reversal and extra-dimensional shifts', *J. Exp. Psychol.*, 1967, **75**, pp. 180–187.

Newson, E. *The development of line figure discrimination in preschool children.* Doctoral thesis: University of Nottingham, 1955.

Norcross, K. J. 'Effects of discrimination performance of similarity of previously acquired stimulus names', *J. Exp. Psychol.*, 1958, **56**, pp. 305–309.

Norcross, K. J. and Spiker, C. C. 'The effects of type of stimulus pre-training on discrimination performance in preschool children', *Child Dev.*, 1967, **28**, pp. 79–84.

Oetjen, F. 'Die Bedeutung der Orienterung des Lesestoffes für das Lesen und der Orienterung von sinnlosen Formen für das Wiedererkennen derselben', *Z. Psychol.*, 1915, **71**, pp. 321–355.

Ogden, R. M. 'Insight', *Amer. J. Psychol.*, 1932, **44**, pp. 350–356.

Oléron, P. 'Le développement des réponses à la relation identité-dis-semblance. Ses rapports avec le langage', *Psychol. Franç.*, 1962, **7**, pp. 4–16.

Oléron, P. 'Sur les effets assimilateurs et différenciateurs des étiquettes verbales', *J. Psychol. Norm. Pathol.*, 1967a, **64**, pp. 431–450.

Oléron, P. 'Sur la médiation verbale'. In: *Hommage à André Rey*, Brussels: C. Dessart, 1967b, pp. 151–176.

Oléron, P. and Gumusyan, S. 'Analyse perceptive et langage. Applica-tion d'une épreuve de Poppelreuter à des enfants sourds et entendants', *Psychol. Franç.*, 1964, **9**, pp. 47–96.

Olver, R. R. and Hornsby, J. R. 'On equivalence', In: J. S. Bruner, R. R. Olver and P. M. Greenfield (eds), *Studies in cognitive growth*, New York, London, Sydney: John Wiley and Sons, 1966, pp. 68–85.

Orton, S. T. *Reading, writing and speech problems in children*, London: Chapman and Hall, 1937; New York: Norton, 1937.

Osgood, C. E. *Method and theory in experimental psychology*, New York: Oxford University Press, 1953.

Over, R. 'Detection and recognition measures of shape discrimination', *Nature*, 1967, **214**, pp. 1272–1273.

Page, E. I. 'Haptic perception: a consideration of one of the investiga-tions of Piaget and Inhelder', *Educ. Rev.*, 1959, **11**, pp. 115–124.

Pavlov, I. P. *Les réflexes conditionnels. Étude objective de l'activité nerveuse supérieure des animaux.* Translated from the Russian. Paris: Félix Alcan, 1927.

Pêcheux, M. G. 'Etude génétique de la reproduction de figures geometriques simples isolées ou associées', *Personal communication*, 1969.

Pêcheux, M. G. and Stambak, M. 'Essai d'analyse de l'activité de reproduction de figures géométriques complexes', *Année Psychol.*, 1969, **69**, pp. 55–66.

Perkins, C. C., Hershberger, W. A. and Weyant, G. R. 'Difficulty of a discrimination as a determiner of subsequent generalization along another dimension', *J. Exp. Psychol.*, 1959, **57**, pp. 181–186.

Piaget, J. *Le langage et la pensée chez l'enfant*, Neuchâtel, Paris: Delachaux & Niestlé, 1923 (5th edition, 1962).

Piaget, J. *La naissance de l'intelligence chez l'enfant*, Neuchâtel, Paris: Delachaux & Niestlé, 1936 (4th edition, 1963).

Piaget, J. *La construction du réel chez l'enfant*, Neuchâtel, Paris: Delachaux & Niestlé, 1937 (3rd edition, 1963).

Piaget, J. 'Essai d'une nouvelle interprétation probabiliste des effets de centration, de la loi de Weber, et de celle des centrations relatives', *Arch. de Psychol.* (Geneva), 1955, **35**, pp. 1–24.

Piaget, J. *Les mécanismes perceptifs*, Paris: Presses Universitaires de France, 1961.

Piaget, J. 'Le développement des perceptions en fonction de l'âge', In: P. Fraisse and J. Piaget (eds), *Traité de psychologie expérimentale, Section VI: La Perception*, 1963 (2nd edition 1967), pp. 1–62.

Piaget, J. and Inhelder, B. *Le développement des quantités chez l'enfant (conservation et atomisme)*, Neuchâtel, Paris: Delachaux & Niestlé, 1941.

Piaget, J. and Inhelder, B. *La représentation de l'espace chez l'enfant*, Paris: Presses Universitaires de France, 1948.

Piaget, J. and Inhelder, B. *La genèse des structures logiques élémentaires (classification et sériations)*, Paris: Presses Universitaires de France, 1959.

Piaget, J. and Inhelder, B. *L'image mentale chez l'enfant*, Paris: Presses Universitaires de France, 1966.

Piaget, J. and Lambercier, M. 'Recherches sur le développement des perceptions: II. La comparaison visuelle des hauteurs à distances variables dans le plan fronto-parallèle'. *Arch. de Psychol.* (Geneva), 1943a, **29**, 173–253.

Piaget, J. and Lambercier, M. 'Recherches sur le développement des perceptions: III. Le problème de la comparaison visuelle en profondeur (constance de la grandeur) et l'erreur systématique de l'étalon', *Arch. de Psychol.* (Geneva), 1943b, **29**, pp. 253–308.

Piaget, J. and Lambercier, M. 'Recherches sur le développement des perceptions: XII. La comparaison des grandeurs projectives chez l'enfant et chez l'adulte', *Arch. de Psychol.* (Geneva), 1951, **33**, pp. 81–130.

Piaget, J. and Lambercier, M. 'Grandeurs projectives et grandeurs réelles avec étalon éloigné', *Arch. de Psychol.* (Geneva), 1956, **35**, pp. 257–280.

Piaget, J. and Morf, A. 'Note sur la comparaison de lignes perpendiculaires égales', *Arch. de Psychol.* (Geneva), 1956, **35**, pp. 233–255.

Piaget, J. and Morf, A. 'Les isomorphismes partiels entre les structures logiques et les structures perceptives', In: J. S. Bruner, F. Bresson, A. Morf and J. Piaget, *Logique et perception*, Paris: Presses Universitaires de France, 1958, pp. 49–116.

Piaget, J., Sinclair, H. and Vinh-Bang. *Epistémologie et psychologie de l'identité*, Paris: Presses Universitaires de France, 1968.

Piaget, J. and Stettler-von Albertini, B. 'Observations sur la perception des bonnes formes chez l'enfant par l'actualisation des lignes virtuelles', *Arch. de Psychol.* (Geneva), 1954, **34**, pp. 203–242.

Piaget, J. and Szeminska, A. *La genèse du nombre chez l'enfant*, Neuchâtel, Paris: Delachaux & Niestlé, 1941.

Piaget, J. and Voyat, G. 'Recherche sur l'identité d'un corps en développement et sur celle d'un mouvement transitif', In: J. Piaget, H. Sinclair and Vinh-Bang, *Epistémologie et psychologie de l'identité*, Paris: Presses Universitaires de France, 1968, pp. 1–82.

Piaget, J. and Vinh-Bang. 'Comparaisons des mouvements oculaires et des centrations du regard chez l'enfant et chez l'adulte', *Arch. de Psychol.* (Geneva), 1961a, **38**, pp. 167–200.

Piaget, J. and Vinh-Bang. 'L'enregistrement des mouvements oculaires en jeu chez l'adulte dans la comparaison de verticales, horizontales ou obliques et dans les perceptions de la figure en équerre', *Arch. de Psychol.* (Geneva), 1961b, **38**, pp.89–141.

Pick, A. D. 'Improvement of visual and tactual form discrimination', *J. Exp. Psychol.*, 1965, **69**, pp. 331–339.

Pick, A. D., Pick, H. L. and Thomas, M. L. 'Cross-modal transfer and improvement of form discrimination', *J. Exp. Child Psychol.*, 1966, **3**, pp. 279–288.

Pick, H. L. 'Some Soviet research on learning and perception in children'. In: J. C. Wright and J. Kagan (eds), 'Basic cognitive processes in children', *Monogr. Soc. Res. Child Dev.*, 1963, **28**, Monogr. 86, pp. 185–190.

Pick, H. L. 'Perception in Soviet Psychology', *Psychol. Bull.*, 1964, **62**, pp. 21–35.

Pinard, A. and Laurendeau, M. 'Le caractère topologique des premières représentations spatiales de l'enfant. Examen des hypothèses de Piaget', *Internat. J. Psychol.*, 1966, **1**, pp. 243–255.

Pineau, A. 'Influence de la force des configurations dans une épreuve de différentiation perceptive chez des enfants d'âge préscolaire', *Mémoire de psychologie expérimentale*. Master's thesis, Paris, Sorbonne, 1969.

Poincaré, H. *La science et l'hypothèse*, Paris: Flammarion, 1902 (new edition, 1968).

Polidora, V. J. and Fletcher, H. J. 'An analysis of the importance of S-R spatial contiguity for proficient primate discrimination performance', *J. Comp. Physiol. Psychol*, 1964, **57**, pp. 224–230.

Pollack, R. H. 'Figural after-effects as a function of age', *Acta Psychol. Amst.*, 1960, **17**, pp. 417–423.

Poppelreuter, W. *Die psychischen Schädigungen durch Kopfschuss im*

*Kriege 1914–1916 mit besonderer Berucksichtigung der patho-psychologischen, pädagogischen, gewerblichen und sozialen Beziehungen,* Leipzig: Leopold Voss, 1917.

Poppelreuter, W. 'Zur Psychologie und Pathologie der optischen Wahrnehmung', *Z. gesam. Norm. u. Pathol.,* 1923, **83**, pp. 26–152.

Porter, E. L. H. 'Factors in the fluctuation of fifteen ambiguous phenomena', *Psychol. Rec.,* 1938, **2**, pp. 231–253.

Poulton, E. C. 'Peripheral vision, refractoriness, and eye movements in fast oral reading', *Brit. J. Psychol.,* 1962, **53**, pp. 409–419.

Pritchard, R. M., Heron, W. and Hebb, D. O. 'Visual perception approached by the method of stabilized images', *Canad. J. Psychol.,* 1960, **14**, pp. 67–77.

Pubols, B. H. Jr. 'The facilitation of visual and spatial discrimination reversal by overlearning', *J. Comp. Physiol. Psychol.,* 1956, **49**, pp. 243–248.

Pupura, D. P., Carmichael, M. W. and Housepian, E. M. 'Physiological and anatomical studies of development of superficial axodendritic synaptic pathways in neocortex', *Exp. Neurol.,* 1960, **2**, pp. 324–347.

Rapoport, J. L. 'Attitude and size judgment in school-age children', *Child Dev.,* 1967, **38**, pp. 1187–1192.

Rapoport, J. L. 'Size-constancy in children measured by a functional size-discrimination task', *J. Exp. Child Psychol.,* 1969, **7**, pp. 366–373.

Reid, L. S. 'The development of non-continuity behaviour through continuity learning', *J. Exp. Psychol.,* 1953, **46**, pp. 107–112.

Reiser, O. L. 'The logic of gestalt psychology', *Psychol. Rev.,* 1931, **38**, pp. 359–368.

Renan, E. *L'avenir de la science,* Paris, 1890.

Renshaw, S. 'The errors of cutaneous localization and the effect of practice on the localizing movement in children and adults', *J. Genet. Psychol.,* 1930, **38**, pp. 223–238.

Rey, A. *Étude des insuffisances psychologiques. I. Méthodes et problèmes,* Neuchâtel, Paris: Delachaux & Niestlé, 1947 (2nd edition, 1962).

Rice, C. 'The orientation of plane figures as a factor in their perception by children', *Child Dev.,* 1930, **1**, pp. 111–143.

Riggs, L. A., Ratcliff, F., Cornsweet, J. C. and Cornsweet, T. M. 'The disappearance of steadily fixated visual test objects', *J. Opt. Soc. Amer.,* 1953, **43**, pp. 495–501.

Rudel, R. G. and Teuber, H. L. 'Discrimination of direction of line in children', *J. Comp. Physiol. Psychol.,* 1963, **56**, pp. 982–898.

Rudel, R. G. and Teuber, H. L. 'Cross-modal transfer of shape discrimination by children', *Neuropsychologia,* 1964, **2**, pp. 1–8.

Rush, G. P. 'Visual grouping in relation to age', *Arch. Psychol.,* 1937, **31**, No. 217.

Ruzskaya, A. G. 'Orienting-exploratory activity in the formation of elementary generalisations in children. In: *Orientirovochny reflex i orientirovchno-issledovatelskaya deyatelnost,* Moscow, 1958, Izd. Akademii Pedagogicheskikh U.S.S.R.

Salapatek, P. 'Visual scanning of geometric figures by the human new-born', *J. Comp. Physiol. Psychol.*, 1968, **66**, pp. 247–258.

Salapatek, P. H. and Kessen, W. 'Visual scanning of triangles by the human newborn', *J. Exp. Child Psychol.*, 1966, **8**, pp. 155–167.

Santa Barbara, J. F. Jr, and Paré, W. P. 'Information processing in preschool children', *Psychon. Sci.*, 1965, **2**, pp. 143–144.

Schadé, J. P. and Baxter, C. F. 'Changes during growth in the volume and surface area of cortical neurons in the rabbit', *Exp. Neurol.*, 1960, **2**, pp. 158–178.

Schafer, R. and Murphy, G. 'The role of autism in a visual figure-ground relationship', *J. Exp. Psychol.*, 1943, **32**, pp. 335–343.

Schober, G. and Schober, A. 'Ueber Bilderkennungs und Unter-scheidungsfähigkeit bei kleinen Kindern', *Bh. z. ang. Psychol.*, 1919, **19**, pp. 94–137.

Schonell, F. J. *Backwardness in the basic subjects*, Edinburgh: Oliver and Boyd, 1942.

Schopler, E. *Visual and tactical receptor preference in normal and schizophrenic children*, Doctoral thesis, University of Chicago, 1964.

Scott, K. G. and Christy, M. 'Dependent measures of children's dis-crimination learning, *Psychon. Sci.*, 1968, **12**, pp. 53–54.

Segers, J. E. 'Recherches sur la perception visuelle chez des enfants ages de 3 à 12 ans et leur application à l'éducation', *J. Psychol. Norm. Pathol.*, 1926a, **23**, pp. 608–636; 723–753.

Segers, J. E. *Les perceptions visuelles et la fonction de globalisation chez les enfants*, Brussels: Ed. M. Lamertin, 1926b.

Sekuler, R. W. and Rosenblith, J. F. 'Discrimination of direction of line and the effect of stimulus alignment', *Psychon. Sci.*, 1964, **1**, pp. 143–144.

Selinka, R. 'Der Uebergang von der ganzheitlichen zur analytischen Auffassung im Kindesalter', *Z. padag. Psychol.*, 1939, **40**, pp. 256–278.

Simon, Th. 'Observation d'un timbre-poste à l'école maternelle et con-clusions générales sur l'observation des enfants', *Bull. Soc. Libre pour Étude Psychol. de l'Enfant*, 1913, **13**, pp. 208–218; 231–233.

Sinclair, H. and Piaget, J. 'Sondage sur l'identité. Les formes d'équiva-lence et la conservation lors de la rotation d'un carré'. In: J. Piaget, H. Sinclair and Vinh-Bang. *Epistémologie et psychologie de l'identité*. Paris: Presses Universitaires de France, 1968, pp. 123–144.

Smith, N. B. 'Matching ability as a factor in first grade reading', *J. Educ. Psychol.*, 1928, **19**, pp. 560–571.

Sokhina, V. P. 'Sur l'isolement de la figure par rapport au fond chez des enfants d'age préscolaire', *Doklady Akademii Pedagogicheskikh Nauk*, U.S.S.R., 1962, Nos 1–2.

Sokolov, Y. N. *Vospriiate i uslovny refleks*. Moscow University Press, 1958. Translated into English: *Perception and the conditioned reflex*. Oxford, London, New York, Paris: Pergamon Press, 1963.

Sokolov, Y. N. 'Orienting reflex as information regulator'. In: *Psycho-logical research in the U.S.S.R.*, Moscow: Progress Publishers, 1966, pp. 334–360.

Spence, K. W. 'The nature of discrimination learning in animals', *Psychol. Rev.*, 1936, **43**, pp. 427–449.

Spence, K. W. 'The differential response in animals to stimuli varying within a single dimension', *Psychol. Rev.*, 1937, **44**, pp. 430–444.

Spence, K. W. 'Continuous versus non-continuous interpretations of discrimination learning', *Psychol. Rev.*, 1940, **47**, pp. 271–288.

Spence, K. W. 'Theoretical interpretations of learning'. In: S. S. Stevens (ed.), *Handbook of experimental psychology*, New York: John Wiley and Sons, 1951, pp. 690–729.

Spence, K. W. 'The nature of the response in discrimination learning', *Psychol. Rev.*, 1952, **59**, pp. 89–93.

Spiker, C. C. 'Verbal factors in the discrimination learning of children'. In: J. C. Wright and J. Kagan, 'Basic cognitive processes in children', *Monogr. Soc. Res. Child Dev.*, 1963, **28**, Monogr. 86, pp. 53–69.

Spiker, C. C. and Norcross, K. J. *The effects of previously acquired stimulus names on discrimination performance.* Unpublished paper, University of Iowa, 1957, quoted in Spiker, 1963.

Spitz, R. A. *La première année de la vie de l'enfant*, Paris: Presses Universitaires de France, 1954 (2nd edition, 1963).

Staples, R. 'The responses of infants to color', *J. Exp. Psychol.*, 1932, **15**, pp. 119–141.

Stern, W. L. 'Ueberverlagerte Raumformen', *Z. angrew. Psychol.*, 1909, pp. 498–526.

Stevenson, H. W. and Iscoe, I. 'Transposition in the feeble-minded', *J. Exp. Psychol.*, 1955, **49**, pp. 11–15.

Street, R. F. *A gestalt completion test,* Teachers   College, Contrib. Educ., 1931, No. 481.

Sully, J. *Études sur l'enfance*, Paris: Félix Alcan, 1898.

Sutherland, N. S. 'Visual discrimination of orientation and shape by *Octopus*', *Nature*, London, 1957a, **179**, pp. 11–13.

Sutherland, N. S. 'Visual discrimination of orientation by *Octopus*', *Brit. J. Psychol.*, 1957b, **48**, pp. 55–71.

Sutherland. N. S. 'Visual discrimination of the orientation of rectangles by *Octopus vulgaris* Lamarck', *J. Comp. Physiol. Psychol.*, 1958, **51**, pp. 452–458.

Sutherland, N. S. 'Stimulus analysing mechanisms'. In: *Proceedings of a symposium on the mechanization of throught processes*, Vol. 2. London, England: H.M.S.O., 1959, pp. 575–609.

Sutherland. N. S. 'Visual discrimination of orientation by *Octopus*. Mirror images', *Brit. J. Psychol.*, 1960a, **51**, pp. 9–18.

Sutherland, N. S. 'Theories of shape discrimination in *Octopus*', *Nature*, London, 1960b, **186**, pp. 840–844.

Sutherland, N. S. 'Discrimination of horizontal and vertical extents by *Octopus*', *J. Comp. Physiol. Psychol.*, 1961, **54**, pp. 43–48.

Sutherland, N. S. 'Shape discrimination and receptive fields', *Nature*, London, 1963, **197**, pp. 118–122.

Sutherland, N. S. and Mackintosh, J. 'Discrimination learning: non-additivity of cues', *Nature*, London, 1964, **201**, pp. 528–530.

Sutherland, N. S., Mackintosh, N. J. and Mackintosh, J. 'Simultaneous discrimination training of *Octopus* and transfer of discrimination along a continuum', *J. Comp. Physiol. Psychol.*, 1963, **56**, pp. 150–156.

Tarakanov, V. B. and Zinchenko, V. P. 'Sravnitelnyi analiz osyazaniya i zreniya. Soobschenie: VI. Proizvol'noe i neproizvolnoe zapomenanie formy v doshkol'nom vozrasti (Comparative analysis of touch and vision: VI. Voluntary and involuntary recall of forms in preschool children)', *Dokl. Akad. Nauk. U.S.S.R.*, 1960, **4**, pp. 49–52.

Teegarden, L. 'Tests for the tendency to reversal in reading', *J. Educ. Res.*, 1933, **27**, pp. 81–97.

Thirion, A. N. 'Étude expérimentale de la représentation spatiale chez l'enfant de 3 à 6 ans', *Scientia paedogogica experimentalis*, 1969, **6**, pp. 121–183.

Terman, L. M. *The measurement of intelligence*, London: G. G. Harrap & Co., 1916.

Thomas, E. L. 'Eye-movements in speed reading'. In: *Speed reading: practices and procedures*, 1962, **10**, pp. 104–112.

Thomas, E. L. 'Eye-movements and fixations during initial viewing of Rorschach cards', *J. Project. Tech. Person. Assess.*, 1953, **27**, pp. 345–353.

Thomas, E. L. and Lansdown, E. L. 'Visual search patterns of radiologists in training', *Radiology*, 1963, **81**, pp. 288–292.

Thompson, G. G. *Child psychology*, Boston: Houghton Mifflin, 1952 (2nd edition, 1962).

Thurstone, L. L. *A factorial study of perception*, Chicago: University of Chicago Press, 1944.

Tighe, L. S. 'The effect of perceptual pretraining on reversal and non-reversal shifts', *J. Exp. Psychol.*, 1965, **70**, pp. 379–385.

Tighe, L. S. and Tighe, T. J. 'Overtraining and discrimination shift behavior in children', *Psychon. Sci.*, 1965, **2**, pp. 365–366.

Tighe, L. S. and Tighe, T. J. 'Discrimination learning: two views in historical perspective', *Psychol. Bull.*, 1966, **66**, pp. 353–370.

Tighe, T. J. 'Reversal and nonreversal shifts in monkeys', *J. Comp. Physiol. Psychol.*, 1964, **58**, pp. 324–326.

Tighe, T. J., Brown, P. L. and Youngs, E. A. 'The effect of overtraining on the shift behaviour of albino rats', *Psychon. Sci.*, 1965, **2**, pp. 141–142.

Tighe, T. J. and Tighe, L. S. 'Discrimination shift performance of children as a function of age and shift procedure', *J. Exp. Psychol.*, 1967, **74**, pp. 466–470.

Tobie, H. 'Die Entwicklungun der teilinhaltlichen Beachtung von Farbe und Form im vorschulpflichtigen Alter', *Z. angew. Psychol.*, 1926, *Suppl.* 38.

Tolman, E. C. 'Prediction of vicarious trial and error by means of the schematic sow-bug', *Psychol. Rev.*, 1939, **46**, pp. 318–336.

Tolman, E. C. 'Cognitive maps in rats and men', *Psychol. Rev.*, 1948, **55**, pp. 189–208.

Van der Torren, I. 'Ueber das Auffassungs und Unterscheidungsvermogen fur optische Bilder bei Kindern', *Zeit. angew. Psychol.*, 1907, 1, pp. 189–232.

Uttal, W. B. and Smith, P. 'Recognition of alphabetic characters during voluntary eye-movements', *Percept. Psychophys.*, 1968, **3**, pp. 257–264.

Venger, L. A. 'Discrimination between forms of objects by children of preschool age', *Doklady Akademii Pedagogischekikh Nauk*, 1962, No. 2, quoted in Zaporozhets and Zinchenko, 1966.

Vereecken, P. *Spatial development. Constructive praxia from birth to the age of seven*, Groningen: J. B. Wolters, 1961.

Vernon, M. D. *Backwardness in reading. A study of its nature and origin*, Cambridge University Press, 1957.

Volkelt, H. 'Fortschritte der experimentellen Kinderpsychologie', *Ber. uber d. IX Kongress f. exp. Psychol. in Munchen*, Jena: Fischer, 1926, pp. 80–135.

Vurpillot, E. 'Details caracteristiques et reconnaisance de formes familières', *Psychol. Franç.*, 1972, **7**, pp. 147–155.

Vurpillot, E. 'La materialité du trace figural chez l'enfant'. In: Vinh-Bang, P. Greco, J.-B. Grize, Y. Hatwell, J. Piaget, G. N. Seagrim and E. Vurpillot. *L'epistémologie de l'espace*, Paris: Presses Universitaires de France, 1964a, pp. 93–112.

Vurpillot, E. 'Perception et représentation dans la constance de la forme', *Année Psychol.*, 1964b, **64**, pp. 61–82.

Vurpillot, E. 'Données expérimentales récentes sur le développement des perceptions visuelles chez le nourrisson', *Année Psychol.*, 1966, **66**, pp. 213–230.

Vurpillot, E. 'The development of scanning strategies and their relation to visual differentiation', *J. Exp. Child Psychol.*, 1968, **6**, pp. 632–650.

Vurpillot, E. 'Contribution à l'étude de la différenciation perceptive chez l'enfant d'âge préscolaire', *Année Psychol.*, 1969a, **69**, pp. 37–54.

Vurpillot, E. 'Influence de la nature d'une différence sur la détection par des enfants d'âge préscolaire', *Enfance*, 1969b, **22**, pp. 149–164.

Vurpillot, E. 'Activité oculo-motrice et activités cognitives', *Bull. de Psychol.*, 1969c, **22**, pp. 660–668.

Vurpillot, E. *Les perceptions du nourrisson*, Paris: Presses Universitaires de France, 1972.

Vurpillot, E. and Berthoud, M. 'Evolution génétique de la localisation dans un cadre de référence rectangulaire', *Année Psychol.*, 1969, **69**, pp. 393–406.

Vurpillot, E. and Florès, A. 'La genèse de l'organisation perceptive: I. Rôle du contour et de la surface enclose dans la perception des figures'. *Année Psychol.*, 1964, **64**, pp. 375–395.

Vurpillot, E., Lécuyer, R., Moal, A. and Pineau, A. 'Perception de déplacements et jugements d'identité chez l'enfant d'âge préscolaire', *Année Psychol.*, 1971, **71**, pp. 31–52.

Vurpillot, E. and Moal, A. 'Evolution des critères d'identité chez des enfants d'âge préscolaire dans une tâche de différenciation perceptive' *Année Psychol.*, 1970, **70**, pp. 391–406.

Vurpillot, E. and Zoberman, M. 'Rôle des indices communs et des indices distincts dans la différenciation perceptive', *Acta. Psychologica*, 1965, **24**, pp. 49–67.

Walk, R. D. and Gibson, E. J. 'A comparative and analytical study of visual depth perception', *Psychol. Monogr.*, 1961, **75** (Monogr. 519), pp. 1–44.

Wapner, S. 'Age changes in perception of verticality and of the longitudinal body axis under body tilt', *J. Exp. Child Psychol.*, 1968, **6**, pp. 543–555.

Wapner, S. and Werner, H. *Perceptual development: An investigation within the framework of sensory-tonic field*, Worcester, Mass.: Clark University Press, 1957.

Watson, J. B. *Psychology from the standpoint of a behaviorist*, Philadelphia, London: Lippincott, 1919.

Van Wayenburg, G. 'Ontwikkeling van het kinderlijk denken of jongen leeftüd, met proveven toegelicht', *Eerste Nederlandsche Congres voor Kinderstudie*, 1913, p. 41.

Wekker, L. M. 'On the basic properties of the mental image and a general approach to their analogue simulation'. In: *Psychological research in the USSR*, Moscow: Progress Publishers, 1966, pp. 310–333.

Werner, H. *Comparative psychology of mental development* (Revised edition), New York: International Universities Press, Inc., 1957.

Wertheimer, M. *Untersuchungen zur Lehre von der Gestalt: II. Psychol. Forsch.*, 1923, **4**, pp. 301–350. English translation in: W. D. Ellis (ed.), *A souce book of gestalt psychology*, London: Routledge and Kegan Paul, 1950, pp. 71–88.

Wever, E. G. 'Figure and ground in the visual perception of form', *Amer. J. Psychol.*, 1927, **38**, pp. 194–226.

White, B. L. and Held, R. 'Plasticity of sensorimotor development in the human infant'. In: J. F. Rosenblith and W. Allinsmith (eds), *The causes of behavior: Readings in child development and educational psychology*, Boston: Allyn and Bacon Inc., 1966, pp. 60–70.

White, C. and Ford, A. 'Eye-movements during simulated radar search', *J. Opt. Soc. Amer.*, 1960, **50**, pp. 909–913.

White, S. H. *Research on attentional processes in learning*. Progress Report USPHS Grant M-3639, 1962.

White, S. H. 'Age differences in reaction to stimulus variation', *Paper presented at an ONR Conference on adaptation to complex, changing environments*, Boulder, Colorado, 1964.

White, S. H. 'Evidence for a hierarchical arrangement of learning processes'. In: L. P. Lipsitt and C. C. Spiker (eds), *Advances in child development and behavior, Vol. 2*, New York, London: Academic Press, 1965, pp. 187–220.

White, S. H. 'The hierarchical organization of intellectual structures'. *Paper presented to a symposium on 'The role of experience in intellectual development', American Association for the Advancement of Science*, Washington, 1966.

## 362  *The Visual World of the Child*

White, S. H. 'The learning-maturation controversy: Hall to Hull', *Merrill-Palmer Quart.*, 1968, **14**, pp. 187–196.

White, S. H. 'Some general outline of the matrix of developmental changes between five and seven years'. *Paper presented to the 19th International Congress of Psychology*, London, 1969.

White, S. H. and Plum, G. E. 'Eye-movement photography during children's discrimination learning', *J. Exp. Child Psychol.*, 1964, **1**, pp. 327–338.

Wiesel, T. N. and Hubel, D. H. 'Single-cell responses in striate cortex of kittens deprived of vision in one eye', *J. Neurophysiol.*, 1963, **26**, pp. 1003–1017.

Witkin, H. A. 'Individual differences in ease of perception of embedded figures', *J. Person.*, 1950, **19**, pp. 1–15.

Wittling-Lauret, M. 'Quelques aspects génétiques de l'intégration sensori-motrice, *Psychol. Franç.*, 1966, **11**, pp. 127–148.

Wohlwill, J. F. ' "Overconstancy" in space perception'. In: L. P. Lipsitt and C. C. Spiker (eds), *Advances in child development and behavior,* Vol. 1, New York, London: Academic Press, 1963, pp. 265–312.

Wohlwill, J. and Wiener, M. 'Discrimination of form orientation in young children', *Child Dev.*, 1964, **35**, pp. 1113–1125.

Wolff, P. H. 'Observations on the early development of smiling'. In: B. M. Foss (ed.), *Determinants of infant behavior,* Vol. II, London: Methuen and Co. Ltd., 1963, pp. 113–134.

Wolff, P. H. and White, B. L. 'Visual pursuit and attention in young infants', *J. Amer. Acad. Child. Psychiat.*, 1965, **4**, pp. 473–484.

Woodworth, R. S. and Schlosberg, H. *Experimental psychology*, New York: Holt and Co., 1954.

Wright, J. C. 'Acquired relevance of cues and ritualistic attention to irrelevant cues in children's learning'. *Paper presented to the American Psychological Association*, Los Angeles, 1964.

Wright, J. C. and Daehler, M. W. 'Shaping children's observing behavior for an oddity problem learning set'. *Paper presented to the Psychonomics Society*, Saint-Louis, 1966.

Wright, J. C. and Gliner, C. M. 'Relevance of observing response set and distinctiveness of cues in children's haptic discrimination learning', *Personal communication*, duplicated paper, 1967.

Wright, J. C. and Smothergill, D. 'Observing behavior and children's discrimination learning under delayed reinforcement', *J. Exp. Child Psychol.*, 1967, **5**, pp. 430–440.

Wursten, H. 'L'évolution des comparaisons de longeurs de l'enfant à l'adulte', *Arch. de Psychol.* (Geneva), 1947, **32**, pp. 1–144.

Wyckoff, L. B. Jr. 'The role of observing responses in discrimination learning, Part 1.' *Psychol. Rev.*, 1952, **59**, pp. 431–442.

Young, J. Z. 'The visual system of Octopus: I. Regularities in the retina and optic lobes of octopus in relation to form discrimination', *Nature*, London, 1960, **186**, pp. 836–839.

Youniss, J. and Furth, H. G. 'Reversal learning in children as a function of overtraining and delayed transfer', *J. Comp. Physiol. Psychol.*, 1964, **57**, pp. 155–157.

Zaporozhets, A. V. *Razvitie proizvol' nykh dvizhenii* (The development of voluntary movements), Moscow, Acad. Pedag. Sci., 1960.

Zaporozhets, A. V. 'The origin and development of the conscious control of movements in man'. In: N. O'Connor (ed.), *Recent Soviet psychology*, Oxford, London, New York, Paris: Pergamon, 1961, pp. 273–289.

Zaporozhets, A. V. 'The development of perception in the preschool child'. In: P. E. Mussen (ed.), 'European research in cognitive development', *Monogr. Soc. Res. Child Dev.*, 1965, **30**, Monogr. 100, pp. 82–101.

Zaporozhets, A. V. 'The development of perception and activity'. In: *Transactions of the 18th International Congress of Psychology, Symposium on perception and action*, Moscow, 1966, pp. 45–53.

Zaporozhets, A. V. and Zinchenko, V. P. 'Development of perceptual activity and formation of a sensory image in the child'. In: *Psychological research in the U.S.S.R.*, Progress Publishers: Moscow, 1966, pp. 393–421.

Zeaman, D. and House, B. J. 'The role of attention in retardate discrimination learning'. In: N. R. Ellis (ed.), *Handbook in mental deficiency: psychological theory and research*, New York: McGraw Hill, 1963, pp. 159–223.

Zeaman, D., House, B. J. and Orlando, R. 'Use of special training condition in visual discrimination learning with imbeciles', *Amer. J. Ment. Def.*, 1958, **63**, pp. 453–459.

Zeigler, H. P. and Leibowitz, H. 'Apparent visual size as a function of distance for children and adults', *Amer. J. Psychol.*, 1957, **70**, pp. 106–109.

Zinchenko, V. P. 'Sravnitel'nyi analiz osyazaniya i zreniya: Soobschenye: II. Osobenesti orientirovochno issledo vatel'skikh dvzhenii glaza u detei doshkolnogo vazrasta (Comparative analysis of touch and vision; II. Characteristics of eye-movements of orientation and investigation in preschool children)', *Dokl. Akad. Ped. Nauk. U.S.S.R.*, 1960, 4(2), pp. 53–60.

Zinchenko, V. P. and Ruzkaya, A. G. 'Svravnitel'nyi analiz osyazaniva i zreniya: Coobschenie: III. Zritel' no-gapticheskii perenos v doshkol'nom vozraste (Comparative analysis of touch and vision: III. Visual-haptic transfer at the preschool age-level)', *Dokl. Akad. Ped. Nauk. U.S.S.R.*, 1960a, 4, 95–98.

Zinchenko, V. P. and Ruzskaya, A. G. 'Sravnitel'nyi analiz osyazaniya i zreniya: Soobschenie: VII. Nalychnye unroveni vospriyatiya formy u detei doshkolnogo vozrasta. (Comparative analysis of touch and vision. VII. The observed level of form perception in children of preschool age)', *Dokl. Akad. Ped. Nauk. U.S.S.R.*, 1960b, 4, pp. 85–89.

Zinchenko, V. P., van Chizi-Tsin, V. and Tarakanov, V. V. 'Stavrovlenie i razvitie pertstivnykh deistvii (The formation and development of perceptual activity)', *Vop. Psikhol.*, 1962, **8**, pp. 1–14. (Translated into English in: *Soviet Psychology Psychiat.*, 1963, **1**, pp. 3–12.)

Zusne, L. and Michels, K. M. 'Nonrepresentational shapes and eye movements', *Percept. Mot. Skills*, 1964, **18**, pp. 11–20.

# Index

abstraction of a dimension of differentiation 154–9, 166
acquired distinctiveness of cues 168–9, 171, 173, 215
acquired equivalence of cues 169, 173
adaptation 21, 25
Amato, M. R. d' 185
ambiguous figures 153
Ames, E. W. 274
AMO problems 46
analysers 182, 183, 186, 211, 259, 260, 261, 262
Ananiev, B. G. 263–4, 272
Anderson, I. H. 252
Andrieux, C. 34
animal form-perception 85–8
animal psychology 11
Antonovsky, H. F. 89, 92
articulation between whole and parts 61, 132–45, 269
associationism 33, 124, 148, 288
attention defined: 175; selective Ch. 7 *passim*
Attneave, F. 172, 196, 233
Aubert effect 73

Babska, Z. 290–2, 308
behavioural psychology 11
Bender, L. 334
Benton, A. L. 334
Berlyne, D. E. 188, 261, 263
Berthoud, M. 303–5
Beyrl, F. 67
Bijou, S. W. 81
Binet, A. 126, 128, 321
Bingham, H. C. 85, 281
Birch, H. G. 220
Bloom, B. S. 333
Bobbitt, J. M. 52–3
Botha, E. 49, 60
Botzum, W. A. 53
Bower, T. G. R. 60, 66, 283, 324
Braine, L. 89, 95, 97
Brandner, M. 105
Brandt, H. F. 232
Brault, H. 70
Brian, C. R. 209

Broadbent, D. E. 182
Bruner, J. 9, 10, 26, 48, 146, 195–6, 273, 282–3, 306, 324, 327
Brunswik, E. 61
Burzlaff, W. 68
Buss, A. H. 156
Busse, K. 125
Buswell, G. T. 253, 255

CA problems 40, 42–4, 46
Campione, J. 157, 159
Cantor, G. N. 169, 170, 171, 215
Capaldi, E. J. 185
categorial identity 283–4
categories 195–6, 283–4, 292, 306, 324, 330, 332, 336
cell-assemblies, genesis of 61
centration 51, 57, 62, 236, 277, 321–2
Chase, W. P. 154, 212, 324
Chow, K. L. 321
circles, displacement of single component of 110–13
Claparède, E. 125–8, 132–3, 137, 148, 288
closed forms 99, 101–2
closure 52–63 *passim*
cognitive structures *see* structures
Colby, M. C. 209
colouring 39, 45, 47
comparison strategies 236ff
Compayré 126
completion test 58
component of a configuration, displacement of a 110–13
conceptual experience replacing perceptual experience 73
conceptual systems 24–5
configurations, irregular 143
configurations used in investigating displacement of a single component 111–12
connectionist learning models 159–61
conservation of relevant dimension *see* relevant dimension
*Construction of Reality* 133
Cook, F. M. 212, 324
Corah, N. L. 141–2, 209–10

Cramaussel, E. 99, 126, 129, 132, 135, 146
critical dimension 191–2, 195
curvilinear and rectilinear forms, differentiation between 99–101
'cut-into' figures 58

Dalcroze 126
Davidson, H. P. 77
Debot-Sevrin, M. R. 243
Decroly, O. 126
Demoor, J. 126, 128
Denis-Prinzhorn, M. 67–8
Denner, B. 266
Descoeudres, A. 209–10
detection of differences 203–8
development, evolution of 37–8, 43–44
Dickerson, D. J. 157–60, 199–200, 202
difference 292: judgments of 284–5
differences, sensitivity to 288–9
differences caused by component permutation, perception of 114–21: 'singularity' of components 118–120
different orientations: differentiation of forms presented in 75–81; recognising an identical form in 81–4
differentiation Ch. 5 *passim*, 277–9, 282, 284–5, 287–90, 306, 314, 323–4, 328–9, 336–7; and identification 278–86; Gibsons' theory of 188–95; tasks 229–32
differentiators 153–5, Ch. 8 *passim*
dimensions of differentiation 154–9, 195ff, 202, 209–10, 212, 325
direction of internalised exploration 93–6
discrimination learning Ch. 6 *passim*, 175–8, 181, 187–8, 195, 201, 213–14, 269, 287, 290, 319, 321, 325, 329, 335
displacement of a single component of a configuration 110–13
distance constancy 69
distinctive features 190–1
Djang, S. S. 34
dominant dimensions 211
drawing, reproduction by 100–4, 269–271, 327–8
Dreyfus-Brisac, C. 312

Dworetzki, G. 51, 133–4, 136–8, 146–147, 153, 325–6

Eimas, P. D. 156
elementarism 126
Elkind, D. 51, 136–9, 145, 147, 153, 243–5, 313, 319
embedded figures, discrimination of 32–47, 153, 269, 314
enactive representation 195–6, 272
enclosed figures 102
Enoch, J. M. 253
environment 21–2, 24, 60, 189, 332
equivalence 278, 280, 283–6
errors of localisation 108–9
Euclidean relationships 98–103, 122, 123
Euclidean space 98, 213
exploration: influence of training on visual 267–9; internalised 93–6, 263, 327; perceptual 261–3; sequential 88–91, 94, 191; spontaneous visual 176–8, 180–1; tactile 263–4
exploration, Visuo-motor Ch. 9 *passim*; complete 295–6, 299–300, 302, 309–10; differentiation task 223ff; insufficient 229–32, 295–6, 298–301, 304, 306, 330; strategies of 235–56, 274–6, 320; task adaptation 226ff
extra-dimensional shifts 156–60, 162–164, 199–202; *see also* non-reversal shifts
eye-hand co-ordination 27
eye-movements 221ff, 236ff

familiar forms, identification of 53–5
familiarisation tasks 221–3
Fantz, R. L. 113, 154, 192, 274, 284, 318, 324
FE problems 40, 42–4, 46
Fellows, B. J. 75, 77, 82, 87–8, 281
'field effect' 277
figure-ground discrimination 26, 31, 50
first learning 154, 156, 158, 160, 163, 182
fixations 176, 177, 221, 223–9, 237, 243–6, 248–51, 273–4, 295, 302, 318, 321–2, 328: concentration of 233–5; distribution of 232–5; duration of 251–5, 275; information value of 233

FJ problems 40, 42–4
Florès, A. 36, 37, 40, 43, 45–6
focal points 89–97
form 281–2, 324: and structure 135; constancy 70–3
form orientation, perception of 75–97 *passim*: interpretation of children's performances 84–97 *passim*
form representation, topological and Euclidean relationships in 98–103
foveal vision 322
Fraisse, P. 13, 181, 235
frame of reference, localisation of a part within 105–10, 117: errors of 108–9
Francès, R. 34
functionalism 9
Furth, H. G. 157–9, 194, 200

Gaines, R. 209
Galifret-Granjon, N. 64
Gassel, M. M. 243
Gaydos, H. F. 222, 266–7
Gellermann, L. W. 56, 63, 80, 281
Gennep, A. Van 125
Gesell, A. 105, 249
Gestalt theories 32–4, 47, 57, 60, 66, 134–5, 146, 153, 196, 277, 324
Ghent, L. 37, 38, 83–4, 89, 90–7, 122, 134, 153, 326
Gibson, E. J. 10, 60, 80, 154, 188–9, 191–4, 197, 201, 207–8, 212, 273
Gibson, J. J. 9, 10, 71, 188, 192–4, 213–4, 331
Ginevskaya, T. O. 264
globalism 126, 127, 128–9, 134–5, 148, 277, 323, 326
Gollin, E. S. 53–6, 59, 63
'good' continuity 35
'good' forms 35, 55–8
Goodwin, W. R. 182
Gorman, J. J. 284
Gottschaldt, K. 33–5, 62, 314, 326
Gottschalk, J. 243
Gouin-Décarie, Th. 282
Gould, J. D. 232, 253
Graham, C. H. 48
Guignot, E. 72
Guilford, J. P. 48
Guillaume, P. 146
Gumusyan, S. 38

habituation 274
Haeckel's law of recapitulation 125

Hanawalt, N. G. 34
Harrow, M. 156
Harway, N. I. 67
Hebb, D. O. 12, 26, 61, 88–9, 97, 219, 324, 327
Hebb's theory of form-perception 88–9
Hecaen, H. 78
Heckenmueller, E. G. 251
Heilbronner, K. 129
Helson, H. 53
Hermelin, B. 220
Hershenson, M. 154, 324
Hertz, M. 113
Hill, M. B. 77
homologous comparisons 241–3, 246
Honkavaara, S. 209
Hooker, D. 220
Horn, G. 181
House, B. J. 182, 187–8
Hubel, D. H. 12, 61, 88
Hull, C. L. 159, 168
Huttenlocher, J. 77–80, 87, 122

iconic representation 195–6
identification Ch. 5 *passim*, 277, 279–280, 326–7
identification and differentiation, relationships between 278–86
identification tasks 229
identity 278–9, 281, 292: child's concept of 283; judgment of 39, 284–5, 314, 330; relationship of 280, 295–6, 289–306, 329, 331
identity criteria of equivalence and difference Ch. 11 *passim*
image, theory of 257–63, 271
imaginary lines 55–8
incomplete drawings: identification and differentiation experiments with 129–30; recognition of 53–7, 63
individual identity 279, 282–3
information theory 196, 258
intelligence 21
intermodal transfer 264–6
internalised exploration 93–6
intra-dimensional change 157–60, 199–202
intra-dimensional reversal *see* reversals
intrafigural relationships, conservation of set of 281

intrafigural relationships and the perceived form 103–5
intrafigural spatial relationships Ch. 4 *passim*
inversions in space 75–6, 78–81, 87, 96, 122
irregular forms 102, 143

Jackson, H. 333
Jakobson, R. 190
James, W. 186, 187
Janet, P. 134
Jenkin, N. 67
Johannsen, D. E. 49, 60
Johnson, M. S. 76
Jonckheere, T. 126–8, 132, 288
juxtaposed figures 36, 39–40, 102

Kagan, J. 209, 274
Katz, D. 209
Katz, P. A. 172–3
Kelleher, R. T. 156, 159
Kendall's W 43
Kendler, H. 161, 163, 164, 166–8, 175–6, 184–5, 186, 201–2, 211, 214, 312, 325
Kendler, T. S. 156, 159, 161–3, 166–168, 184–6, 194–5, 201–2, 210–11, 214, 287, 312, 317, 325
Kessen, W. 31, 89, 233, 318
Klimpfinger, S. 70
knowledge 23
Köhler, W. 12, 48–52, 82, 85–7
Köhler's satiation theory of reversal 50–2
Koffka, K. 52
Kohs' blocks 140
Komaki, J. 185
Krechevsky, I. 315
Kretshmar, J. 125
Kuenne, M. R. 167
Kurtz, K. H. 155, 159, 172, 175

Lambercier, M. 68–9
Lamprecht, K. 125
Lang, A. 113
*Language and Thought* 134
language intervention in discrimination learning 161–74, 214–5
Lashley, K. S. 85–6, 155, 175–6, 315
Lavrentyeva, T. V. 267
Lawrence, D. H. 155, 159, 169, 175, 182
learning: connectionist models 159–

161; involving conservation of relevant dimension 155; involving reversals and non-reversal shifts 155–9; to read 76; uniformity of 22; *see also* under specific aspects, e.g. discrimination learning
Lécuyer, R. 118–20, 308
left-right relationship 105–6
Leibowitz, L. 70
Leontiev, A. N. 219, 257, 271, 327
Lépine, D. 284, 292, 306
Lesèvre, N. 243, 246, 248–50, 253–5, 274, 302
Levine, M. 316, 319
Lévy-Bruhl, L. 125
Lévy-Schoen, A. 233
Lewis, M. 274
line, privileged role of the 61
line-drawings, perception of 65–6
Lipsitt, L. P. 323
localisation 204–5, 212, 232, 245, 251, 273, 318, 322; errors of 108–9; of a part within a frame of reference 105–10, 117, 121, 122; of component permutation 116–17
Lovell, K. 99, 101
Luquet, G. H. 125–6, 257, 327
Lurçat, L. 101
Luria, A. R. 167, 287

MacCaslin, E. F. 188
Mackintosh, N. J. 155, 175–6, 181–4, 186–8, 211, 335
Mackintosh's hypothesis 182–6
Mackworth, N. H. 232–3, 253–6, 321–2
Mandès, E. J. 89, 97
Marsh, G. 185
maturation 12, 23–4, 26–7, 332–4
mediational generalisation 169, 173
mediational learning model 161
mediational responses 161–8, 184, 186, 189, 335
mediational theories of learning Ch. 6 *passim*, Ch. 7 *passim*
Meili, R. 132, 134–6, 146–8
memory 21, 23
Meneghini, K. A. 70, 72
metric relationships 65–6, 98, 101–3, 105, 270
Miller, G. 182, 317
Miller, N. E. 161, 168, 171
Miller, S. 313
Milner, E. 334

MO problems 46
Moal, A. 116, 308
Monroe, M. 76
Mooney, C. M. 53, 58–9
Moses 128
motor activity 23–4
Mouchly, R. 82, 85
multiple transfer 12
Mumbauer, C. C. 157, 159, 210, 214

neonate, behaviour of 26
nervous system, immaturity of 23, 24
neural receptors *see* sensory organs
neurones, specialised 87–8
neurophysiological development 12
Newson, E. 77, 80
non-relevant dimension 156–7, 164, 167, 178
non-reversal shifts 155–7, 160–3, 165–6, 184–6, 194–5, 201, 312, 337; *see also* extra-dimensional shifts
non-selective responses 162–6, 186
Norcross, K. J. 170–1

Oetjen, F. 82, 85
observing responses 175–81
Ogden, R. M. 53
Oléron, P. 38, 173, 185, 286–7, 290–2
Olver, R. R. 324
open forms 99, 101–2
operative structures 262
optional shift 162–3, 168, 186, 202
ordered differentiation 191
organisation Ch. 5 *passim*, 323, 336: Gestalt theories of *see* Gestalt theories; level of 39–40, 45–7, 62–3; rigidity of perceptual 134ff
orientation 183, 184, 187, 192, 194, 261–2, 274, 326
orientations, different: differentiation of forms presented in 75–81; recognising an identical form in 81–4
Orton, S. T. 78
Over, R. 81
over-constancy in perceiving irregular forms 72
overlapping figures 32–3, 35–40, 102: adult discrimination of 33
overlearning 159, 184–6, 193, 202, 213–4

Page, E. I. 99
parts, exclusive perception of 134–48
part-whole confusion 132–4

part-whole relationships 105–21 *passim*
Pavlov, I. P. 187, 258, 261
Pêcheux, M. G. 102, 269–71
perceived form, intrafigural relationships and 103–5
perceived identity 279–80
perception, Gestalt theories of *see* Gestalt theories
perception of differences caused by component permutation 114–21: 'singularity' of components 118–20
perception of displacement of single component of a configuration 110–113
perceptual activities in the child, evolution of 262–3
perceptual activity and representational structures Ch. 10 *passim*
perceptual constancies 65–73, 280–1, 283, 285
perceptual differentiation *see* differentiation
perceptual exploration 261–3
perceptual invariants 280–2, 329
perceptual organisation *see* organisation
perceptual space 64, 121
perceptual structures *see* structures
Perkins, C. C. 188
permutation of components, perception of differences caused by 114–21: localisation of permutation 116–17; 'singularity of components 118–20
perseveration errors in localisation 108
phenomenal instructions 72
physical identity 279–80
physical properties of stimuli 34, 48, 60, 72, 113, 132, 147, 154, 186, 264, 273, 325
Piaget, J. 9, 10, 37–8, 49–51, 55, 57, 58, 63–4, 66–7, 84, 98–103, 106, 110, 123, 133, 146–8, 154, 219, 232, 234–6, 246, 248, 253, 254–5, 257–8, 271, 273, 275, 277, 282–4, 312, 316–18, 321, 323, 327–8, 336
Piaget's theory of reversal 50–2
Pick, A. 196, 198–9, 273
Pick, H. 263, 266
picture books, upside-down 82
Pinard, A. 99–101
Pineau, A. 110–12, 142–4, 307–8

plasticity of perception 34, 51, 61, 137
Poincaré, H. 281
pointillism 126, 128–9, 148, 326
Polidora, V. J. 182
Pollack, R. H. 52
Poppelreuter, W. 33
Porter, E. L. H. 48
Poulton, E. C. 253, 255
predictions of perceptual organisation 34–6, 47
predominance of whole or parts 125–132
pretraining *see* training for learning
preverbal stage 167–8
primary area structures 35, 37, 40, 45
primary contour structures 34–7, 40–42, 44–5, 141–2
primary structures 24–5, 31, 34–7, 39, 320, 324, 326–8
Pritchard, R. M. 61
privileged structures 36–7
prototypes 196
proximity, law of 61
proximity factor 105, 109
Pubols, Jr., B. H. 185
Pupura, D. P. 88

Rapoport, J. L. 68
reaction time, visuo-motor 246, 248
reactive inhibition 55
reading 76, 243–6, 252, 254, 322
recapitulation, Haeckel's law of 125
recognition 265–8, 272, 284–5
recognition tasks 221–3, 229
recording of visuo-motor activity 221ff
rectilinear and curvilinear forms, differentiation between 99–101
reflexes 258, 274, 313, 315, 318
regular forms 102
Reid, L. S. 185
Reiser, O. L. 53
relevant dimension 155–6, 158–61, 163–4, 167, 178, 180–1, 186–8, 194–196, 201, 211
Renan, E. 125–6, 137, 148
Renshaw, S. 220
repetition, its influence on differentiation performance 192–3, 214
representation 21, 37–8, 48, 195–6, Ch. 10 *passim*, 327
representation of forms, topological

and Euclidean relationships in 98–103
representational space 64, 121
representational structures, genesis of Ch. 10 *passim*
reproduction techniques 39, 45, 269–271
retarded children 187
retinal frame of reference 92–3, 103–105
retinal orientation 86–7
'reversals' 76–7, 155–60, 162–4, 166, 168, 184–6, 193–5, 199–202, 312, 337
reversible and ambiguous figures, perception of 47–52, 136–9
Rey, A. 53
Rice, C. 80
Riggs, L. A. 248
right-left relationship 105–6
rigidity of perceptual organisation 134ff
Rorschach test 233
rotations in a single plane 75–7, 80
Rudel, R. G. 77–8, 80, 87, 122, 265–6
Rush, G. P. 60
Ruzskaya, A. G. 269

Salapatek, P. H. 31, 89, 233, 274
'same' or 'not the same' judgments 142–4, 236ff, 286–90, 292–311, 316, 320, 329–31
Santa Barbara, Jr., J. F. 213, 321
satiation theory 12, 50–2
Schadé, J. P. 88
Schafer, R. 48
Schober, G. and A. 129–30, 132, 136, 145
Schonell, F. J. 76
Schopler, E. 220
Schroeder staircase 48
Scott, K. G. 178, 269
Sechenov 258
second learning 156–8, 160, 165–70, 181, 184–6, 199–201
secondary area structures 35–6, 42
secondary contour structures 35–6, 39–40, 42, 44–5, 142
secondary structures 35, 37, 327–8
Segers, J. E. 127–9, 131–2, 135, 288
segmented circle figure 48–9
Sekuler, R. W. 78
selective attention Ch. 7 *passim*, 211
Selinka, R. 140

semiotic function 312, 318
sensori-motor variables 246–51, 271, 318, 337
sensory organs 22–4, 124, 182, 189, 221, 259–61, 274, 320: sensitivity of 22–3, 211–12, 309, 328–9, 332–3
'sensory tableau' 154, 257, 283, 321
sequential exploration 88–91, 94, 191
shape 281
similarities, sensitivity to 288–9
Simon, Th. 128
Sinclair, H. 103
single-stage connectionist learning model 159–61
single-stage learning 155, 188, 211
'singularity' of components 118–20
size constancy, development of 66–70
size perception 328
Skinner 335
Smith, N. B. 77
Snedecor's F 224
Sokhina, V. P. 269
Sokolov, Y. N. 196, 261
space, perceptual 64, 121
space, representational 64, 121
spatial frame of reference, role of 84–5
spatial localisation *see* localisation
spatial relationships: awareness of 27; intrafigural Ch. 4 *passim*; between structures in three-dimensional space 64–74 *passim*
spatial transformations 75–8, 80, 96, 207–8
Spence, K. W. 159–61, 163, 167, 175–176, 288, 202
Spiker, C. C. 169–71
Spitz, R. A. 323
spontaneous visual exploration 221–3
S-R learning 11, 160–1, 184, 186, 188, 202, 315, 318
stability of perception 48
Staples, R. 212
stereognostic tasks 98–100
Stern, W. L. 82
Stettler-von Albertini, B. 37, 38
Stevenson, H. W. 187
stimulus-bound actions 318
stimulus-patterns, repeated presentation of 33
Street, R. F. 58
strong and weak structures 135–6
structure and form 135

structures 134, 137, 146, 153: acquisition of 211–12; evolution of Ch. 1 *passim*; models of 24–5; primary 24–5, 31, 34–7, 39, 320, 324, 326–8; primary area 35, 37, 40, 45; primary contour 34–7, 40–2, 44–5, 141–2; privileged 36–7; rigidity of 31, 37, 277, 325–6; secondary 24; strong and weak 135–6
subjective orientation 90–7, 122
substitution differences 294–5, 303
subtractive mediation theories 182ff
Sully, J. 125
Sutherland, N. S. 87, 175, 182–4, 187, 211–12, 281
symbolic function 64
symbolic representation 195–6
symmetrical localisation errors 108–9
syncretism Ch. 5 *passim*, 288, 326

tactile exploration 263–4
tactile modality 198–9, 263ff
tactile models 263–7, 273
tactile-kinaesthetic system 99, 198, 220, 262–3, 266
Tarakanov, V. B. 267
Teegarden, L. 243
Terman, L. M. 288
Thirion, A. N. 102
Thomas, E. L. 233, 253, 255
Thompson, G. G. 220
three-month-old child, behaviour of 27
Thurstone, L. L. 34, 39, 45
Tighe, L. 182, 185–6, 194, 202–3, 214, 325
Tighe, T. J. 156, 159, 185, 194
Tobie, H. 209–10
Tolman, E. C. 177, 317
topological relationships 65–6, 98–103, 105
Torren, I. Van der 129–30, 132, 136, 145
tracing 39, 45–6, 139–40
training for learning 155–8, 165, 168, 171–2, 178–81, 183, 185, 187–8, 193–5, 198–9, 267–9
training in recognising incomplete drawings 53–5, 59
TRAMO problems 40, 42–6
transfer along a continuum 186–8
TRMO problems 40, 43–4, 46
TRO problems 40, 42–5
tunnel vision 322

two-stage learning 184, 186, 188, 201

uniform destiny, law of 53
Uttal, W. B. 221

Venger, L. A. 268
verbal deficiency 167–8
verbal labels 168–73, 215
verbal mediation 167, 214–5, 317
verbal mediators in discrimination
  ¯ learning Ch. 6 *passim*
verbalisation 165–7, 173–4, 213
Vereecken, P. 96, 105–6, 109, 122
Vernon, M. D. 77
verticality, perception of 73–4
Vinh-Bang 246, 248–9
visual models 263–7, 273
visual structures analysed in terms of
  their properties Part Two *passim*
visual structures and spatial relationships Part One *passim*
visuo-motor exploration Ch. 9 *passim*: complete 295–6, 299–300, 302,
  309–10; differentiation task 223ff;
  insufficient 229–32, 295–6, 298–
  301, 304, 306, 330; strategies of
  235–6, 274–6, 320; task adaptation
  226ff
visuo-motor reaction time 246, 248
Volkelt, H. 126, 209
voluntary displacement of gaze 249
Vurpillot, E. 9–10, 12, 26, 36–7, 40,
  43, 45–6, 70–2, 99, 107–8, 110,
  112–18, 134, 142, 147, 153, 172,
  203–7, 212, 223–4, 229–30, 232,
  235, 237–8, 242, 244, 253–5, 273,
  275, 289–90, 292, 294, 301–2,
  304–5, 307–9, 313–14, 323, 326, 331

Walk, R. D. 60
Wapner, S. 93, 122

Watson, J. B. 11, 315
Wayenburg, G. van 132
weak and strong structures 135–6
Wekker, L. M. 219, 257–9, 271, 273,
  327
Wekker's hypothesis 258–61
Werner, H. 323
Wertheimer, M. 35, 52–3, 112
Wever, E. G. 26
White, B. 274
White, C. 252–3, 255
White, S. H. 175–8, 188, 220, 269,
  315, 318, 333–4
whole, exclusive perception of 134–48
whole or parts, predominance of
  125–32
whole-part confusion 132–4
Wiesel, T. N. 12, 321
Witkin, H. A. 34, 37
Wittling-Lauret, M. 101
Wohlwill, J. 69, 78–80, 96
Wolff, P. H. 220, 318
Woodworth, R. S. 252
Wright, J. C. 179–82, 269, 319
Wursten, H. 84
Wyckoff, Jr., L. B. 175–6

Young, J. Z. 87
Youniss, J. 158–9, 194, 200

Zaporozhets, A. V. 219–21, 223, 257–
  258, 261–2, 267–9, 271, 273, 307,
  316–17, 327
Zeaman, D. 175, 182, 187–8, 211
Zeigler, H. P. 67
Zinchenko, V. P. 221–2, 229, 237,
  254–5, 264, 266, 268, 272–3, 275,
  321
Zusne, L. 233, 253, 263
Zutphen, Van 105–6